Rheumatology and Orthopaedics

For UKMLA and Medical Exams

First and second edition authors

Annabel Coote

Paul Haslam

Daniel Marsland

Sabrina Kapoor

Third edition authors

Cameron Elias-Jones

Martin Perry

Fourth edition authors

Marc Joseph Aitken

Anthony Gibson

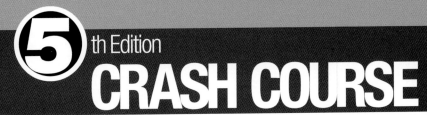

5th Edition
CRASH COURSE

SERIES EDITOR

Philip Xiu
MA (Cantab), MB BChir, MRCP, MRCGP, MScClinEd, FHEA, MAcadMEd, RCPathME
Honorary Senior Lecturer
Leeds University School of Medicine
PCN Educational Lead
Medical Examiner
Leeds Teaching Hospital Trust
Leeds, UK

FACULTY ADVISORS

Anthony Gibson
MBBS, FRCS
National Spine Fellow, Leeds General Infirmary
Honorary Clinical Lecturer
University of Glasgow, UK

Martin Perry
MBChB, BSc(Hons), MRCP(UK), FHEA, MMEd
Clinical Director Medicine Clyde
Consultant Physician & Rheumatologist
Hospital Subdean & Honorary Senior Lecturer
University of Glasgow, UK

Rheumatology and Orthopaedics

For UKMLA and Medical Exams

ELSEVIER

Elspeth Murray
MBChB, MRCS
Trauma and Orthopaedics Registrar, West of
Scotland Deanery
Honorary Clinical Lecturer
University of Glasgow, UK

Anna Bradford
BSc (Hons)
Medical Student
University of Glasgow, UK

First edition 1998

First edition 2004

Second edition 2008

Third edition 2013

Updated Third edition 2015

Fourth edition 2019

Notices

Practitioners and researchers must always rely on their own experience and knowledge in evaluating and using any information, methods, compounds or experiments described herein. Because of rapid advances in the medical sciences, in particular, independent verification of diagnoses and drug dosages should be made. To the fullest extent of the law, no responsibility is assumed by Elsevier, authors, editors or contributors for any injury and/or damage to persons or property as a matter of products liability, negligence or otherwise, or from any use or operation of any methods, products, instructions, or ideas contained in the material herein.

ISBN: 978-0-443-11535-6

Content Strategist: Trinity Hutton
Content Project Manager: Taranpreet Kaur
Design: Miles Hitchen
Marketing Manager: Deborah Watkins

Printed in India

Last digit is the print number: 9 8 7 6 5 4 3 2 1

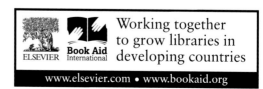

Series editor's foreword

With great honour and pride, we present the latest edition of the *Crash Course* series. This series has traversed a journey of nearly a quarter-century, stemming from the vision of Dr. Dan Horton-Szar, and his legacy continues to walk with us on this pathway of knowledge.

The series has been popular with students worldwide, selling over **1 million copies** and being translated into more than **8 languages**, reinforcing our commitment to global learning.

We remain extremely grateful for your unwavering trust. The series has once again been refreshed and fully upgraded in accordance with the rapidly changing medical guidelines, ensuring the content is comprehensive, accurate and fully up-to-date.

This latest series continues our tradition of integrating clinical practice with basic medical sciences, tailored meticulously for today's medical undergraduate curriculum. A central highlight of this instalment is our emphasis on high-yield exam content designed specifically for the UKMLA curriculum.

The addition of the **Rapid UKMLA Index** at the beginning of the book enhances this offering, serving as a valuable aid to students to track their exam preparation efficiently. We have also revised all self-assessment questions to align with the single best answer format in line with the latest UKMLA examination style. We have also added ***High-Yield Association Tables***. These are essential tools designed to aid students in recognizing clinical patterns and acing vignette-style exam questions. By condensing complex medical scenarios into digestible, manageable insights, these tables ensure efficient learning. They connect symptoms, diagnosis and treatment, bolstering understanding and confidence in tackling the rigorous UKMLA exams. This comprehensive approach makes these tables an indispensable asset in your exam preparations.

Utilizing student feedback, we have strived to maintain the core principles of this series: delivering precise and readable text that brings together depth and clarity. The authors are experienced junior doctors who successfully navigated these exams recently, ensuring practical and tested guidance. A team of expert faculty advisors from across the United Kingdom ensures the content's accuracy, making it resilient and reliable.

As we turn a new chapter with the latest edition, we honour the past, cherish the present, and embrace the promise of the future. We wish you every success in your journey of learning and growth and hope that this series adds value to your life, both as students and as future medical professionals.

Philip Xiu

Prefaces

Authors

Musculoskeletal problems affect a large number of patients. It is also an area of emerging treatments and therapies. I hope that this textbook will help students to gain a good understanding of the most common musculoskeletal problems and their treatments. Furthermore, I hope that this textbook will be a useful aid to exam revision and will help students to achieve their desired grades.

Elspeth Murray and Anna Bradford

Faculty advisors

Musculoskeletal problems represent an increasing problem in primary and secondary care as a result of an ageing population, the anticipated obesity epidemic and active sporting young adults. It is inevitable that all doctors will encounter patients with orthopaedic and rheumatological problems. Musculoskeletal medicine is a rapidly changing field, subject to much clinical and basic science research.

This *Crash Course* has been redesigned, rewritten and reformatted to help medical students develop a basic knowledge of diseases that affect the musculoskeletal system and the new understanding that underlies their pathologies and treatments.

We hope you enjoy reading and learning from this book and that it will help you pass your exams, and perhaps stimulate you toward a career in orthopaedics or rheumatology.

Anthony Gibson and Martin Perry

Acknowledgements

To my husband Kevin for his enthusiasm, support and sense of humour, whilst I was working on this book.

Elspeth Murray

I would like to thank Dr. Martin Perry for giving me the opportunity to be involved in the writing of this textbook. I would also like to thank my Mum and Dad for their continuous love and support.

Anna Bradford

Thanks to Alison and Leon for their patience and help.

Anthony Gibson

To the late Dr Marjorie Allison, instrumental in the development of the Glasgow Medical School and renal service, a generous and gifted clinician and teacher.

Martin Perry

Series editor's acknowledgement

We would like to express our sincere gratitude to those who have provided their support and expertise in preparing this fifth edition of the *Crash Course* series. Our junior doctor contributors' participation in crafting the manuscript has been indispensable. Their first-hand experience and current medical knowledge have infused realism and practicality into our content.

Our faculty editors deserve a special note of thanks. They have extensively validated the correctness of the information, ensuring that the content is not just accurate but also contemporaneous, credible, and aligns with the latest medical standards.

We extend our heartfelt thanks to our publisher, Elsevier. Their staff have demonstrated an unwavering commitment to quality, maintaining the high standards set since the first edition. Their insights have routinely enriched the content and process alike.

Our Commissioning Editor, Jeremy Bowes, deserves a special mention for his consistent support and guiding hand throughout the development process. His directions and advice have bettered this edition and spurred us on our quest for excellence.

We are greatly indebted to Alex Mortimer for her wisdom, practical insights and valuable guidance. A big thank you to our Content Strategists, Trinity Hutton and Cloe Holland-Borosh, who need special acknowledgement for meticulously outlining the direction and scope of the content. They've managed to mix details with a strategic plan, keeping our readers in mind.

Lastly, much gratitude is owed to our Content Product Managers, Taranpreet Kaur, Ayan Dhar, Shivani Pal and Tapajyoti Chaudhuri, who have juggled the numerous day-to-day tasks with utmost dedication and perseverance. Despite the ever-approaching deadlines, they have shown remarkable patience and steadfast determination, ensuring that each step of the book's development was accomplished seamlessly.

In conclusion, we sincerely thank each of these wonderful people for their outstanding contributions and support, without which this work wouldn't have been achieved. Their passion, commitment and collaborative effort have helped us bring this edition together.

Philip Xiu

Rapid UKMLA Index

The UKMLA Curriculum Conditions Priority levels have been based on the below:

Level 1: Conditions that a newly qualified doctor should have a good knowledge of and be able to recognise and manage.

Level 2: Conditions requiring knowledge for recognising and confirming diagnosis and planning first-line management in straightforward cases.

Level 3: Conditions where recognition of clinical presentation and describing principles of management are important.

continued

continued

continued

Table 2 UKMLA Presentations and Where to Find Them—cont'd

Contents

Contents

Taking a history

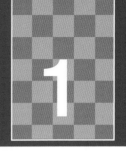

Taking a good history is vital in making a correct diagnosis and assessing the impact of a disease on a patient's life. A clear history can often give many clues to diagnosis long before you have examined the patient or ordered any tests. It is important to establish a rapport and make the patient feel at ease: patients will find it easier to share information if they feel comfortable.

COMMUNICATION

Begin your history taking with open questions, e.g., 'Tell me about your pain', then ask closed questions if necessary, e.g., 'Does your knee swell up?'

HINTS AND TIPS

Politely introduce yourself to the patient using your name and grade. Remember to ask for the patient's consent, particularly if you plan to take notes.

The first points to document in your history are:

- The patient's full name, date of birth, sex and hospital number.
- The time, date and place of the consultation (e.g., Accident and Emergency Department).
- The source of the referral, e.g., GP referral.

It is a good idea to ask the patient how they would like to be addressed during the consultation. This can help to make the patient feel more comfortable and will allow you to build rapport.

PRESENTING COMPLAINT

This is a short statement summarizing the patient's presenting symptoms, for example:

- Painful right knee
- Stiffness and swelling in both hands

HISTORY OF THE PRESENTING COMPLAINT

This should contain details of the patient's presenting symptoms from their onset to the current time. The following areas are important to discuss when taking a history:

Symptom onset

- Date and time of symptom onset
- Speed of onset: was it acute or insidious?
- Presence of precipitating and relieving factors such as trauma, other illnesses, medication use, etc.

Pain, swelling and stiffness

It is important to establish the following points:

- Site and radiation
- Character, e.g., whether it is sharp or dull
- Periodicity: is it continuous or intermittent?
- Exacerbating and relieving factors
- Timing: is it worse at any particular time of day?

As a rule, pain and stiffness due to inflammatory conditions such as rheumatoid arthritis are worse first thing in the morning and improve as the day progresses. The duration of early morning stiffness (minutes-to-hours) is a good guide to the severity of the inflammation. By contrast, pain due to mechanical or degenerative problems tends to be worse later in the day, is associated with less severe stiffness and is worse with activity.

HINTS AND TIPS

If pain is involved in the patient's presenting complaint, the **SOCRATES** acronym can be useful in taking a detailed pain history:

Site: e.g., 'Where is it painful?'.
Onset
Character
Radiation

Warmth/erythema

Inflamed joints may appear red and feel warm to touch.

Deformity

Some patients consult their doctor because they have developed deformity and are concerned. These often occur in patterns associated with specific conditions. This may or may not be associated with pain.

Weakness

It is important to ascertain whether any weakness is localized or generalized. Localized weakness suggests a focal problem, such as a peripheral nerve lesion, whereas generalized weakness is more likely to have a systemic cause.

Fatigue

Many inflammatory conditions are associated with varying degrees of patient fatigue; this may even be the reason for the patient consulting a doctor in the first place.

Numbness

The distribution of numbness or paraesthesia should be documented, as well as any precipitating factors. For example, if the numbness affects the radial 3.5 fingers and is worse at night, it is probably due to carpal tunnel syndrome. If it affects all the digits, is associated with skin colour changes and is provoked by cold weather, Raynaud phenomenon is more likely.

Functional loss and disability

Loss of function refers to a person's inability to perform an action, such as gripping an object or walking. This is often why a person goes to see their doctor. Disability is a measure of the impact that loss of function has on a patient's ability to lead a full and active life.

SYSTEMIC ENQUIRY

This should be brief but should include symptoms affecting other parts of the body. This is particularly relevant if you think the patient has a connective tissue disease.

MEDICAL HISTORY

Ask about all current and past medical and surgical disorders, including musculoskeletal problems. In certain situations it is worth asking about specific illnesses. For example, a patient with carpal tunnel syndrome may have underlying diabetes or hypothyroidism or, if a patient has one autoimmune condition (e.g., diabetes mellitus), they are more likely to have another such as rheumatoid arthritis.

DRUG HISTORY

A patient's drug history is always important and sometimes has great relevance to orthopaedic and rheumatological problems. Acute gout can be precipitated by diuretic use and long-term corticosteroids can cause osteoporosis. It is important to

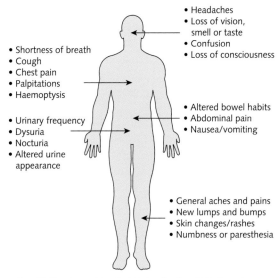

- Headaches
- Loss of vision, smell or taste
- Confusion
- Loss of consciousness

- Shortness of breath
- Cough
- Chest pain
- Palpitations
- Haemoptysis

- Urinary frequency
- Dysuria
- Nocturia
- Altered urine appearance

- Altered bowel habits
- Abdominal pain
- Nausea/vomiting

- General aches and pains
- New lumps and bumps
- Skin changes/rashes
- Numbness or paresthesia

Constitutional symptoms to enquire about: weight change, fevers, fatigue, night sweats

Fig. 1.1 Systemic enquiry.

ask about over-the-counter medications that the patient may be taking as well as prescribed medications. At this point, it is essential to ask the patient if they have any drug allergies.

SOCIAL HISTORY

Record relevant information about the patient's occupation, smoking history and alcohol intake. It is important to enquire about the patient's domestic situation and if they have support at home. This is important if a rheumatological or orthopaedic problem is affecting the patient's ability to live independently at home. Ask about drugs and sexual history if appropriate. Record the patient's dominant hand.

FAMILY HISTORY

Ask about any family history of musculoskeletal disorders. For example, ankylosing spondylitis and psoriasis are diseases that can be inherited.

Ideas, concerns and expectations

Asking about the patient's ideas, concerns and expectations (ICE) allows you to understand what the patient hopes to gain from the consultation. Furthermore, this helps the patient to feel understood and that their concerns have been addressed.

SUMMARY

Summarizing the key points of the consultation back to the patient allows them to add any important facts that you may have missed out.

After summarizing, thank the patient for their time and close the consultation.

Chapter Summary

- An accurate history is vital to arriving at a correct and sensible differential diagnosis.
- Use open and closed questions to investigate a presenting complaint.
- Remember to ask about pain, swelling and stiffness: these often help to differentiate between mechanical and inflammatory causes.
- Complete a thorough systemic enquiry to ensure no important symptoms are missed. Remember to explore the patient's ideas, concerns and expectations.

UKMLA Condition
Rheumatoid arthritis

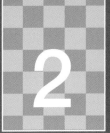
GENERAL PRINCIPLES

It is important to establish a rapport with patients. Dress smartly, be polite and carry identification.

Introduce yourself, explain the examination that is about to be carried out and gain informed consent. Then, ask if the patient is in any pain before beginning the examination. It is important to first generally inspect the patient from the end of the bed. Note any walking aids or medications that belong to the patient. Look for missing digits or limbs and for any neurological signs such as a tremor or muscle fasciculations.

- Start with adequate exposure of the joint.
- Stand and walk the patient. Watch how they walk. Pathological gait patterns are shown in Table 2.1.
- Position the patient for the joint(s) to be examined. Ensure the patient is comfortable.

Remember that some musculoskeletal conditions are part of multisystem diseases. In the case of polyarthritis and those with inflammatory arthritis, it may be necessary to examine the cardiovascular system, respiratory system and the abdomen. For those with widespread aches and pain, examination of the nervous system may be required.

Table 2.1 Pathological patterns of gait

Gait	Features	Cause
Trendelenburg	Waddling gait	Loss of hip abductor function
Antalgic (painful)	The patient tries to offload the painful limb by quickening and shortening the weight-bearing stance phase of the gait cycle	Any painful condition
Short-leg gait	Dipping of shoulder on affected side	Any condition causing significant leg length discrepancy
High stepping	Knee is flexed and foot is lifted high to avoid foot dragging on the floor	Nerve palsy (peroneal or sciatic)
Stiff knee	Knee cleared off floor by swinging out away from the body	Fusion of knee

HINTS AND TIPS

As a general principle, always examine the joints above and below the affected joint.

CLINICAL EXAMINATION

Examination of a patient should be performed systematically and in a structured way. Use the following method:

- Look: check for swelling, muscle wasting, scars, skin changes, erythema and deformity.
- Feel: palpate the joint, noting any effusions, tenderness and heat. Note any other prominent features.
- Move: demonstrate joint movement actively and passively.
- Special tests: each joint has tests that can be performed to assist in arriving at a diagnosis.
- Examine areas above and below the joints.

Practice this routine on your friends; note how normal joints look, feel and move.

HINTS AND TIPS

Remember to check active and passive movement. In active movement, the patient moves the joint; in passive movement, the examiner moves the joint.

Peripheral nervous examination

Abnormalities of the structures of the back such as intervertebral disc prolapse can cause abnormalities of the peripheral nerves due to compression of the nerve roots. The most commonly affected are the L5 and S1 nerve roots. In the upper limbs, the most common peripheral neuropathies typically involve compression of the median nerve as it travels through the wrist (carpal tunnel syndrome).

Prior to commencing the examination of the peripheral nervous system, it is important to inspect the patient from the end of the bed and to look for signs that may suggest an underlying neurological condition. For example, this could be muscle wasting suggesting a lower motor neuron lesion or a resting tremor suggesting Parkinsonism.

Lower limb

Tone

Lower limb tone is usually normal. However, increased tone will suggest an upper motor neuron lesion while decreased tone will suggest a lower motor neuron lesion. The findings in an upper motor neuron lesion in comparison to a lower motor neuron lesion are summarized in Table 2.2.

Power

Power is assessed by Medical Research Council grades:

0: Nothing
1: Flicker
2: Power to move limb with gravity eliminated
3: Power to move limb against gravity
4: Reduced from normal
5: Normal

Test muscle functions are shown in Table 2.3.

Reflexes

Always compare the reflexes between the two limbs and make sure the patient is relaxed. Reflexes can be present, reduced, brisk or absent.

Three reflexes are commonly tested:

- Knee L3–L4: flex both knees over the couch or your arm and tap lightly on the patellar tendon.
- Ankle L5–S1: dorsiflex the ankle with the knees flexed and the leg externally rotated. Tap the Achilles tendon.
- Plantar or Babinski reflex: this is performed by stoking the handle of the tendon hammer from the heel, up the lateral

aspect of the foot and then medially towards the big toe (Fig. 2.1). If the first movement of the toe is extension, this is abnormal and is 'upgoing', indicating an upper motor neuron lesion.

Sensation

Ask the patient whether the sensation is normal for them and the same as the other side. Use the sternum as a reference point for sensation. The patient should have their eyes closed when testing sensation. Dermatomes of the lower limb are shown in Fig. 2.2.

It is important to assess the different sensory pathways. The dorsal column pathways can be tested by using cotton wool (fine touch) and a tuning fork (vibration). The spinothalamic pathway can be tested using a neurotip (pinprick sensation).

Anal tone and perianal sensation

In cauda equina syndrome, anal tone is lost and perianal sensation reduced; therefore, a per rectal examination is an important part of any spinal examination.

Table 2.3 Testing lower-limb muscle function (myotomes)

Muscle action	Nerve roots tested
Hip flexion (iliopsoas)	L1, L2
Knee flexion (quadriceps)	L3
Ankle dorsiflexion (tibialis anterior)	L4
Great toe extension (extensor hallucis longus)	L5
Ankle plantar flexion (soleus/gastrocnemius)	S1

Table 2.2 Findings in upper versus lower motor neuron lesions

Findings	Lower motor neuron lesion	Upper motor neuron lesion
Inspection	Muscle wasting and/or fasciculations may be present	No obvious muscle wasting or fasciculations
Tone	Decreased muscle tone	Increased muscle tone
Power	Decreased	Decreased. Flexor muscles will be stronger than extensor muscles in the upper limbs and the opposite can be said for the lower limbs
Reflexes	Hyporeflexia or areflexia	Hyperreflexia

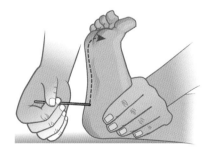

Fig. 2.1 The Babinski reflex. (From Menche N, Bender A, Keller C. *PFLEGEN Gesundheits- und Krankheitslehre, 2. Auflage*. Elsevier; 2021.)

If a full neurological exam were to be carried out, it would be important to test proprioception and coordination, although this can be left in a peripheral nervous examination.

Upper limb

Tone
This is usually normal unless there is a lesion in the cervical spine or injury to the brachial plexus.

Power
Upper limb function can be tested as shown in Table 2.4. The innervation of the upper limb muscles is more complex than in the lower limb.

Reflexes
Three reflexes are commonly tested:

- Biceps C5–C6: place your finger over the biceps brachii tendon as it passes through the cubital fossa at the elbow. Tap your finger with the tendon hammer.

- Triceps C7: with the elbow at 90 degrees, place your finger over the triceps tendon and tap lightly with the tendon hammer.
- Brachioradialis C6–C7: tap the brachioradialis tendon about 4 inches proximal to the base of the thumb as it inserts into the radial styloid process.

Sensation
Ask the patient if sensation is the same on both sides, use the sternum as a reference point and have the patient close their eyes. The dorsal column and spinothalamic pathways should be tested as explained previously. Upper limb dermatomes are shown in Fig. 2.3.

Table 2.4 Testing upper-limb function (myotomes)

Muscle action	Nerve root tested
Shoulder abduction	C5
Shoulder adduction	C6, C7
Elbow flexion	C5, C6
Elbow extension	C7, C8
Wrist flexion/extension	C6, C7
Metacarpophalangeal/interphalangeal flexion/extension	C7, C8
Metacarpophalangeal abduction/adduction	T1

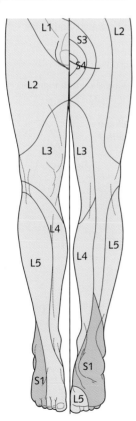

Fig. 2.2 Dermatomes of the lower limb. *L,* Lumbar; *S,* sacral.

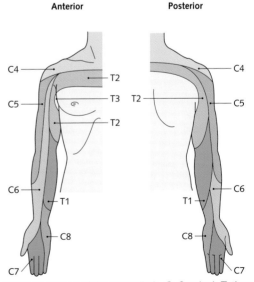

Fig. 2.3 Dermatomes of the upper limb. *C,* Cervical; *T,* thoracic.

EXAMINATION OF THE HIP

Hip disease is common and examination follows the pattern of look, feel, move and special tests. True hip pain is often felt in the groin and may radiate to the knee on movement.

The examiner starts by observing the patient walk from the waiting area. A Trendelenburg (waddling) gait is due to failure of the hip abductors to elevate the pelvis on weight bearing, causing a dipping or rolling gate (Fig. 2.4). To compensate for this, the trunk is thrown over the weight-bearing hip, which maintains balance.

Failure of hip abduction can be due to pain or as a complication following surgery.

The patient may also have an antalgic gait (see Table 2.1).

Look

Scars from previous surgery could be present anteriorly, laterally or medially. Look for erythema, obvious deformity and muscle wasting, particularly over the gluteal or quadriceps muscles. As the hip is a deep joint, swelling can be difficult to see. Look at both sides of the hip by turning the patient to the prone position.

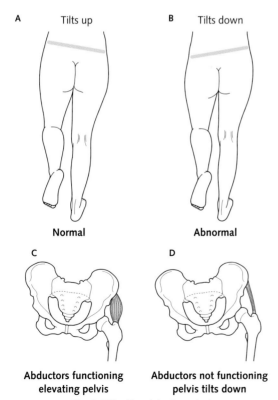

| A | Tilts up | B | Tilts down |

Normal **Abnormal**

C D

Abductors functioning elevating pelvis **Abductors not functioning pelvis tilts down**

Fig. 2.4 The Trendelenburg test.

True leg-length discrepancy

Ensure the patient is lying comfortably on the examination couch with both knees straight. Firstly, determine if this is a true leg length discrepancy or an apparent leg length discrepancy. If there is visible shortening of the leg but the pelvis is straight, this suggests a true leg length discrepancy that can be recorded by measuring the distance from the anterior superior iliac spine to the medial malleolus. An apparent leg length discrepancy occurs when the pelvis is tilted. This can be recorded by measuring the distance from the xiphisternum to the medial malleolus. Remember to measure each side and compare.

With the hips and knees flexed and the knees placed together, look from side to side to determine the position of knees.

If one knee is higher than the other, this suggests tibial shortening. However, if one knee lies behind the other, it suggests a femoral discrepancy (Fig. 2.5).

Feel

The hip is deeply situated and few features are palpable. The greater trochanter is easily felt laterally, over which bursitis may be present. Assess the temperature around the joint using the back of the hand and compare both sides.

Move

Normal movements are shown in Fig. 2.6.

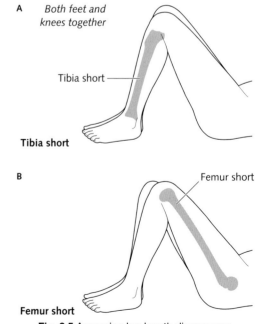

A *Both feet and knees together*

Tibia short

Tibia short

B Femur short

Femur short

Fig. 2.5 Assessing leg-length discrepancy.

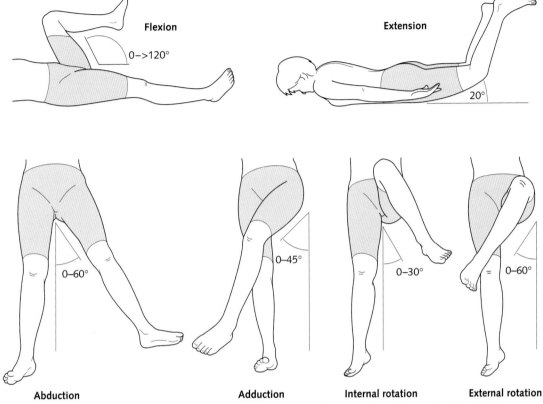

Fig. 2.6 Movements of the hip (note that all ranges are approximate and vary from patient to patient).

Special tests

Trendelenburg test

This is used to assess the function of the hip abductors.

Stand face-on to the patient and put your hands on the patient's pelvis, then ask the patient to place their hands on your forearms lightly to steady themselves. Ask the patient to lift each leg in turn and watch for pelvic tilting. Remember that you are testing the standing leg and the patient should lift their other leg up behind them by flexing the knee. Flexing the hip can tilt the pelvis.

If the abductors on the standing leg are not working properly, the pelvis tilts towards the unsupported leg (Fig. 2.4B and D).

Thomas test

This is a test for fixed flexion of the hip.

The purpose of the test is to abolish the natural lordosis of the lumbar spine and to visualize the true degree of flexion deformity at the hip.

To perform the test, the patient is positioned supine (flat on the back) and the opposite hip is flexed fully. The manoeuvre fully corrects the lordosis that is felt by placing the hand under the spine. Now simply observe any degree of flexion (if any) in the opposite hip (Fig. 2.7).

EXAMINATION OF THE KNEE

The knee lies superficially and many landmarks are easily palpable.

Look

- Look for quadriceps wasting, which can be assessed by measuring the thigh circumference and comparing with the other side.
- Localized swelling anteriorly and posteriorly may be visible.
- Note any effusions (which can be seen by loss of the normal skin dimples at the joint line), scars, erythema or evidence of psoriasis.
- Look for surgical scars.
- Ask the patient to stand and walk; note any gait abnormalities.
- Deformities (varus, valgus and fixed flexion) are more obvious on standing. See Fig. 2.8 for the general appearance of knee deformities.

> **COMMON PITFALLS**
>
> Posterior swelling of the knee is easily missed. Ask the patient to stand and examine them from behind.

Feel

Flexing the knee to 90 degrees allows structures to be palpated more easily. Feel for warmth in the knees with the back of the hand.

Be methodical, starting distally over the tibial tuberosity and moving proximally, palpating in turn the patellar tendon,

proximal tibia, medial and lateral joint lines, femoral condyles, patella and quadriceps tendon (Fig. 2.9). The collateral ligaments are also palpable.

> **RED FLAG**
>
> Remember to palpate the posterior aspect of the knee. A Baker's cyst or bursa may be present!

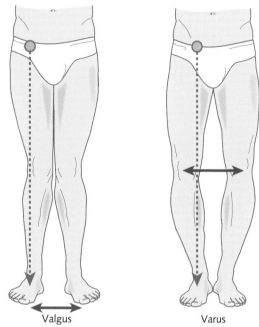

Valgus   Varus

Fig. 2.8 The general appearance of knee deformities. (From Bowen WT, Dennis M, Cho L. *Mechanisms of Clinical Signs*. 3rd ed. Elsevier; 2020.)

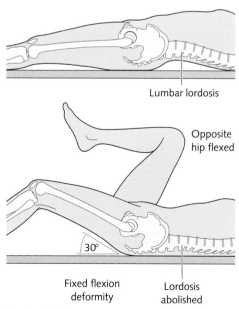

Lumbar lordosis

Opposite hip flexed

30°

Fixed flexion deformity   Lordosis abolished

Fig. 2.7 The Thomas test for fixed flexion of the hip.

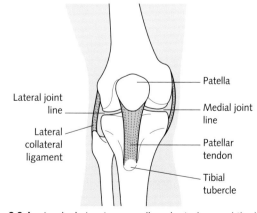

Patella

Lateral joint line

Medial joint line

Lateral collateral ligament

Patellar tendon

Tibial tubercle

Fig. 2.9 Anatomical structures easily palpated around the knee.

It is important to recognize a knee effusion (Fig. 2.10), as it always indicates pathology. There are two tests commonly used to confirm this: the patellar tap and the swipe test.

Patellar tap

Fluid is forced from the suprapatellar pouch, which lifts the patella away from the femur. The patella is then pushed down on the femur, producing a palpable tap (Fig. 2.11).

Sweep test

Fluid is forced out of the medial compartment. The examining hand then sweeps fluid from the lateral side of the knee, refilling the medial compartment with a visible bulge.

Move

Both active and passive movements should be tested. The normal range of movement is shown in Fig. 2.12. Note any fixed

flexion or hyperextension of the knee. Feel for patellar crepitus during flexion.

Medial and lateral collateral ligaments

Patients have differing degrees of laxity of the ligaments. It is therefore important to compare your findings with the healthy side. Flex the knee to 15 degrees and alternately stress the joint line on each side. Place one hand on the opposite side of the joint line to that which is being tested and apply force to the lower tibia (Fig. 2.13).

Anterior cruciate ligament

Anterior draw test

This is a test for anterior cruciate ligament (ACL) deficiency but can be misleading because it can also be positive after medial

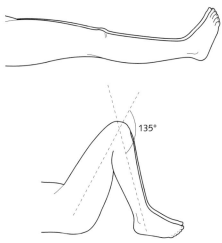

Fig. 2.12 Range of movement of the knee.

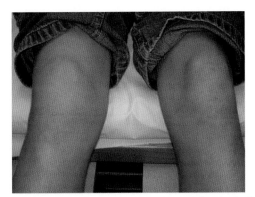

Fig. 2.10 Right knee effusion. Note the loss of dimples in the thigh and under the patella.

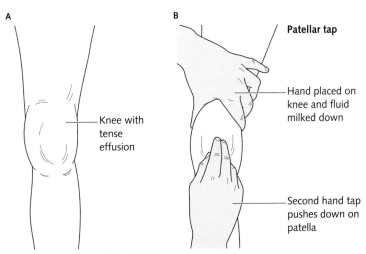

Fig. 2.11 The patellar tap sign.

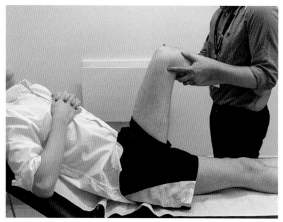

Fig 2.13 Collateral ligament examination.

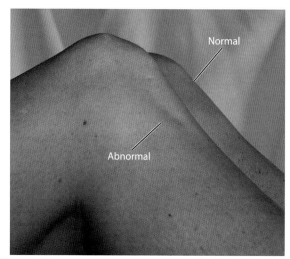

Fig. 2.14 Posterior sag sign. The right knee shows the positive sign. Note that the tibial tuberosity is more prominent on the left.

meniscectomy or in posterior cruciate ligament (PCL) deficiency. The knee is flexed to 90 degrees and the hamstrings are relaxed. The examiner carefully sits on the patient's foot and both thumbs are placed on the proximal tibia and over both joint lines. The tibia is pulled forward and, if movement is excessive, the test is positive.

> **COMMUNICATION**
>
> Testing the anterior cruciate ligament can be uncomfortable for patients. Remember to explain clearly the test before performing it.

Posterior cruciate ligament

The posterior drawer test is performed exactly the same way as the anterior drawer test, but the knee is pushed backwards.

The classic sign of PCL rupture is posterior sag. This is demonstrated by flexing both knees to 90 degrees and comparing the knee contour (Fig. 2.14). A sag occurs because the tibia falls posteriorly and the tibial tuberosity becomes less prominent.

EXAMINATION OF THE ANKLE AND FOOT

Look

Inspect the ankle and foot with the patient in both resting and weight-bearing positions. Observe nails and skin for psoriatic changes. Look at the distribution of any swelling. Synovitis of the ankle usually produces diffuse swelling, obscuring

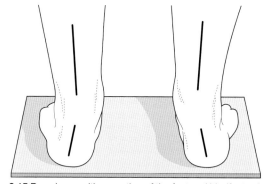

Fig. 2.15 Pes planus with pronation of the feet and hindfoot valgus.

the contours of the medial and lateral malleoli. Swelling in the region of the Achilles tendon is more likely to be due to Achilles tendinopathy or tendon rupture.

Disease of the subtalar joint or abnormalities of the longitudinal arch of the foot may disrupt the alignment of the heel and Achilles tendon. This should be vertical and is easily seen when observing from behind a standing patient. Pes planus (flat foot) can cause pronation of the foot and valgus deformity of the heel (Fig. 2.15). Note that pes planus may be corrected by having the patient stand on the tips of their toes.

Forefoot issues are common. Hallux valgus is a deformity of the great toe, which becomes abducted at the metatarsophalangeal (MTP) joint. Excessive pressure on the medial side can lead to formation of a bursa, often called a bunion. Look at the patient's footwear for signs of excessive wear. Fig. 2.16 shows other common forefoot deformities. These deformities can occur due to a variety of reasons including trauma, rheumatoid arthritis and diabetic neuropathy.

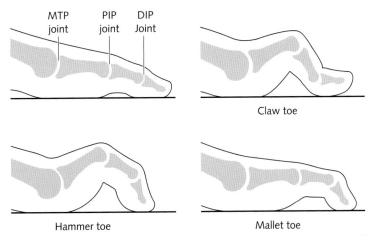

Fig. 2.16 Common deformities of the forefoot. *DIP*, Distal interphalangeal; *MTP*, metatarsophalangeal; *PIP*, proximal interphalangeal.

Feel

Feel for warmth. Palpate the ankle joint, subtalar joint and forefoot and squeeze the MTP joints to elicit any discomfort. Palpate the dorsalis pedis and posterior tibial pulses and assess capillary refill time. Note that this should be less than 2 seconds.

> **HINTS AND TIPS**
>
> Do not forget to feel the Achilles tendon and check its integrity. This can be done by elevating the leg and gently squeezing the calf muscle, observing for plantarflexion of the foot.

Move

Test plantar flexion and dorsiflexion of the ankle with the knee flexed. The subtalar joint allows inversion and eversion of the hindfoot. This is tested by stabilizing the tibia with one hand and turning the calcaneus inward and outward with the other.

Midtarsal movements contribute to plantar flexion, dorsiflexion, inversion and eversion. These are tested by stabilizing the heel with one hand and moving the foot with the other. Movements of the MTP joints, proximal interphalangeal (PIP) joints and distal interphalangeal (DIP) joints are best examined actively while the patient is lying or sitting.

EXAMINATION OF THE SPINE

When examining the spine, remember to perform a peripheral nervous system examination.

Look

Assess the patient's posture. Check for cervical lordosis, thoracic kyphosis and lumbar lordosis. If the patient has sciatica, the affected leg is often flexed and the posture stooped. Muscle wasting, asymmetry and scoliosis may be present.

> **HINTS AND TIPS**
>
> In scoliosis, the rib hump deformity is more clearly seen when the patient bends forward.

Feel

Palpation is performed with the patient standing and lying prone.

Feel the spinous processes, the paraspinal muscles and the sacroiliac joints for tenderness.

Move

Cervical spine
Movements of the cervical spine (Fig. 2.17) are usually stated as percentage loss when compared with normal.

Flexion
Ask the patient to bend their head forward to put their chin on their chest.

Extension
Ask the patient to look towards the ceiling.

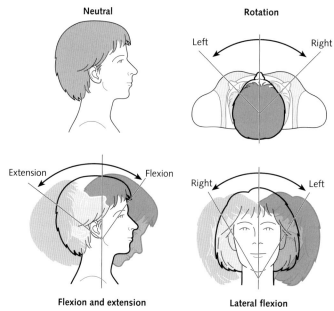

Fig. 2.17 Movements of the cervical spine.

Lateral flexion

Ask the patient to put their ear down towards their shoulder.

Rotation

Ask the patient to look to either side.

Thoracolumbar spine (Fig. 2.18)

Flexion

Patients are often reluctant to flex the spine if it is acutely tender. Ask the patient to bend over, keeping their knees extended and reach as far as they can.

Look and feel for movement of the lumbar spine. This can be done by marking two points on the lumbar spine and observing the increase in distance between them on flexion. This is known as the Schober's test (discussed further in Chapter 13).

Extension

Ask the patient to arch their back backwards. In conditions such as spinal stenosis, this can exacerbate pain.

Rotation

With the patient sitting on a bed to fix the pelvis and with their arms crossed in front, ask the patient to turn from side to side.

Lateral flexion

Ask the patient to slide one hand down the side of their leg and observe.

Temporomandibular joint

The integrity of the temporomandibular joint can be assessed by having the patient open and close their mouth and move their jaw from side to side.

Special tests

Straight-leg raise

Straight-leg raising is a test for radiculopathy (nerve root irritation).

With the patient supine, elevate the affected leg passively, keeping it straight and dorsiflex the foot. If the patient complains of pain down the leg, look at the angle that the leg makes with the couch, e.g., 30 degrees. The next step is to bend the knee, as this will abolish the symptoms by relieving tension on the nerve.

For the test to be positive, the pain must radiate to the foot (often patients will complain of back pain when raising the leg). This test stretches the sciatic nerve and elicits pain with lumbar disc disease.

EXAMINATION OF THE SHOULDER

Movement of the shoulder is complex and occurs at four joints (Fig. 2.19). The majority of the total range of movement arises from the glenohumeral and scapulothoracic joints.

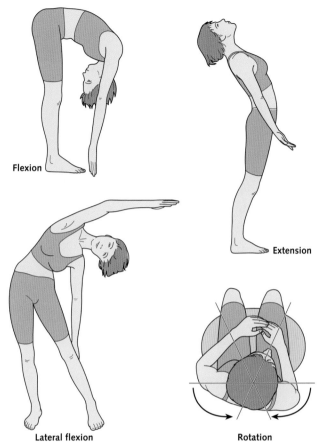

Fig. 2.18 Thoracolumbar spinal movements.

Look

Look at the position and contours of the shoulder from the front, side and behind and compare with the opposite side.

- Swelling of the shoulder is uncommon but is best seen anteriorly.
- Muscle wasting may occur due to chronic shoulder pathology, such as rotator cuff tendinopathy or deltoid muscle wastage due to axillary nerve damage.
- Scars from shoulder replacement are usually anterior.
- Deformity most commonly presents as winging of the scapula. This can be best viewed from behind with the patient standing straight with their hands placed flat against a wall.

Feel

Palpate for tenderness over the acromioclavicular, sternoclavicular and glenohumeral joints. A gap on palpation of the acromioclavicular joint indicates dislocation. Palpate the spine of the scapula. Feel for warmth, comparing both sides. Palpate the surrounding muscles for tenderness.

Move

Examine active and passive movements.

A normal range of passive movements means glenohumeral disease is unlikely.

The shoulder movements to be assessed are:

- flexion
- extension
- abduction
- adduction
- external rotation
- internal rotation (have the patient reach behind their back with their thumb. Measure how far the thumb can reach, e.g., the greater trochanter, sacroiliac joint, mid-scapular level, etc.)

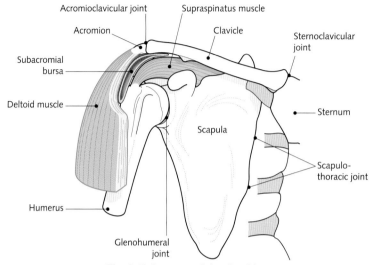

Fig. 2.19 Anatomy of the shoulder.

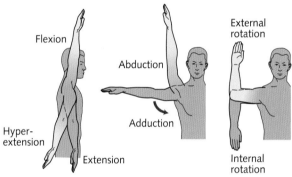

Fig .2.20 Movements of the shoulder joint. (From Remmert LN, Sorrentino SA, Remmert. *Mosby's® Essentials for Nursing Assistants*. 7th ed. Elsevier; 2023.)

These movements are shown in Fig. 2.20.

> **HINTS AND TIPS**
>
> Normal passive movement with painful or restricted active shoulder movements suggests a muscle or tendon problem.

A hitch-up of the shoulder on active abduction of the arm is a sign of reduced glenohumeral range (Fig. 2.21).

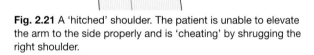

Fig. 2.21 A 'hitched' shoulder. The patient is unable to elevate the arm to the side properly and is 'cheating' by shrugging the right shoulder.

- Loss of passive external rotation and abduction are highly indicative of adhesive capsulitis (frozen shoulder).
- Scapular movements should be assessed from behind during the range of movements. 'Winging' is a common sign of serratus anterior dysfunction caused by damage to the long thoracic nerve.

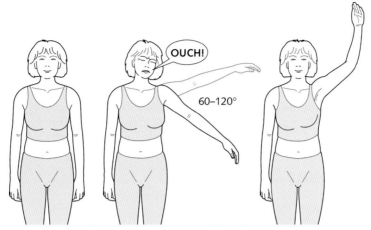

Fig. 2.22 Demonstration of the painful arc.

Special tests

The rotator cuff

The supraspinatus, infraspinatus, teres minor and subscapularis muscles make up the rotator cuff. They hold the head of the humerus in the glenoid cavity, maintain stability and initiate shoulder abduction. Rotator cuff inflammation, injury and degeneration are common. Disease of the supraspinatus especially causes pain on abduction when the tendon becomes depressed beneath the acromion. The pain is felt at between 60 and 120 degrees of abduction. This is what is referred to as a 'painful arc' (Fig. 2.22).

Resisted shoulder movement should be examined. Pain or weakness on resisted movements suggests involvement of the rotator cuff muscles and tendons.

- Supraspinatus is tested with the arm abducted to 30 degrees, flexed to 30 degrees and internally rotated with the thumb pointing down. Abduction is then resisted.
- Subscapularis is tested with resisted internal rotation.
- Infraspinatus and teres minor are tested with resisted external rotation.

Shoulder impingement

Shoulder impingement can be assessed by carrying out the Hawkins-Kennedy test. The patient's shoulder should be flexed to 90 degrees and the elbow should be rotated to 90 degrees. The patient should stay relaxed as their arm is passively internally rotated. Reproducible pain is a positive sign for shoulder impingement. The Hawkins-Kennedy test is seen in Fig. 2.23.

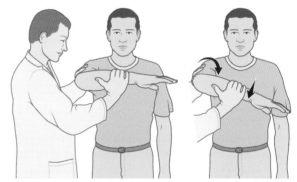

Fig. 2.23 The Hawkins-Kennedy test. (From Innes JA, Dover AR, Fairhurst K. *Pemeriksaan Klinis Macleod, Edisi Fourteen.* Elsevier; 2020.)

EXAMINATION OF THE ELBOW

The elbow consists of two articulations. The first is between the humerus, radius and ulna, which allows flexion to 150 degrees. The second is the superior radioulnar joint, which allows rotation of the wrist through 180 degrees.

Look

Examine the elbow in flexion and extension looking for scars, muscle wasting, fixed flexion, swelling, erythema, rheumatoid nodules and psoriatic plaques. Olecranon bursitis may be seen as a 'golf-ball' swelling over the elbow. Look for elbow deformity such as cubitus varus or cubitus valgus.

Feel

Feel for warmth. Palpate the olecranon process and medial and lateral epicondyles. The medial will be tender in golfer's elbow; the lateral is tender in tennis elbow. The radial head is usually felt easily in the lateral aspect of the joint and its movement can be assessed in pronation and supination. Flex the elbow to 90 degrees and look for an effusion between the lateral epicondyle, radial head and olecranon.

Move

Test flexion and extension, pronation and supination. Extension of the elbow to 180 degrees and beyond is normal. The inability to straighten the elbow to 180 degrees is therefore considered pathological, even if pain-free. Many people can extend a further 5 to 10 degrees, therefore, true hypermobility is defined as extension beyond 190 degrees.

It is best to assess pronation and supination with the elbow flexed at 90 degrees and held close to the body. If you suspect the patient may have epicondylitis, examine resisted movements of the wrist for pain. Assess active movement before assessing passive movement. While assessing passive movement, feel for crepitus.

Special tests

- Tennis elbow (lateral epicondylitis): palpate the lateral epicondyle and stabilize the humerus while pronating the patient's forearm. Then, palmar flex the wrist and fully extend the elbow. If the patient complains of pain at the lateral epicondyle, this is positive for tennis elbow.
- Golfer's elbow (medial epicondylitis): palpate the medial epicondyle and stabilize the humerus while supinating the patient's forearm. Then, extend the patient's wrist and fully extend the elbow. If the patient complains of pain at the medial epicondyle, this is positive for golfer's elbow.

Functional testing

Assess if the patient can easily move their hand to their mouth.

EXAMINATION OF THE WRIST AND HAND

Rest the patient's hands on a pillow for comfort.

Look

Inspection of the hands is an important part of the musculoskeletal examination. Look at the skin, nails, joints and muscles.

Skin

Check for psoriasis, rheumatoid nodules and tightening of the skin (scleroderma) or skin thinning (steroid use). Nail fold infarcts, haemorrhages and digital ulcers can occur as a consequence of vasculitis and systemic sclerosis. Scars from carpal tunnel decompression are seen on the volar aspect of the wrist. Redness, or erythema, is often seen when inflammation is present.

Nails

Look for pitting or onycholysis in psoriasis and splinter haemorrhages in vasculitis.

Joints

Look for deformity (e.g., to ganglion cysts), swelling and scars of joint replacement. The pattern of deformity aids in diagnosis:

- Osteoarthritis tends to affect the DIP/PIP joints.
- Rheumatoid arthritis mainly affects the PIP/MCP and wrist joints.

Other deformities seen in the hands in rheumatoid arthritis include ulnar deviation, swan neck deformity, z-thumb deformity or a boutonniere deformity (this will be explained in more detail in Chapter 12).

Muscles

Wasting of the thenar and hypothenar eminences suggests median (carpal tunnel) or ulnar nerve pathology, respectively, or disuse due to joint disease.

Atrophy of the dorsal interossei occurs in rheumatoid arthritis.

Feel

Palpate each joint systemically for the boggy and spongy feeling of synovitis. Bony overgrowth, such as osteophytosis, will feel hard. A bimanual approach is best with the examiner's fingertips placed at either side of the joint, feeling for soft-tissue swelling.

Tenosynovitis of the finger flexors can be associated with tendon nodules, which can be felt moving on finger flexion.

Remember to feel the metacarpophalangeal joints for warmth and to squeeze them to elicit tenderness. Perform the piano key test. Pronate the wrist and apply pressure to the head of the ulna. Pain elicited would suggest pathology at the distal radio-ulnar joint.

Check sensation in the distribution of the radial, median and ulnar nerves.

Assess capillary refill and palpate the radial pulse.

Move

It is important to assess hand function. Active and passive movements of the wrist and digits should be performed and the patient's ability to perform certain tasks should be assessed. The muscles responsible for various movements are shown in Table 2.5.

- The prayer sign is useful when assessing hand and wrist function. Ask the patient to extend both wrists and place the palms together as if praying (see Fig. 2.24). Patients with limited wrist extension, deformities and synovitis of the MCP or PIP joints will find this difficult. Next 'reverse' the prayer sign so that the fingers point down towards the floor.
- Ask the patient to make a fist, tucking fingers into the palm.
- Ask the patient to straighten their fingers against resistance.
- Abduct fingers and check power with the corresponding finger of the examiner's hand pressing against the patient's finger.
- Check interossei by asking the patient to hold a sheet of paper between the fingers.
- Abduction of the thumb against resistance checks median nerve function.

HINTS AND TIPS

Ask the patient to pick up a penny from the table or fasten a button. This will give you a good idea of the hand function.

Table 2.5 Muscles responsible for hand and wrist movements

Movement	Muscle(s) responsible (nerve supply)
Wrist flexion	Flexor carpi radialis (median) Flexor carpi ulnaris (ulnar) Palmaris longus (median)
Wrist extension	Extensor carpi radialis longus and brevis (both radial) Extensor carpi ulnaris (radial)
DIP joint flexion	Flexor digitorum profundus (median and ulnar)
PIP joint flexion	Flexor digitorum superficialis (median)
MCP joint flexion and IP joint extension	Lumbricals (median and ulnar)
Finger abduction	Dorsal interossei (ulnar)
Finger adduction	Palmar interossei (ulnar)
Extension of MCPs, PIPs and DIPs	Extensor digitorum (radial)
Thumb abduction	Abductor pollicis brevis (median)
Thumb adduction	Adductor pollicis (ulnar)
Thumb opposition	Opponens pollicis (median)
Thumb extension	Extensor pollicis longus (radial)

DIP, *Distal interphalangeal*; IP, *interphalangeal*; MCP, *metacarpophalangeal*; PIP, *proximal interphalangeal*.

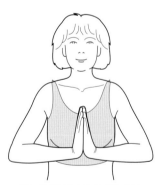

Fig. 2.24 The 'prayer' sign.

Special tests

Tinel and Phalen tests should be performed in patients who have symptoms suggestive of carpal tunnel syndrome.

Chapter Summary

- Joint examination should be undertaken using a look, feel and move approach.
- You should always consider examining the joints above and below the affected joint.
- Gait observation gives vital clues to pathology in the lower limbs.
- When examining the hip, remember to stabilize the pelvis during movement.
- Examination of the knee should always involve testing for an effusion, which can be done using the patellar tap and swipe tests.
- Testing ligament stability using the anterior and posterior draw test can be painful, but it is necessary during knee examination.
- The straight-leg raise test is a quick way to test for nerve root irritation in the lumbosacral spine.
- A painful shoulder arc is typical of a supraspinatus rotator cuff injury, which is a common cause of shoulder pain.
- The patterns of joint involvement in the small joints of the hands give vital clues to the aetiology: PIP and DIP joint involvement in osteoarthritis, PIP, MCP and wrist joint involvement in rheumatoid arthritis.

UKMLA Conditions
Bursitis
Rheumatoid arthritis

UKMLA Presentations
Musculoskeletal deformity
Soft tissue injury

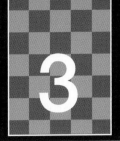
BLOOD TESTS

Many different blood tests are taken when evaluating rheumatic and orthopaedic problems. The following are most useful.

Full blood count

Full blood count (FBC) is a measure of the different constituent cells of the blood sample. Anaemia refers to a state of low haemoglobin (Hb). Once it has been established that the patient has anaemia, the size of the red blood cells should be determined by measuring the mean corpuscular volume (MCV). This will help to ascertain the cause of anaemia.

Microcytic anaemia may be due to iron deficiency anaemia, anaemia of chronic disease or thalassaemia. Iron deficiency anaemia may arise from the use of nonsteroidal antiinflammatory drugs (NSAIDs) causing chronic gastrointestinal blood loss. Normocytic anaemia is more likely due to acute blood loss or anaemia of chronic disease. Macrocytic anaemia is usually secondary to a vitamin deficiency (most commonly vitamin B^{12} or folate). Haemolytic anaemia typically presents as a macrocytic anaemia that can occur as a result of autoinflammatory disease. Investigations for a patient with anaemia should include Hb, MCV, vitamin B^{12}, folate, ferritin and in some cases, a blood film.

- A high white cell count may be due to infection, inflammation or due to steroid use.
- A leukopenia can be a feature of systemic lupus erythematosus (SLE), connective tissue disease or from bone-marrow suppression from antirheumatic drugs.
- Thrombocytosis often occurs in active inflammatory disease. In this case, it is referred to as a reactive thrombocytosis. Thrombocytopenia can be seen in SLE and antiphospholipid syndrome.

> **RED FLAG**
>
> A normal or low white cell count does not exclude infection if the clinical situation suggests otherwise. Patients who are immunosuppressed, or who are elderly, often present in this way.

Erythrocyte sedimentation rate

Erythrocyte sedimentation rate (ESR) is the rate at which red blood cells sediment over an hour and is a marker of inflammation.

- The measurement increases with higher levels of plasma proteins such as immunoglobulins and fibrinogen.
- The upper limit of ESR increases with advancing age and in those who are overweight.

C-Reactive protein

C-Reactive protein (CRP) is an acute phase protein that is manufactured in the liver.

- Its level rises in a nonspecific way as a result of inflammation and infection.
- It typically takes 6 to 10 hours after an inflammatory event to increase.

> **HINTS AND TIPS**
>
> C-Reactive protein responds more rapidly than erythrocyte sedimentation rate to changes in inflammation.

Urea and electrolytes

Renal impairment may occur in gout or connective tissue disease. NSAIDs can cause interstitial nephritis.

Liver function tests

- Alkaline phosphatase (ALP) is found in both the liver and bone; some tests can differentiate between the isoenzymes.
- A raised ALP is seen in Paget's disease.
- Some drugs used for musculoskeletal problems are hepatotoxic, such as methotrexate and sulfasalazine, and require routine monitoring.

Uric acid

Uric acid levels are high in many patients with gout, but they can be normal during an attack of gout.

Calcium

- Hypocalcaemia occurs in osteomalacia and vitamin D deficiency.
- Hypercalcaemia can be a feature of malignancy, sarcoid and excess parathyroid hormone production.

Creatine kinase

Creatine kinase is a muscle enzyme that increases in response to muscle injury (trauma, hypoperfusion or inflammation). A raised creatine kinase would be seen in rheumatic conditions such as polymyositis and dermatomyositis as well as rhabdomyolysis, acute kidney injury or a myocardial infarction.

Procalcitonin

Procalcitonin is a relatively new test performed when a patient's joint is hot. It can be useful in combination with ESR, CRP and the FBC to establish whether patients have joint infections or joint inflammation. A high procalcitonin is indicative of bacterial infection and sepsis.

Rheumatoid factor

Rheumatoid factor is an antibody directed against the Fc fragment of human immunoglobulin G (IgG). It may be of any class, but IgM anti-IgG is the most commonly measured. Around 75% of patients with RA have a positive rheumatoid factor antibody. It is sensitive for RA but not very specific.

Cyclic citrullinated peptide antibody

Cyclic citrullinated peptide antibody (anti-CCP) is an antibody found in patients with RA. It is more specific than rheumatoid factor and when strongly positive, it has a high predictive value in the risk of developing RA. Anti-CCP is associated with an increased risk of joint erosions and more aggressive disease.

Antinuclear antibodies

Antinuclear antibodies (ANAs) are antibodies to nuclear antigens. They are detected in blood using labelling methods such as indirect immunofluorescence. A positive ANA means there are antibodies present in the blood that will bind to a sample cell used in the test. It is important that detected ANAs are interpreted in the context of the patient and their symptoms. They may be detected in a variety of autoimmune conditions and in healthy patients.

If an ANA test is positive, it is important to examine which nuclear antigens the antibodies bind to. The pattern of

Table 3.1 Antinuclear antibodies against specific nuclear antigens and their associated diseases

Autoantibody	Associated disease
Anti–double-stranded DNA (anti-dsDNA)	SLE
Histone	Drug-induced lupus
Ro, La	Sjogren syndrome, SLE
Anticentromere	Limited cutaneous systemic sclerosis
Scl-70 (topoisomerase)	Diffuse systemic sclerosis
RNP	Mixed connective tissue disease
Jo-1	Antisynthetase syndrome (polymyositis and dermatomyositis)
Anti-Sm	SLE

SLE, *Systemic lupus erythematosus.*

immunofluorescence gives a clue, such as speckled, nucleolar or homogenous. The titre of the antibody also offers valuable information; the significance of the positive result is increased if the antibody is detectable after multiple dilutions (e.g., 1/2560 is more significant than 1/40).

Table 3.1 shows the ANAs directed against specific nuclear antigens and the diseases they are associated with. Antibodies to double-stranded DNA are very specific for SLE and are useful measures of disease activity.

Antineutrophil cytoplasmic antibodies

Antineutrophil cytoplasmic antibodies (ANCA) are antibodies directed against enzymes present in neutrophil granules. They are associated with inflammatory and vasculitic conditions. Two main immunofluorescent patterns are seen: cytoplasmic (c-ANCA) and perinuclear (p-ANCA).

c-ANCA and p-ANCA bind to several neutrophil enzymes, the most common being proteinase-3 (PR3) in the case of c-ANCA and myeloperoxidase (MPO) in the case of p-ANCA. Antibodies to PR3 are found in around 80% of patients with granulomatosis with polyangiitis (GPA), formerly known as Wegener's granulomatosis. Those against MPO are found in microscopic polyangiitis and eosinophilic granulomatosis with polyangiitis (EGPA, formerly Churg-Strauss syndrome).

Antiphospholipid antibodies

Lupus anticoagulant Beta-2 glycoprotein 1a and anticardiolipin antibodies are found in antiphospholipid syndrome. There is an association with venous and arterial thrombosis and recurrent miscarriages.

Complement

Complement molecules are small proteins activated in response to injury and inflammation. They bind to vessel walls and tissue when activated. This can lead to low serum levels of C3 and C4, as seen in active SLE and some forms of vasculitis.

Urine tests

- A quick urine dip test gives a guide to protein and blood in the urine.
- Microscopic haematuria is often seen in vasculitis affecting the kidneys.
- Proteinuria can suggest glomerulonephritis found in connective tissue disease, vasculitis and amyloidosis.
- Free light chains can be detected in multiple myeloma.
- Antistreptolysin-O (ASO) titre can be a useful way of detecting recent streptococcal infection in cases of reactive arthritis.

SYNOVIAL FLUID ANALYSIS

Synovial fluid analysis is the most useful test for investigating potential cases of septic or crystal arthropathies. Synovial fluid can be aspirated from most peripheral joints and many departments have microscopy facilities for quick analysis.

Macroscopic appearance

Normal fluid is a pale yellow, straw-like colour. Changes in the colour of the fluid can give clues to the underlying pathology (see Table 3.2).

Gram stain and culture

This should be performed if there is any suspicion of septic arthritis.

RED FLAG

The absence of organisms on microscopy does not exclude infection. It may be more difficult to detect organisms if antibiotics have been given before an aspirate is obtained.

Polarized light microscopy

To assess accurately the presence of crystals in fluid, the sample should be examined under polarized light. Urate crystals are

Table 3.2 Macroscopic appearance of synovial fluid and associated pathology

Synovial fluid appearance	Pathology
Yellow and clear	Normal
Blood stained	Haemarthrosis or trauma from aspiration
Cloudy	Increased numbers of white cells from infection or inflammation
Frank pus	Infection or occasionally crystal arthropathy
Chalky	Gout crystals, occasionally cholesterol crystals

needle-shaped and show strong negative birefringence: this means that crystals parallel to the plane of light appear yellow, while those at right angles appear blue. Calcium pyrophosphate dihydrate crystals are small and rhomboid-shaped and show weak positive birefringence. Urate crystal arthropathy is indicative of gout while calcium pyrophosphate crystal arthropathy is indicative of pseudogout. Fig. 3.1 shows the difference in polarized light microscopy appearance between gout and pseudogout. These conditions will be discussed further in Chapter 17.

NERVE CONDUCTION STUDIES AND ELECTROMYOGRAPHY

Nerve conduction studies (NCS) and electromyography (EMG) are electrophysiological tests used to diagnose and assess neuromuscular problems. They help to differentiate between primary muscle disease and neuropathic disorders, for example, carpal tunnel syndrome, myositis and steroid myopathy. NCS measure the velocity of motor and sensory nerve signals and can localize and assess the severity of peripheral nerve lesions. EMG records the spontaneous and voluntary electrical activity of muscles.

BIOPSY

Biopsies are occasionally performed to help with the investigation of musculoskeletal disorders. They are important in the assessment of bony lesions in suspected cancer. Vasculitis can often be diagnosed based on skin, blood vessel or nerve biopsies. For example, a temporal artery biopsy will be taken to assess for multinucleated giant cells if giant cell arteritis is suspected. Muscle biopsies are sometimes necessary in cases of suspected myositis. Renal biopsies may be taken in cases where glomerulonephritis is suspected. Occasionally, synovial biopsies are undertaken in cases of unexplained monoarthritis.

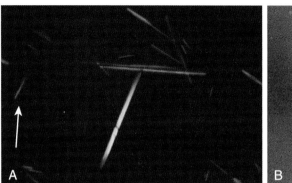
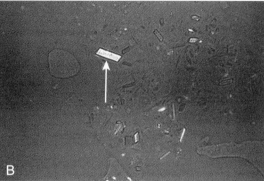

Fig. 3.1 Polarized light microscopy showing sodium urate crystals in gout (A) and calcium pyrophosphate crystals in pseudogout (B). (A from Henry JB. *Clinical Diagnosis and Management by Laboratory Methods*. 20th ed. Philadelphia, Saunders, 2001; Plate 19-7. B from Kjeldsberg CR, Knight JA. *Body Fluids: Laboratory Examination of Amniotic, Cerebrospinal, Seminal, Serous, and Synovial Fluids*. 3rd ed. Chicago. American Society for Clinical Pathology; 1993.)

Nailfold capillaroscopy

Nailfold capillaroscopy involves visualizing the small capillaries of the nailbed under a microscope. Raynaud's phenomenon and peripheral ischaemic changes are seen in almost all patients with systemic sclerosis. Nailfold capillaroscopy will show nailbed capillary destruction which will help to determine disease progression.

IMAGING

X-ray examinations

A plain X-ray (radiograph) examination is usually the first line of investigation in most musculoskeletal disorders. X-rays are good at visualizing bone but not soft tissue. To investigate ligaments and tendons, an ultrasound or MRI is often required.

Using X-rays involves the use of electromagnetic radiation produced by electrons striking a rotating metal target in an X-ray tube. A narrow beam of X-rays is produced, which then passes through the patient, and the image is formed when these rays hit an X-ray sensitive film placed behind the patient (Fig. 3.2).

Two views are required to assess for fractures, usually taken at 90 degrees to each other (usually anteroposterior and lateral). Sometimes specific views are required, such as a scaphoid view.

Ultrasound

Ultrasound is widely used and has the advantage of being safe, cheap and portable. It allows a dynamic assessment of joints and surrounding structures.

The image is produced using a transmitter that emits a beam of high-frequency sound (ultrasound) and detects the

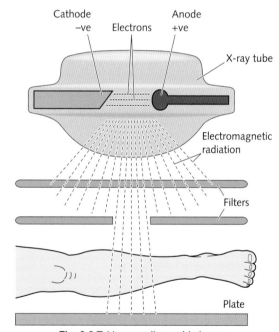

Fig. 3.2 Taking a radiographic image.

sound waves reflected from the soft tissues of the patient. The different tissues absorb and reflect varying amounts of the beam and the reflections are analyzed to produce a greyscale image.

Over recent years, the detection of synovitis and early erosions by ultrasound has helped to tailor therapy in RA (see Figs. 3.3 and 3.4). Other commonly imaged areas include shoulders looking for rotator cuff tears and the hip joint looking for evidence of effusions.

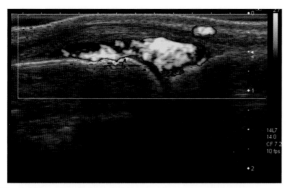

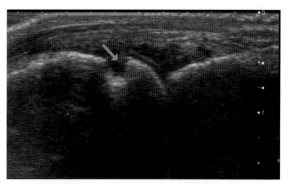

Fig. 3.3 Doppler ultrasound image showing synovitis of a metacarpophalangeal joint in a patient with rheumatoid arthritis. The high orange/yellow signal indicates increased blood flow within the synovium. (Provided by Dr Anna Ciechomska, Consultant Rheumatologist, Wishaw General Hospital.)

Fig. 3.4 Ultrasound image showing early erosion on the head of the metacarpal bone at the metacarpophalangeal joint in a patient with rheumatoid arthritis. The arrow indicates the 'bitten out' appearance of the erosion. (Provided by Dr Anna Ciechomska, Consultant Rheumatologist, Wishaw General Hospital.)

Ultrasound can also be used for guidance in joint injection and aspiration.

Computed tomography

Computed tomography (CT) uses the principles of an X-ray machine but the images are obtained when the X-ray tube is circled around the patient. Instead of an X-ray plate, the CT scanner has detectors within the machine to collect images. A large number of images are required by the computer software to build up the cross-sectional images taken in different planes.

The main role of CT in musculoskeletal disorders is in the study of bones, although contrast studies can be useful in conditions such as vasculitis.

CT scans also allow three-dimensional images to be reconstructed, which can be useful in complex fractures.

> ### COMMUNICATION 💬
>
> Remember computed tomographies and X-rays can carry a significant radiation exposure, dependent on the anatomical site to be imaged. Always communicate clearly why an investigation is required and gain consent.

Magnetic resonance imaging

Magnetic resonance imaging (MRI) gives excellent imaging of soft tissues and bone marrow.

Images are generated using a powerful magnet and radio waves. The electromagnetic field of the scanner causes the

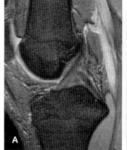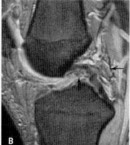

Fig. 3.5 Magnetic resonance imaging scans of the knee. (A) Normal. (B) Rupture of both cruciate ligaments (*arrows*).

protons in the body to line up with the field. Short bursts of radio waves are then directed at certain parts of the body, causing the protons to be knocked out of alignment. When the radio waves are turned off, the protons realign, sending out radio waves that are picked up by the receiver within the machine. Different tissue protons realign at differing speeds, which allows the computer to generate detailed images.

As the machine uses a large magnet, caution must be taken with metal components. Patients with cardiac pacemakers, intracranial aneurysm clips or with a suspicion of intraocular foreign bodies must not have an MRI examination unless first discussed with a radiologist.

MRI is commonly used to look at the knee (Fig. 3.5), the shoulder and the spine. In rheumatology, it can be used to assess synovitis and erosive damage (see Chapter 11, Fig. 11.10).

Isotope bone scan

An isotope bone scan involves the use of radioactive tracers injected into the body and taken up physiologically by bone.

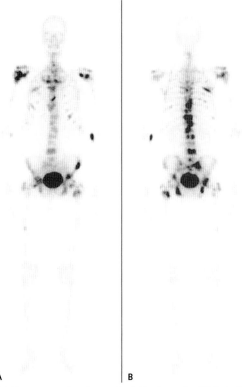

A   B

Fig. 3.6 Bone scan showing metastatic deposits. (A) Anterior view. (B) Posterior view.

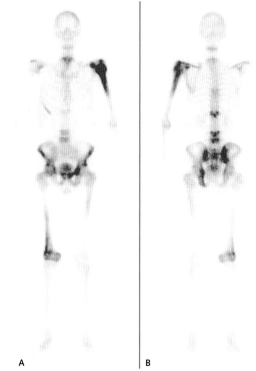

A   B

Fig. 3.7 Bone scan showing Paget's disease. (A) Anterior view. (B) Posterior view.

The most commonly used tracer is technetium-99m and its decay is measured using a gamma camera. The procedure is divided into three stages: blood flow (initial), blood pool (30 minutes) and delayed (4 hours).

The images show an outline of the body with areas highlighted where the isotope has accumulated.

Bone scans are a useful tool for identifying the presence of a disease process in bone (sensitive) but not in giving a diagnosis (nonspecific). Increased uptake typically occurs in growth plates, arthritis, fractures, metastases, infection and Paget's disease. Fig. 3.6 shows multiple metastatic deposits. Fig. 3.7 shows active lesions in Paget's disease.

Decreased uptake occurs in some tumours (haemopoeitic) and also in avascular bone.

Bone mineral density assessment

Bone densitometry (DEXA scanning) uses two X-ray beams to determine the density of bone relative to age- and sex-matched controls and is used in assessing and diagnosing osteoporosis. It is further explained in Chapter 15.

Positron emission tomography

Positron emission tomography (PET) is a nuclear medicine scanning technique that can be used to observe metabolic activity within the body. Radiolabelled tracers are injected into patients who are then scanned to observe specific concentrations within the tissues. This can be a very useful imaging modality for identifying active inflammation in specific tissues, such as large vessel vasculitis or for localizing occult infections.

Chapter Summary

- Various blood tests are used in investigating rheumatological and orthopaedic disorders.
- Many autoantibodies are disease-specific, such as anti-CCP antibody for rheumatoid arthritis and anti–double-stranded DNA antibody for SLE.
- Joint aspiration with fluid microscopy is the gold-standard test for a hot, swollen joint.
- Plain X-rays are useful for visualizing bone, while MRI and ultrasound are useful for examining soft tissues.
- Ultrasound has an emerging role in the detection of early synovitis and erosions in inflammatory arthropathies.

UKMLA Conditions

Crystal arthropathy
Osteomalacia
Osteoporosis
Rheumatoid arthritis
Septic arthritis
Systemic lupus erythematous

Regional musculoskeletal pain

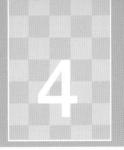

4

This chapter outlines how to approach patients with musculoskeletal pain in different areas of the body, highlighting indicators that point towards certain diagnoses. More in-depth discussions on these different diagnoses, are given later in the book.

NECK PAIN

As with all types of musculoskeletal pain being described in this chapter, there are many different causes that can usually be determined by a good history and examination. Remember to consider not only musculoskeletal aetiologies but also other relevant aetiologies such as cardiac and neurological.

DIFFERENTIAL DIAGNOSIS OF NECK PAIN

Mechanical neck pain
Cervical spondylosis
Cervical disc prolapse
Metastatic vertebral deposits (see Chapter 21)
Discitis (see Chapter 20)
Referred pain from
    Local structures (e.g., carotid dissection,
      lymphadenopathy, thyroiditis)
    Distant structures (e.g., ischaemic heart disease)

History

Acute trauma or high-impact injuries to the neck require careful assessment to exclude neurological damage, vascular damage or c-spine fracture (see Chapter 19), whereas chronic pain may suggest a degenerative or inflammatory cause. Pain may be accompanied by radiculopathy (injury or entrapment of a specific nerve root observable on examination) or myelopathy (injury to or compression of the spinal cord). Shooting pain radiating down the arms suggests nerve entrapment, whereas weakness or clumsiness in the legs, with/without bladder or bowel disturbance suggests cord compression.

Dizziness may occur in severe degenerative disease due to vertebral artery compression.

Fever, weight loss and general malaise raise the prospect of malignancy or infection.

A chronic bilateral ache in the neck and shoulders with high erythrocyte sedimentation rate (ESR) suggests a systemic, inflammatory disease, for example, polymyalgia rheumatica.

Examination

Examination of the neck is described in Chapter 2. Any patient with neck pain should have a full neurological examination of the cranial nerves and the peripheral nerves of all four limbs.

RED FLAG

In a patient with neck pain following trauma, the neck should be immobilized to protect the spinal cord until further imaging can be performed. You should not proceed to examine the neck further until imaging can rule out an unstable fracture.

Investigations

In acute neck pain following trauma, radiographs and computed tomography (CT) scans may be required to exclude a fracture. The Canadian C-spine Rule and NEXUS (National Emergency X-Radiography Utilisation Study) criteria can help to identify patients who require immobilization and further imaging.

In chronic neck pain, radiographs may show degenerative disease as in cervical spondylosis.

Magnetic resonance imaging (MRI) is used to assess for a cervical disc prolapse and nerve compression. Bloods are not usually helpful in neck pain, however if infection or malignancy is suspected, inflammatory markers and tumour markers should be obtained, respectively.

Nerve conduction studies may be used where a cervical radiculopathy is suspected and can differentiate between the neck being the source of pathology as opposed to a more distal nerve pathology.

SHOULDER PAIN

Shoulder pain similarly has many different aetiologies including trauma, age-related degeneration and inflammation. Pain in the shoulder can also commonly be referred pain from the neck or abdomen.

DIFFERENTIAL DIAGNOSIS OF SHOULDER PAIN

Rotator cuff pathology (impingement, tear or tendinopathy)
Subacromial bursitis (see Chapter 23)
Adhesive capsulitis
Arthritis of the acromioclavicular joint
Arthritis of the glenohumeral joint
Bicipital tendinopathy
Polymyalgia rheumatica (see Chapter 14)
Rheumatoid arthritis (see Chapter 12)
Referred pain from
  Neck pathology
  Cardiac ischaemia
  Pancoast tumour
  Intraabdominal pathology; Kehr's sign (e.g.,
    subphrenic abscess, splenic rupture)

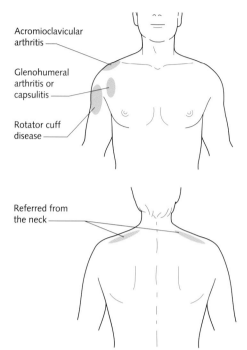

Fig. 4.1 Many structures can give rise to shoulder pain. These diagrams show how the site of pain varies with the origin.

History

Important features in a history of shoulder pain include:

- The site of pain; Fig. 4.1 shows how the site of shoulder pain varies depending on the cause. Remember that pain can be referred to the shoulder tip from the abdomen.
- Range of passive movement; reduction in passive range of movement and functional ability with pain may occur in frozen shoulder. In a rotator cuff tear, active movement will be reduced, especially in abduction (painful arc), but passive movement will be preserved.
- Timing of pain; osteoarthritis will typically cause pain that is worse with activity and worse at the end of the day, whereas inflammatory disorders will cause pain that is worse on waking and better with activity.

Examination

Shoulder examination is also described in Chapter 2. Typical appearances indicating specific pathologies include:

- 'Squaring off' of the shoulder, and an obvious bulge anteriorly indicates an anterior dislocation.
- Muscle wasting of supraspinatus and infraspinatus suggests a chronic rotator cuff tear.
- Global restriction in all directions of movement at the shoulder joint is seen in osteoarthritis or in adhesive capsulitis.
- A reduction in active range of movement but preserved passive movement is seen in a rotator cuff tear.

Investigations

Radiographs may show features of osteoarthritis or suggest a rotator cuff tear with a high-riding humeral head in the glenohumeral joint. Soft tissue injuries such as a rotator cuff tear or proximal biceps tendon rupture, can be further investigated with an MRI or ultrasound scan.

ELBOW

The elbow while a relatively small joint, can cause significant problems which impact a patient's quality of life, and ability to perform at work.

DIFFERENTIAL DIAGNOSIS OF ELBOW PAIN

Lateral epicondylitis (tennis elbow)
Olecranon bursitis (see Chapter 23)
Septic arthritis (see Chapter 20)
Crystal arthropathy (e.g., gout, pseudogout) (see Chapter 16)
Osteoarthritis (see Chapter 11)
Inflammatory arthritis (see Chapters 12 and 13)
Medial epicondylitis (golfer's elbow)
Referred pain from the neck or shoulder

History

The mechanism of injury is key in the history. A history of repetitive movements can trigger lateral epicondylitis (tennis

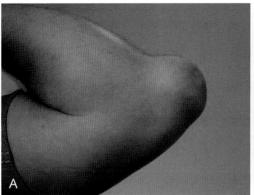
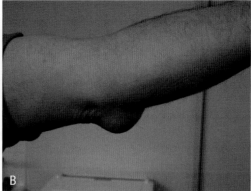

Fig. 4.2 A patient with large chronic olecranon bursitis. (From Reilly D, Kamineni S. *Olecranon bursitis*. J Shoulder and Elbow Surg. Jan; 25[1]:158-167; 2016.)

elbow) or medial epicondylitis (golfer's elbow). Prolonged time spent leaning on the elbow can cause an egg-like swelling over the elbow as in olecranon bursitis.

Examination

Elbow examination is also described in Chapter 2.

- Swelling over the olecranon with a near normal range of motion is seen in olecranon bursitis (see Fig. 4.2). This can be contrasted with septic arthritis where the swelling is generalized around the elbow joint and any movement is resisted by the patient.
- Palpating over the lateral epicondyle and performing resisted dorsiflexion commonly exacerbates the pain of tennis elbow, while golfer's elbow gives localized tenderness over the medial epicondyle and pain in supination and resisted wrist flexion.

Investigations

Once again, radiographs can be used to assess for osteoarthritis. Ultrasound scanning can be used when the diagnosis of tendinopathy is in doubt, but largely this is a clinical diagnosis. In septic arthritis, a joint aspirate should be obtained and sent for microscopic analysis. This is contrasted with olecranon bursitis, where every attempt should be made to maintain the integrity of the bursa. Once the bursa is breeched (e.g., if an infected bursitis is not settling with antibiotics and must be drained) it can be difficult to encourage the bursa to heal. This is because it is constantly producing bursal fluid and so a chronic sinus can result which may then require excision.

WRIST AND HAND

The wrist and small joints of the hands can be affected by many pathologies which can quickly become disabling.

DIFFERENTIAL DIAGNOSIS IN WRIST AND HAND PAIN

Osteoarthritis (see Chapter 11)
Inflammatory arthritis (see Chapters 12 and 13)
Carpal tunnel syndrome (see Chapter 10)
De Quervain's tenosynovitis
Crystal arthropathy (see Chapter 16)
Ulnar nerve entrapment (see Chapter 10)
Raynaud's phenomenon (see Chapter 14)
Complex regional pain syndrome
Referred pain from the cervical spine, shoulder or elbow

History

Rheumatoid arthritis is most likely to be found in the small joints of the hands and feet. A full history including the patient's family history is essential. Specific triggers for different symptoms are important in forming a differential diagnosis:

- Cold weather typically triggers Raynaud's phenomenon.
- Changes in medication and in diet (high in purines) may trigger gout.
- Repetitive use (e.g., using a keyboard) may exacerbate osteoarthritis.

Examination

Look for:

- Heberden or Bouchard nodes, seen in osteoarthritis (see Fig. 4.3);
- synovial swelling of the small joints of the hand or tendon sheaths, seen in rheumatoid arthritis;
- rheumatoid nodules;

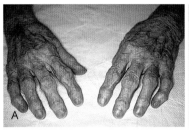
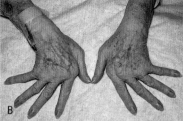
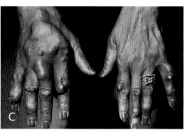

| Osteoarthritis | Rheumatoid arthritis | Gouty arthritis |

Fig. 4.3 Types of arthritis. (A) Osteoarthritis. Note the presence of nodes in the proximal interphalangeal joints (Bouchard nodes) and distal interphalangeal joints (Heberden nodes). (B) Rheumatoid arthritis. Note the marked ulnar deviation. (C) Gouty arthritis. Note tophi (stones) containing sodium urate crystals. (From Swartz MH. *Textbook of physical diagnosis*. 8th ed. Philadelphia, Elsevier; 2021.)

- psoriatic plaques;
- gouty tophi (see Fig. 4.3);
- changes to the nails;
- colour changes to the digits or ulceration as seen in Raynaud's phenomenon (see Fig. 4.4);
- changes in skin colour with atrophy and reduced hair growth as features of complex regional pain syndrome (CRPS);
- wasting of the thenar and hypothenar muscles resulting from median and ulnar nerve compression, respectively.

Palpation of joints helps in assessing causes of swelling. Advanced osteoarthritis can cause hard bony swelling if large osteophytes are present, and is easily distinguishable from the soft, warm, boggy synovial swelling of inflammatory arthritis.

Investigations

Many diagnoses in the hand can be reached without further investigation, such as dull aching hands in a 75-year-old with Heberden nodes and carpometacarpal (CMC) joint pain, indicating osteoarthritis. In a case such as this, plain radiographs will confirm the diagnosis but will not alter the management. Bloods should be taken where inflammation or infection is suspected. Rheumatoid factor and CCP-antibodies should be taken in a patient with suspected rheumatoid arthritis.

COMPLEX REGIONAL PAIN SYNDROME

This is also known as reflex sympathetic dystrophy and is a chronic complex pain syndrome that worsens over time. The pathogenesis is largely unknown, but CRPS can result after trauma or surgery, and is thought to be due to abnormal nervous system functioning. It is an uncommon cause of regional pain that typically affects the extremities, but in particular the distal forearm and hand. The pain experienced is usually severe and out-of-context of the original injury, with accompanying key

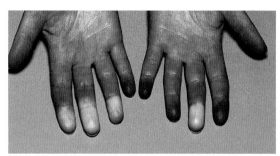

Fig. 4.4 Raynaud's phenomenon. (From Hallett JW et al. *Comprehensive vascular and endovascular surgery*. 2nd ed. Philadelphia, Elsevier; 2009.)

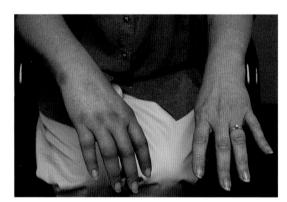

Fig. 4.5 Complex regional pain syndrome (CRPS). (From Mathews AL, Chung KC. *Management of complications of distal radius fractures*. Hand Clin. 31[2] , 205–215. Elsevier Inc.; 2015.)

features of hypersensitivity, skin changes and autonomic disturbance (Fig. 4.5). Allodynia is often present (pain from a stimulus that would not normally produce pain, e.g., light touch).

Treatment is challenging and so usually involves a multidisciplinary team approach with physiotherapy from specialist hand physiotherapists and neuropathic analgesia from a dedicated pain team.

BACK, HIP AND LEG PAIN

Eighty percent of people will suffer from back pain in their life-time. History and examination of patients presenting with pain in the back, hips and lower limbs are both very important. Many patients do not appreciate the anatomy of the hip and commonly point to the greater trochanter or iliac crests when describing 'hip pain'. In addition, because of the complex anatomy of the spinal cord, pain signals can be referred to other regions, and a detailed clinical examination is therefore required. There is often overlap of symptoms and diagnoses and so in this part of the chapter, they will be appreciated together.

There are four common patterns to consider:

- back pain
- back and leg pain
- hip pain, with or without leg pain
- leg pain

Figure 4.6 shows the different patterns of pain around the back, hip and leg.

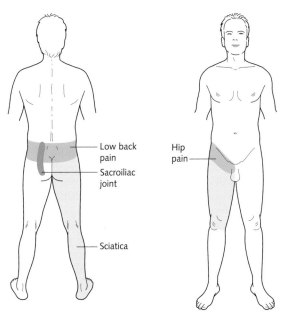

Low back pain
Sacroiliac joint
Sciatica
Hip pain

Fig. 4.6 Patterns of pain around the back, leg and hip.

Back pain can also be referred from the abdomen and associated with a myriad of intraabdominal causes.

BACK PAIN

DIFFERENTIAL DIAGNOSIS IN BACK PAIN

Simple lower back pain (see Chapter 9)
Osteoarthritis (see Chapter 11)
Prolapsed intravertebral disc/degenerative disc disease (see Chapter 9)
Inflammatory spondyloarthropathy (see Chapter 13)
Vertebral crush fracture (see Chapter 15)
Spinal stenosis/spondylolisthesis (see Chapter 9)
Malignancy (see Chapter 21)
Infective discitis (see Chapter 9)

RED FLAG

Red flag symptoms of sinister back pain:
Age of onset <20 or >55 years
History of weight loss
Fevers
Persistent pain not affected by movement
History of malignancy
Associated progressive neurology, bowel/bladder dysfunction or saddle anaesthesia
Pain worse at night

History

Mechanical back pain is the most common cause of acute back pain, usually preceded by a history of lifting or straining the lower back. The pain is band-like, severe and does not usually radiate into the legs.

More concerning features in the history include the presence of night sweats and weight loss, and these raise concerns over 'sinister causes' of back pain (see Fig. 21.10). Have a low threshold for intensive investigation in patients presenting with these signs.

COMMUNICATION

There are many psychosocial factors that increase chronicity of back pain. It is valuable to approach back pain in a biopsychosocial manner, listening to concerns about the disabling nature of back pain, its effects on employment and mobility, as well as the patient's perception of pain, their coping mechanisms and mental state.

BACK AND LEG PAIN

Back pain radiating to the legs suggests nerve root entrapment.

History

Sciatica originates from the lower back and radiates down the leg, past the knee and into the foot. Weakness or numbness may also occur. It might result from an acute event (e.g., when lifting a heaving load), resulting in a disc prolapse onto the nerve root, or from chronic degenerative spinal disease causing compression at the exiting foramen. The pain is usually severe, sharp or shock-like and is constant but with exacerbations. Positions such as standing or activities such as coughing can worsen the pain. Over time, pain from a disc prolapse usually settles.

Pain from spinal stenosis is made worse by walking and relieved by rest and leaning forward, which creates more space around the spinal cord. This is what is referred to as spinal claudication. Patients often adopt a stooped gait.

Facet joint osteoarthritis results from the 'wear and tear' degradation of cartilage between the facet joints in the back. When mobilizing, the lack of cartilage causes pain and stiffness and there is therefore loss of normal range of motion. The pain occurs in the back and may radiate to the top of the leg but does not extend below the knee.

HIP PAIN, WITH OR WITHOUT LEG PAIN

True hip pain is felt in the groin and may radiate down to the knee.

DIFFERENTIAL DIAGNOSIS OF HIP PAIN

Osteoarthritis (see Chapter 11)
Hip fracture (see Chapter 18)
Avascular necrosis of the hip
Trochanteric bursitis (see Chapter 23)
Paget's disease (see Chapter 15)
Hip impingement

History

In hip osteoarthritis the onset of pain is insidious and worsens with movement. The patient may describe this as an ache or a 'grinding' pain.

A hip fracture is a common sequela of a low-energy fall in the frail and elderly. The leg will appear shortened and externally rotated, the pain is sharp and severe and the patient cannot bear weight on the affected leg.

LEG PAIN

History

Occasionally sciatica presents with leg pain only, without the lower back discomfort.

Muscular conditions such as myositis or muscular dystrophy can present with muscle pain, weakness and gradual loss of function.

Peripheral vascular disease causes cramping leg pain on walking (claudication), which is relieved with rest. This should be differentiated from spinal stenosis. Skin changes and ulceration may be present.

CLINICAL NOTES

LOSS OF FUNCTION AND DISABILITY

It is important to explore how pain impacts patients' functional abilities and whether there are limitations on certain activities. Patients may need ergonomic adjustments within the workplace.

Examination

The back, hip and lower limbs should be examined together as in Chapter 2. In back pain, it is essential to perform a neurological examination of the lower limbs and to ask about associated symptoms such as bowel and bladder disturbance. Incontinence suggests a cauda equina syndrome requiring urgent MRI and urgent surgical decompression; this is further explored in Chapter 9.

Investigations

A full set of blood tests including bone profile (calcium, phosphate and albumin) is important. Certain tests, such as a myeloma screen, are important in those over 55 years of age with sinister features to their back pain.

X-ray examination of the back, when suspecting mechanical back pain, is not useful. It exposes the patient to a significant amount of radiation and has a low diagnostic yield. When sacroiliac joint disease or inflammatory spondyloarthropathy is suspected, MRI is the investigation of choice.

The following imaging findings are significant and warrant further investigation to guide management:

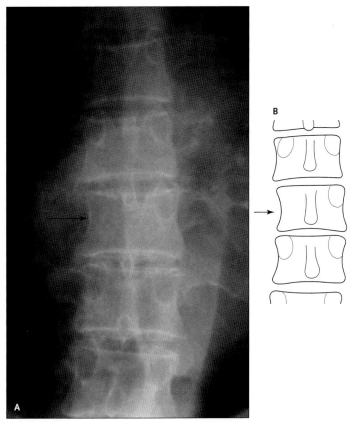

Fig. 4.7 Malignancy of the spine. (A) The 'winking-owl sign' *(black arrow)* occurs when the pedicle is destroyed due to metastasis. (B) The missing 'eye' *(black arrow)* represents bony destruction of the pedicle by tumour, so always look closely at the pedicles.

- 'Squaring' of the vertebral bodies and bridging syndesmophytes in ankylosing spondylitis (see Chapter 13).
- Spondylolisthesis causing neurological symptoms.
- Lytic lesions of the vertebral body, classically the pedicle (winking owl sign; see Fig. 4.7), indicating malignancy.
- Vertebral fracture.
- Erosion of the vertebral body around the disc due to infection.

CT, isotope bone scanning and MRI remain available for situations where doubt remains, especially for infection, malignancy and cord compression.

DIFFERENTIAL DIAGNOSES IN KNEE PAIN
Osteoarthritis (see Chapter 11)
Meniscal injuries (see Chapter 22)
Ligament injuries (see Chapter 22)
Bursitis (see Chapter 23)
Rheumatoid arthritis or other inflammatory arthritis (see Chapters 12 and 13)
Septic arthritis (see Chapter 20)
Patellofemoral disorders
Referred pain from the hip/spine

KNEE PAIN

Knee pain accounts for over a third of all referrals to orthopaedic surgeons.

History

Consider the patient's age, occupation and activity levels. A young athletic patient with a recent injury is more likely to have a meniscal or ligamentous injury, whereas an elderly patient with gradually worsening pain will most likely have osteoarthritis or a degenerative meniscal tear.

Character of the pain

In osteoarthritis, the onset of pain is gradual over months or years. Sudden onset pain is usually due to a ligamentous or meniscal injury, or a fracture if there is significant trauma. Spontaneous atraumatic pain is more likely to be septic arthritis or crystal arthropathy. Pain and stiffness in the morning that gets better as the day goes on suggests inflammatory arthritis. Pain originating from the knee rarely radiates, but children commonly experience pain referred from the hip as knee pain.

Nature of the pain

- Meniscal tears produce sharp, stabbing, easily localized pains.
- Osteoarthritis causes a deep, general, 'gnawing' pain.

Aggravating/relieving factors

Osteoarthritis pain is often worse on movement and relieved by rest; inflammatory pain gets better with use of the joint throughout the day.

Pain from meniscal injury is worse on full flexion or on twisting.

In acute crystal arthropathy or septic arthritis, any movement of the joint produces severe pain.

Pain from prepatellar bursitis is worse on kneeling.

Site of pain

Pain can be generalized or localized. Generalized pain suggests an arthritic process affecting the whole joint. Large, tense effusions, such as after an injury or septic arthritis, also produce pain all over the joint.

Localized pain causes depend on the site of pain. See Fig. 4.8.

- Anterior: patellofemoral pain is felt here. Pain above or below the patella may be due to prepatellar or infrapatellar bursitis, respectively.
- Medial or lateral: localized pain to either side of the joint may be due to osteoarthritis (particularly so in the medial joint line), collateral ligament injury or from meniscal tears.
- Posterior: pain here is less common, but a Baker's cyst may be felt here (although not usually painful) and if large may cause pressure effects around the knee.
- Pain down the front of the thigh and into the knee is typical of referred hip pain.

Loss of function

Patients may have significant disabling symptoms from knee pain. Injuries that affect the ligaments often lead the patient to tell you they 'don't trust the knee' and are worried it will 'give way': a hallmark of joint instability.

Injury

Any history of injury is important. Be sure to ask additional closed questions regarding the injury:

- Ask if the patient heard a 'snap' or 'pop'.
- How long did any swelling take to appear?
- Is there a history of locking? (This might suggest meniscal injury.)

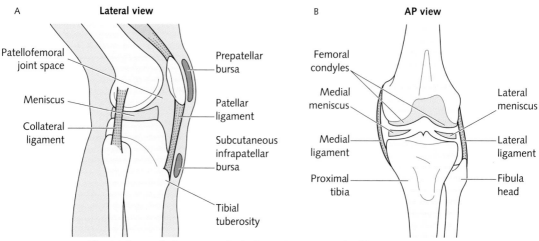

Fig. 4.8 Anatomical structures in the knee that cause pain. *AP,* Anteroposterior.

Investigations

Fig. 4.9 provides an algorithm for investigating knee pain.

Further imaging

This is only warranted in certain conditions:

- MRI: useful for confirming ligamentous or meniscal pathology.
- CT: gives detailed imaging of bony structures such as in an occult tibial plateau fracture.
- Isotope bone scan: useful in showing 'hot spots' of increased metabolic bone activity, but does not give an exact diagnosis. It can be useful for rarer conditions such as bone tumours and osteomyelitis.

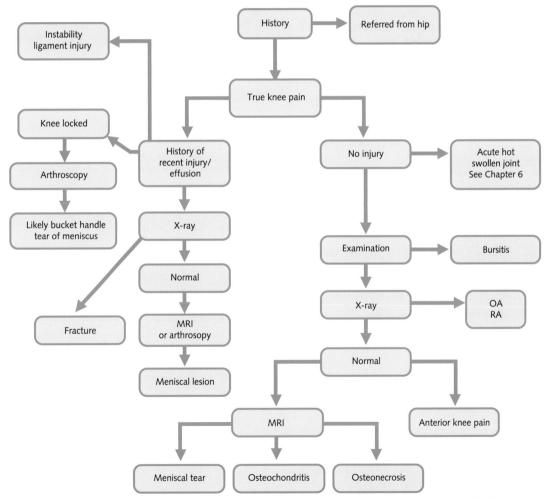

Fig. 4.9 Algorithm for the investigation of knee pain. *MRI*, Magnetic resonance imaging; *OA*, osteoarthritis; *RA*, rheumatoid arthritis.

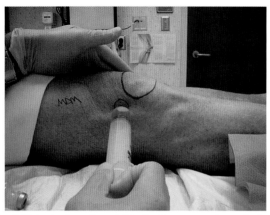

Fig. 4.10 Aspirating a knee joint. Gentle pressure is applied to the plunger to aspirate the fluid. Use of the nondominant hand to compress the opposite side of the joint may be helpful. (From Miller MD, Hart JA, MacKnight JM. *Essential orthopaedics*, Philadelphia, Saunders; 2010.)

- Ultrasound: useful for examining for synovitis and effusions and for guiding injections.

Aspiration

Aspirating a joint is a simple way of getting some specific clues about diagnosis.

Using aseptic technique, feel the upper and lower border of the patella. From roughly the midpoint, feel laterally until you can identify the patellofemoral joint space. This is the easiest landmark to use and the needle should be inserted at 90 degrees to the lateral aspect of the knee, angled slightly proximally to aspirate fluid (Fig. 4.10).

Examine the fluid obtained (Fig. 4.11):

- Normal fluid is yellowish/straw coloured.
- Slightly clouded yellow fluid indicates inflammation.
- A 'milky' appearance can be seen in gout.
- Blood-stained fluid is usually from haemarthrosis after injury or occasionally occurs spontaneously (e.g., patients on warfarin).

Blood and fat are sometimes seen even on a plain radiograph as a haemarthrosis (Fig. 4.12) and can indicate a fracture or an anterior cruciate ligament rupture.

HINTS AND TIPS

Always send joint aspirate fluid for microscopy, culture and sensitivity testing and ask the laboratory to examine for crystals.

Arthroscopy

This involves keyhole surgery into the joint. This is discussed further in Chapter 24.

ANKLE AND FOOT PAIN

The unique complexity of the structure of the foot and ankle combined with the relative difficulty in examining individual joints make diagnosis of ankle and foot disorders more challenging. Biochemical factors play a particularly important role in ankle and foot problems.

Differential diagnosis

The differential diagnosis of pain in the ankle and/or foot is shown in Fig. 4.13.

History

The following points are important to cover when taking a history from patients with ankle or foot pain.

Character of the pain

- Severe, recurrent self-limiting pain (especially of the first metatarsophalangeal joint) suggests crystal arthropathy.
- Chronic dull pain with soft tissue swelling suggests inflammation.
- Posterior pain on walking may be due to Achilles tendinopathy, while discomfort on the sole of the foot suggests plantar fasciitis.

Associated symptoms

- Back or knee pain may suggest referred pain.
- Coldness, pallor or ulcers may be due to peripheral vascular disease.
- Burning and numbness can occur with Morton neuroma, tarsal tunnel syndrome (compression of the tibial nerve passing through the tarsal tunnel) or diabetic neuropathy.
- Plantar fasciitis is associated with spondyloarthropathies so ask about back pain, psoriasis and inflammatory bowel disease.
- Repetitive trauma such as running, jumping or other athletic injuries can result in Achilles tendinopathy. Quinolones, such as ciprofloxacin, can cause spontaneous Achilles tendon rupture.
- A recent illness or starting diuretic therapy can trigger gout.

Loss of function

It is important to enquire about the impact of pain in the foot and ankle on a patient's function and lifestyle. Achilles

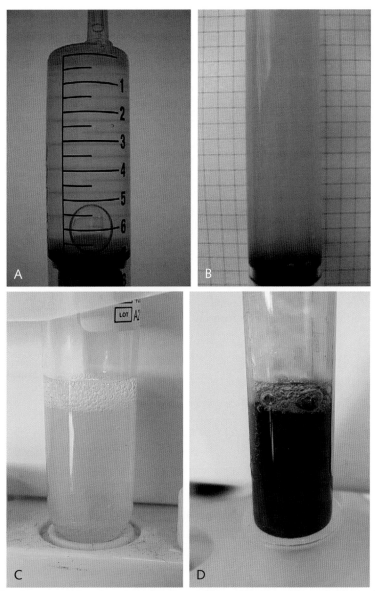

Fig. 4.11 (A) Clear, slightly yellow synovial aspirate (note the clear visibility of the line marks on the back of the syringe); (B) opacity caused by high numbers of cellular content; (C) 'milky' appearance frequently found in gout; (D) bloody synovial fluid (caused by trauma or preceding joint procedures). ((a, b) from Courtney P, Doherty M. *Joint aspiration and injection and synovial fluid analysis. Best Practice & Research Clinical Rheumatology.* 23(2): 161–192; 2009. (c, d) from Hochberg M et al. *Rheumatology.* 8th ed. Elsevier; 2023.)

tendinopathy can ruin the career of an athlete, but a sedentary older patient may not feel significantly impacted by this.

Examination

Examination of the foot and ankle joint is also described in Chapter 2.

Investigations

Plain X-ray images may show inflammatory erosions or degenerative changes.

- Ultrasound images can identify synovitis, effusions, tendinopathy, ligament damage and Morton neuromas.

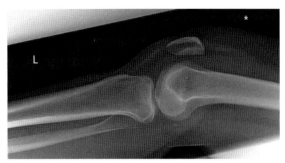

Fig. 4.12 A lipohaemarthrosis in the suprapatellar pouch of the left (L) knee secondary to a subtle tibial plateau fracture. A fluid level is seen as the fat 'floats' on the blood *(white arrow)*. (Courtesy Dr Aziz Marzoug, Radiology Specialist Trainee, Aberdeen Royal Infirmary.)

- MRI can also be used to assess the above and is less user-dependent but more expensive.

Synovial fluid analysis: similar to the knee joint; see above.

Nerve conduction studies: these are useful for confirming diagnoses such as tarsal tunnel syndrome or peripheral neuropathy.

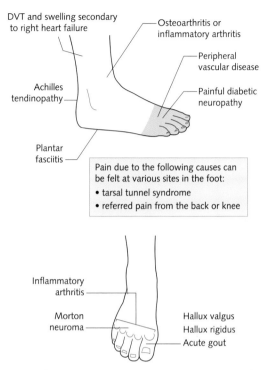

Fig. 4.13 Differential diagnosis of ankle and/or foot pain. *DVT,* Deep vein thrombosis.

Chapter Summary

- The differential diagnoses from regional pain include neurological, musculoskeletal and multisystem causes. Thought must be given to both the clinical history and examination findings in developing a sensible differential diagnosis.
- The important red-flag features of neck and back pain must be considered, particularly in patients with a history of trauma or those whose histories suggest an acute fracture, malignancy, cord compression or infection.
- Pain in the neck, arms and hands typically follows patterns of involvement with specific different triggers.
- Complex regional pain syndrome is an uncommon but debilitating cause of nonspecific regional pain. It requires a multidisciplinary team approach to its management.
- Back pain is a common complaint with many causes and may be associated with pain in the hips or lower limbs.
- Knee and ankle pain differs in different patient populations, the young athlete contrasts to the elderly frail patient.
- Lower limb pain can often be referred from distant proximal sites (back/hip).

Chapter Summary—cont'd

UKMLA Conditions
Bursitis
Crystal arthropathy
Osteoarthritis
Septic arthritis

UKMLA Presentations
Back pain
Bone pain
Chronic joint pain/stiffness
Muscle pain/myalgia
Neck pain/stiffness
Soft tissue injury

Widespread musculoskeletal pain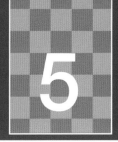

Widespread musculoskeletal pain can be distressing for patients. The differential diagnosis is varied and requires careful examination and investigation to separate causes (see below):

THE DIFFERENTIAL DIAGNOSIS OF WIDESPREAD MUSCULOSKELETAL PAIN

Inflammatory arthritis
Fibromyalgia
Systemic lupus erythematosus
Myositis
Polymyalgia rheumatica
Metabolic bone disease (osteomalacia, Paget's disease)
Paraneoplastic rheumatic syndrome
Widespread skeletal metastases
Vitamin deficiency: B_{12}/folate
Hypothyroidism

The patient's age, gender and race might give important clues about the diagnosis. For example, polymyalgia rheumatica (PMR) rarely affects people under the age of 60 years, fibromyalgia and systemic lupus erythematosus (SLE) are more common in women than men and osteomalacia is more prevalent in the Asian than the Caucasian population.

INVESTIGATING WIDESPREAD PAIN

History

A history should be taken covering the following points:

Site

Patients may struggle to localize pain. Pay close attention to whether the pain is felt in the muscles, joints or along nerve tracts.

Onset of pain

Widespread pain is usually insidious and progressive, but in rare cases SLE and PMR can produce pain that develops over a few days.

Character

Ask the patient to describe their pain. It may be described as a deep aching sensation suggestive of an inflammatory condition such as rheumatoid arthritis or SLE. However, a sharp shooting pain may indicate neuropathy while pain produced upon light palpation in trigger areas may suggest fibromyalgia.

Radiation

Ask the patient if their pain is localized to one area or spreads elsewhere.

Associated symptoms

Ask the patient about symptoms they experience alongside their pain. These could include:

- Stiffness that improves or worsens with activity.
- Temporal headaches, jaw claudication and blurred vision that suggest giant cell arteritis in association with PMR.
- Rashes, mouth ulcers and Raynaud phenomenon that raise the possibility of SLE.
- Psychiatric problems, anxiety and depression that can be features of fibromyalgia.
- Abdominal pain and confusion that can be present in hypercalcaemia.

Timing of pain

Generally, pain that is worse in the morning and eases as the day progresses is typical of inflammation due to SLE or PMR, for example. Pain and stiffness that worsen with activity would be more likely experienced in osteoarthritis. Pain that is constant with episodic periods of worsening without an obvious cause may suggest fibromyalgia.

Exacerbating or relieving factors

Try to determine if there are any factors that are improving or worsening the patient's pain. These could include activity, over-the-counter medications or stress.

Severity of pain

Have the patient rate the severity of their pain on a scale from 1 to 10. This will give you an idea as to the impact the pain is having on the patient's life.

HINTS AND TIPS

Remember the **SOCRATES** acronym for taking a pain history discussed in Chapter 1.

Examination and investigation

Fig. 5.1 gives a suggested algorithm for the examination and investigation of patients with widespread musculoskeletal pain.

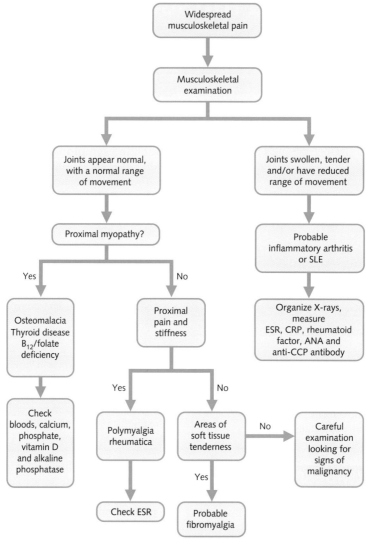

Fig. 5.1 Algorithm for investigation of widespread musculoskeletal pain. ANA, *Antinuclear antibody;* CRP, *C-reactive protein;* ESR, *erythrocyte sedimentation rate;* SLE, *systemic lupus erythematosus.*

Examination

Examination is useful in determining whether pain is coming from the bones and joints or from muscles and soft tissues. Carefully examine the joints for signs of inflammation and palpate the muscles and soft tissues for tenderness. Fibromyalgia triggering spots should also be palpated. Examination of other systems may be required if the history is suggestive of more atypical causes.

Investigations

These are guided by examination findings. It is important to note that many tests can be normal in the early stages of a disease.

Blood tests

- Erythrocyte sedimentation rate (ESR) and C-reactive protein (CRP) may be elevated in PMR, SLE or inflammatory arthritis.
- Calcium levels may be high if there are bony metastases or low in cases of osteomalacia.
- Parathyroid hormone (PTH) levels should be checked in hypercalcaemia to exclude hyperparathyroidism.
- Low vitamin D levels are found in osteomalacia.
- Serum alkaline phosphatase may be elevated in Paget's disease.

- An immune screen including antinuclear antibody (ANA), anti-dsDNA antibodies and complement, may be abnormal in SLE.
- Testing positive for rheumatoid factor and anti-CCP would be indicative of rheumatoid arthritis.
- Testing positive for antineutrophil cytoplasmic antibodies (e.g., p-ANCA or c-ANCA) would suggest vasculitis.

Radiology

Small joint X-ray images may show erosive changes. X-ray examination of the long bones can be useful in osteomalacia, where Looser zones may be seen.

Other radiological tests (chest X-ray examination, bone scans, computed tomography scans) may be required if there is a strong suspicion of malignancy.

FIBROMYALGIA

Definition

Many patients who present to the Rheumatology Department with chronic widespread pain cannot be readily diagnosed. The spectrum of symptoms associated with fibromyalgia is often nonspecific and many patients suffer for a long time between onset of symptoms and establishing a diagnosis. Associated symptoms of fatigue, depression, insomnia, altered bowel habits and poor concentration are accompanied by a widespread soft tissue tenderness localized over a number of trigger points. However, the existence of fibromyalgia as an organic disease remains controversial. Many clinicians recognize the above symptoms and clinical features but feel that labelling patients may reinforce their illness. However, there is evidence that referral rates and investigations lessen once patients have been diagnosed.

Prevalence

Fibromyalgia is common: the prevalence is estimated at between 2% and 5%.

Aetiology

The aetiology of fibromyalgia is poorly understood. Several theories exist, including altered levels of serotonin in the brain and the upregulation of pain receptor sensitivity. However, it has been noted that there is often an event that triggers the onset of symptoms. This event could be a viral infection, bereavement, an operation or the breakdown of a relationship, for example. It is a condition that most commonly affects middle-aged women. There is thought to be a familial element to this condition.

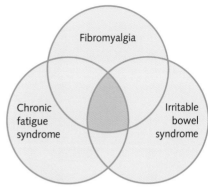

Fig. 5.2 Overlap between fibromyalgia and other syndromes.

There is considerable overlap between fibromyalgia and several other conditions that have a functional component (Fig. 5.2).

Pathogenesis

The roles of various neurotransmitters, pain receptor pathways, hormones and peptides have been examined in fibromyalgia. Unfortunately, in spite of much research, the pathogenesis remains poorly understood. However, there is almost certainly a link between pain, poor sleep and mental health burden in fibromyalgia. This is illustrated in Fig. 5.3.

Clinical features

Fibromyalgia predominantly affects women between the ages of 30 and 60 years. Patients complain of a long history of severe widespread pain that is exacerbated by minimal exertion and responds poorly to analgesia. Other common symptoms are shown in the box below.

COMMON SYMPTOMS IN FIBROMYALGIA
• Fatigue • Sleep disturbance • Poor concentration, sometimes referred to as 'fibro fog' • Headache • Paraesthesia • Anxiety/depression • Altered bowel habit • Widespread pain

The only significant finding on examination is the presence of soft-tissue tenderness, usually in multiple sites. Common sites of tenderness are shown in Fig. 5.4. Pain is often perceived as constant with unpredictable episodic worsening. It is important to note that fibromyalgia may co-exist with other inflammatory rheumatic conditions.

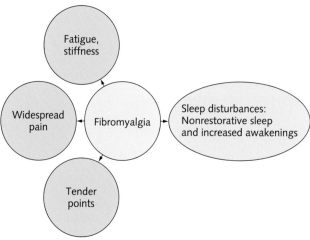

Fig. 5.3 The connection between fibromyalgia pain and sleep disturbances. (From Kryger MH. *Atlas of Clinical Sleep Medicine.* 2nd ed. Elsevier; 2014.)

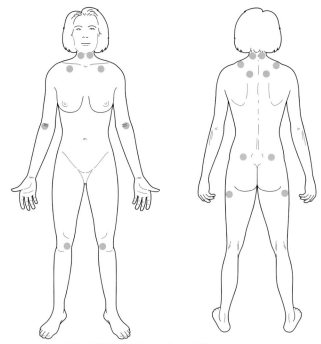

Fig 5.4 The tender points of fibromyalgia.

Investigations

Fibromyalgia is a clinical diagnosis based on recognition of symptoms and tender points. There is no specific diagnostic test for fibromyalgia and the only role of investigations is in the exclusion of other conditions. The diagnosis of fibromyalgia, or, chronic primary pain may have to be reevaluated if the presenting symptoms change.

Management

There is no specific treatment, but some general approaches are advised. Poor quality of life and significant socio-economic impact remain an issue. It is important to understand the effect of pain on different aspects of the patient's life and to discuss with the patient, the skills that they have for managing their pain. Addressing social stressors and depression is essential if better outcomes are to be achieved. The following treatment strategies may help:

Education
- Inform patients about their condition.
- Reassure them they do not have a destructive arthritis.
- Explain why further investigations might not be useful.
- Emphasize that exercise will not cause harm to their joints.
- Direct patients to support groups that may be beneficial.

Physiotherapy/exercise
A graded exercise programme can improve fitness and reduce pain and fatigue.

Cognitive behavioural therapy
This encourages patients to develop coping mechanisms to deal with their symptoms.

COMMUNICATION

It is important to explain a diagnosis of fibromyalgia carefully to patients. Explain that the pain is real and not simply 'in their heads'. It is essential that you acknowledge the difficulties of living with chronic pain while informing the patient that the cause of their pain may never be identified, and ongoing management will likely be required.

Drug therapy
Many types of drugs have been trialled with varying success. Tricyclic antidepressants such as amitriptyline, dual reuptake inhibitors (duloxetine), anticonvulsants (pregabalin, gabapentin) and analgesics such as tramadol are all used with varying success. There is no role for antiinflammatory drugs.

PARANEOPLASTIC RHEUMATIC SYNDROME

This is a rare but serious cause of widespread musculoskeletal pain. Patients with lymphoma, leukaemia or other malignancies might present with rheumatic symptoms. These can mimic inflammatory arthritis or PMR. It is a syndrome that is more commonly seen in patients with haematological malignancies in comparison to solid tumour malignancies. Patients who fail to respond to typical treatment or who have other red flag features should be investigated to rule out an occult malignancy.

Equally, widespread bony metastases can present with widespread, or whole body, pain. Primary tumours that frequently metastasize to bone include breast, lung, kidney, thyroid (follicular) and prostate cancers.

Chapter Summary

- Widespread musculoskeletal pain is a common reason for referral to a rheumatologist.
- Causes are varied, but fibromyalgia is common, particularly amongst middle-aged women.
- Symptoms that are difficult to investigate are often found in conjunction with fibromyalgia, including chronic headache, fatigue, low mood and irritable bowel syndrome.
- Education, reassurance and graded exposure to exercise are key in helping to rehabilitate patients.
- Paraneoplastic rheumatic syndromes are rare, but it is important to consider in patients presenting with apparent inflammatory arthritis that fails to respond to typical therapies.

UKMLA Conditions
Fibromyalgia
Metastatic disease
Osteomalacia
Polymyalgia rheumatica
Systemic lupus erythematous

UKMLA Presentations
Back pain
Chronic joint pain/stiffness
Muscle pain/myalgia
Neck pain/stiffness

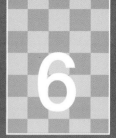

This chapter will give you an overview of how to approach an acutely hot, swollen joint. The differential diagnoses discussed here will be discussed in detail later in the book.

DIFFERENTIAL DIAGNOSIS

The phrase 'acute, hot, swollen joint' implies that the patient has presented with rapid onset of a warm, swollen and painful joint (Figs. 6.1–6.3). Differentials include:

- septic arthritis (pp. 176–177)
- crystal arthropathies (gout, pseudogout) (pp. 133–137)
- inflammatory arthritis (Chapter 12)
- haemarthrosis (bleeding into a joint)
- reactive arthritis (e.g., transient synovitis – more commonly seen in children)

RED FLAG

While there are many causes of a swollen and hot joint, the most important to exclude in an acute setting is septic arthritis. If untreated, this quickly progresses to soft tissue destruction within the joint and in extreme cases, can even go on to cause life-threatening sepsis.

HISTORY FOCUSING ON THE ACUTE, HOT, SWOLLEN JOINT

Pain

Patients with septic arthritis classically present with severe pain that inhibits any movement in the affected joint. It can be difficult to differentiate septic arthritis from alternative diagnoses, as in similar conditions, most patients will present with severe pain which restricts their movement. However, patients with septic arthritis will resist even a few degrees of movement due to pain.

Patient's age and sex

All the above conditions can present in adults, whereas only septic arthritis, reactive arthritis (of which transient synovitis is a type) and inflammatory arthritis, are likely causes in children and young adults. Gout is more common in men and rheumatoid arthritis is more common in women.

Site

Certain joints are more commonly affected by specific disorders (Fig. 6.4):

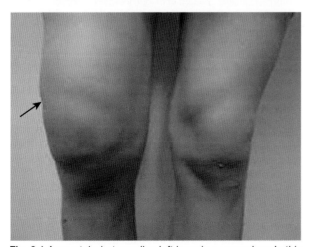

Fig. 6.1 An acutely, hot, swollen left knee in a young boy. In this case, the diagnosis was septic arthritis. (From Miller MD et al. *Review of orthopaedics*. 6th ed. Philadelphia, Saunders; 2012.)

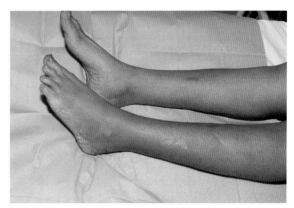

Fig. 6.2 Septic arthritis in the ankle. The ankle is swollen and erythematous, and on palpation was warm and tender. Movement was very painful. (From Herrick AL et al. *Orthopaedics and Rheumatology in Focus*. Elsevier; 2010.)

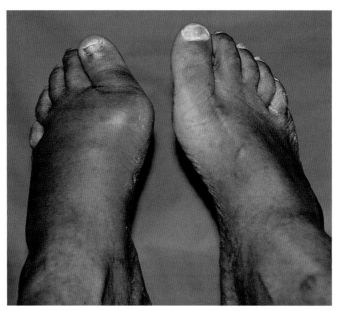

Fig. 6.3 Acute gout, left great toe. (From Swartz MH. *Textbook of physical diagnosis*, 8th ed. Philadelphia, Elsevier; 2021.)

- Septic arthritis most commonly affects the knee, but can also often present in the hip, shoulder, elbow, wrist, ankle, acromioclavicular and sternoclavicular joints. It presents unilaterally.
- Gout most commonly affects the first metatarsophalangeal joint of the foot and presents unilaterally.
- Pseudogout is common in the wrist and knee, again, unilaterally.
- If multiple joints are affected bilaterally, an inflammatory disorder such as rheumatoid arthritis or juvenile idiopathic arthritis is more likely.

Is the patient unwell?

Fever, sweats, rigors and general flu-like symptoms suggest an infection. In the initial stages of septic arthritis, the patient may appear 'well' with a normal blood pressure and heart rate. However, they can quickly progress to becoming septic and proceed on to septic shock. In contrast, a severe flare-up of inflammatory arthritis may cause severe fatigue and patients sometimes feel generally 'run-down', but fevers and rigors are not a feature.

History

Patients with a history of gout or pseudogout are likely to have recurrent episodes (up to 90% of patients), as are those with inflammatory arthritis. Conditions such as septic arthritis usually occur as solitary episodes, unless the patient has a predisposing risk factor such as immunosuppression, diabetes mellitus or sickle cell disease. Recurrent septic arthritis should prompt investigation into an underlying cause.

HINTS AND TIPS

Be careful! Patients with known inflammatory or crystal arthritis can also present with joint infections. Patients on immunosuppressants may not present with the usual inflammatory responses and clinical examination of the joint or the patient's blood tests may not indicate infection.

Associated symptoms

Patients with an inflammatory disorder may have other systemic features of their disease process evident. These include sacroiliitis in ankylosing spondylitis or painful metacarpophalangeal joints in rheumatoid arthritis.

Symptoms affecting the eyes can occur in:

- reactive syndrome (conjunctivitis, uveitis) and patients can also develop urethritis ('can't see, can't pee, can't climb a tree');
- rheumatoid arthritis (keratoconjunctivitis sicca, episcleritis, scleritis);
- juvenile idiopathic arthritis (uveitis).

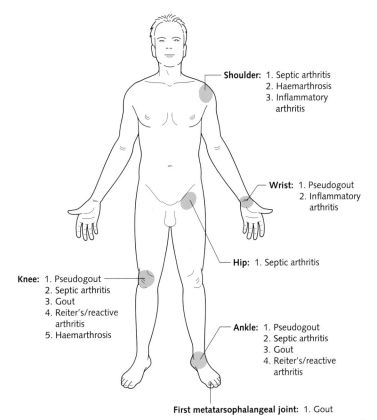

Shoulder: 1. Septic arthritis
2. Haemarthrosis
3. Inflammatory arthritis

Wrist: 1. Pseudogout
2. Inflammatory arthritis

Hip: 1. Septic arthritis

Knee: 1. Pseudogout
2. Septic arthritis
3. Gout
4. Reiter's/reactive arthritis
5. Haemarthrosis

Ankle: 1. Pseudogout
2. Septic arthritis
3. Gout
4. Reiter's/reactive arthritis

First metatarsophalangeal joint: 1. Gout

Fig. 6.4 Likely diagnosis for each joint in a patient presenting with an acute hot swollen joint.

Patients with a history of recent sexually transmitted infection or diarrhoeal illness may have reactive arthritis, so consider this in patients presenting with genitourinary or gastrointestinal symptoms.

Medical history

Some patients are predisposed to developing septic arthritis:

- Patients with diabetes mellitus, rheumatoid arthritis, HIV and IV drug users, are at risk of septic arthritis, as with any other infection.
- Patients with a history of endocarditis or of recent bacteraemia are also at an increased risk.
- Gout is linked with increased cell turnover and therefore any catabolic illness can predispose to a flare. Haematological diseases are particularly likely to cause gout, as are cancers where the patient is given chemotherapy, killing vast numbers of cells (tumour lysis syndrome).
- Patients with bleeding disorders (such as haemophilia) or those taking anticoagulants such as warfarin or direct oral

anticoagulants (DOACs) are at risk of developing acute haemarthrosis (bleeding into the joint). These patients can present with large tense effusions from a seemingly trivial injury. A haemarthrosis will usually self-resolve in time, and doesn't usually need aspirated. Aspiration will give symptomatic relief, but comes with the risk of introducing infection.

Drug history

Diuretics, particularly thiazides, and low-dose aspirin can increase uric acid levels, predisposing to gout.

Patients on steroids or other immunosuppressants are at increased risk of infection.

Social history

Alcohol excess and a high-purine diet (red meat and some fish) predispose to gout.

EXAMINATION OF AN ACUTE, HOT, SWOLLEN JOINT

General

- Most patients presenting with an acute, hot, swollen joint will be in considerable pain, look uncomfortable and may be agitated.
- Pyrexia suggests infection, although a mildly elevated temperature can also be seen in both gout and inflammatory arthritis.
- In severe cases of sepsis, the patient may show signs of cardiovascular instability such as tachycardia and hypotension (septic shock).
- The patient should be examined for signs of inflammatory arthritis, looking for other involved joints and associated systemic signs.
- Patients with chronic gout may have tophi. These can be found on extensor surfaces of the joints.

The joint

- Any affected joint will have a tense effusion and be tender to palpation. Active and passive movement will be painful. Typically, in a septic joint the patient will resist any movement (active or passive). Other causes of arthropathy, while tender, tend not to be as severely painful on movement.

- A full examination of the joint is often not possible on account of pain.
- An examination for other affected joints should be performed.

INVESTIGATION OF AN ACUTE, HOT, SWOLLEN JOINT

An algorithm for investigating a patient with an acute, hot, swollen joint is shown in Fig. 6.5.

Blood tests

The aim of initial investigations is primarily to confirm or to exclude septic arthritis. However, do not rely on blood tests alone because they can be normal in certain situations.

- A raised white cell count (WCC) suggests infection but can also be due to inflammatory causes. The WCC tends not to be elevated, or only very slightly elevated, in cases of crystal arthropathies.
- Inflammatory markers; erythrocyte sedimentation rate (ESR) and C-reactive protein (CRP), can be raised in all conditions due to inflammation or infection.
- In cases of immunosuppression, the usual increases in WCC and inflammatory markers may not be seen. Interpret these results with caution.

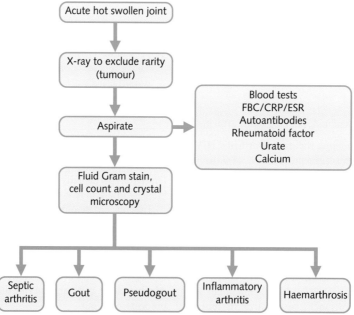

Fig. 6.5 Algorithm for the investigation of an acute hot swollen joint. CRP, *C-reactive protein;* ESR, *erythrocyte sedimentation rate;* FBC, *full blood count.*

- Serum urate may be elevated but can also be normal in patients with acute gout.
- Serum calcium should be checked if pseudogout is suspected, especially if hyperparathyroidism is present.
- If haemarthrosis is suspected, a clotting screen should be performed and patients on warfarin should have their international normalized ratio (INR) level checked.
- A procalcitonin test is useful to determine between infective and inflammatory causes of a hot swollen joint. Procalcitonin levels are high in the presence of a bacterial infection.

X-ray examinations

X-ray images may show:

- a normal appearance;
- chondrocalcinosis (found in pseudogout) (Fig. 6.6);
- bony erosions due to chronic gout or inflammatory arthritis;
- periosteal reaction.

Aspiration/synovial fluid analysis

- A superficial joint such as the knee is simple to aspirate, particularly if a tense effusion is present.
- Deeply situated joints such as the hip must be aspirated using ultrasound or X-ray guidance.
- A native joint may be aspirated in the Emergency Department or Acute Receiving Unit, however a suspected infected prosthetic joint should be aspirated in the 'cleaner' environment of the operating theatre under laminar flow.
- Aspiration should ideally be performed before antibiotics are given to increase the diagnostic yield of the test. Always ask for an urgent Gram stain of the fluid and request culture, sensitivity and microscopy to establish the presence of crystals.
- The general appearance of synovial fluid should be described and documented (see Chapter 4, Fig. 4.11).

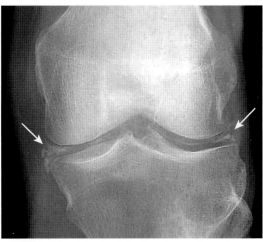

Fig. 6.6 Chondrocalcinosis of the knee in a patient with pseudogout. This is the most common location for chondrocalcinosis. *Arrows* pointing to areas of chondrocalcinosis. (From Herring W. *Learning Radiology.* 5th ed. Elsevier; 2024.)

HINTS AND TIPS

Of all the investigations, joint aspiration is the most important for reaching a diagnosis.

Ultrasound

This can be useful in showing an effusion which is difficult to appreciate, particularly in the hip.

● Chapter Summary

- There are many possible causes for an acute, hot, swollen joint: the most important cause to exclude or to suspect and treat is septic arthritis.
- Septic arthritis can quickly progress to cause cartilaginous destruction and systemic, life-threatening sepsis.
- Patient history, clinical examination and various investigations are important in assessing an acute, hot, swollen joint.
- The suggested investigation algorithm should be followed when investigating a hot swollen joint.
- Joint aspiration with urgent Gram-staining and crystal microscopy is the gold-standard diagnostic test for an acutely hot, swollen joint.
- Procalcitonin is a relatively new test, which is useful for differentiating infective and inflammatory causes of acutely hot, swollen joints.

● Chapter Summary—cont'd

UKMLA Conditions
Crystal arthropathy
Reactive arthritis
Rheumatoid arthritis
Septic arthritis

UKMLA Presentations
Acute joint pain/swelling
Fever
Red eye

A child with a limp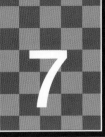

A child can limp for many reasons, but the most important condition to identify is septic arthritis, which can progress to systemic sepsis, cause major morbidity with local tissue destruction or even result in death if not treated. Further explanation of the different diagnoses discussed here can be found in Chapter 17.

DIFFERENTIAL DIAGNOSIS

- Septic arthritis (pp. 176–177).
- Transient synovitis of the hip ('irritable hip').
- Slipped upper femoral epiphysis (SUFE) (pp. 142).
- Developmental dysplasia of the hip (DDH) (pp. 139–141).
- Perthes disease (pp. 141–142).
- Osteomyelitis (pp. 173–175).
- Occult trauma.
- Nonaccidental injury (p. 145).
- Neuromuscular causes.
- Juvenile idiopathic arthritis (JIA; pp. 146–148).
- Malignancy (Chapter 21).

FOCUSED HISTORY

Very young children cannot give an accurate history, and if very unwell, they may be distressed and uncooperative in examination. The collateral history from parent or guardian is of vital importance here.

Age and sex

One of the most important factors in assessing a child with a limp, is their age. Table 7.1 shows the likely differential diagnosis depending on the age of the child. The sex of the child can also give clues to the diagnosis; for example, Perthes disease is much more common in boys than in girls.

Is the child ill?

Children can be well through the initial stages of disease and then become unwell very suddenly. Systemically unwell children will show little interest in play or food and simply will not be themselves. The presence of fever, rigors and sweats indicate that the child is unwell, suggesting infection or JIA (see Chapter 17).

Table 7.1 Diagnosis by age in a child with a limp

All ages	Infection Juvenile idiopathic arthritis Nonaccidental injury
Infant (1–3 years)	Late-presenting DDH Irritable hip Neuromuscular Occult trauma (including nonaccidental injury)
Childhood (3–11 years)	Perthes disease (3–7 years old) Irritable hip Neuromuscular SUFE Nonaccidental injury
Adolescence (12–16 years)	SUFE Infection

DDH, *Developmental dysplasia of the hip*; SUFE: *slipped upper femoral epiphysis.*

Pain

Patterns and timings of pain are a useful tool in differentiating causes.

- Trauma or infection: a rapid onset of pain is more likely.
- Perthes disease: often a vague gradual onset of pain and limp.
- SUFE: commonly a background of hip or knee pain precedes for weeks, followed by a sudden increase in pain.
- Transient synovitis of the hip: pain in the groin and mimics septic arthritis.
- Referred pain: any child complaining of knee pain must be suspected of having possible hip pathology and vice versa.
- Malignancy: should be considered in cases of pain at night or gradually increasing pain not relieved by analgesia (see Chapter 21).

Painless limping

- Late-presenting DDH: limp and leg length discrepancy.
- Neuromuscular disorders: poor gait due to muscle imbalance rather than pain. Cerebral palsy can present as developmental delay but milder forms can present later in childhood as the weakness becomes more apparent. Muscular dystrophy can also present with gradual onset of weakness and limp.

Associated symptoms

Systemic features such as pyrexia, drowsiness and irritability point towards infection as the cause. Polyarthropathy suggests JIA. Neuromuscular signs detected on neurological examination should raise suspicion of a neuromuscular disorder.

> **RED FLAG**
>
> **NONACCIDENTAL INJURY**
>
> Carefully consider nonaccidental injury in any child where the history and examination are incongruous. Signs may include:
> - Multiple/delayed presentations
> - Fractures not in keeping with normal childhood milestones, e.g., a child who is not yet walking is unlikely to have a femoral shaft fracture
> - Inconsistent or changing history in one parent/guardian or between parents and guardians
>
> Any concerns should be acted on immediately (see Chapter 17).

A recent history of upper respiratory tract infection, otitis media or viral gastroenteritis is often found in patients with transient synovitis, although it may be caused by infection or trauma.

Multiple joint aches and pains suggest juvenile arthritis. In JIA, the child's eyes can be involved as part of the systemic effects of the disease. If left untreated, blindness can result (see Chapter 17).

Medical history

Any history of Perthes disease or SUFE is very important as these patients are at increased risk of developing disease in the opposite hip.

Family history

A family history of Perthes disease, DDH and SUFE also leads to an increased risk.

See 'Clinical notes' for a summary of features of a limp requiring urgent assessment in the Emergency Department.

> **CLINICAL NOTES**
>
> Reasons to refer a limping child urgently from the community to the Emergency Department for further assessment:
> - Age <3 years
> - Unable to bear own weight
> - Fever or any other systemic symptoms
> - Severe pain

FOCUSED EXAMINATION OF A CHILD WITH A LIMP

Inspection

Inspect the child as best you can while keeping them as comfortable as possible. You may have to examine them sitting on their parent/guardian's lap or assess them as they play. Examine as you would an adult, initially by inspection, looking for associated joint swelling, erythema and any surgical scars. Then assess both walking and standing.

Gait
- An antalgic gait is present in painful conditions.
- A Trendelenburg gait (see Chapter 2) is present in a toddler with late DDH or some neuromuscular conditions.
- Neuromuscular disorders give a variety of patterns of gait abnormality.
- A worrying sign is if a child is too ill or in too much pain to bear their own weight.

Standing
- An abnormal single large posterior skin crease is present in DDH.
- In SUFE or infection, the hip is often held in an abnormal position of external rotation and flexion (Fig. 7.1).

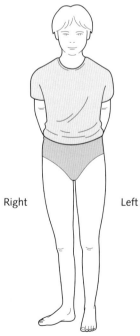

Right   Left

Fig. 7.1 External rotation deformity: a child with externally rotated right leg in slipped upper femoral epiphysis.

Fixed flexion

If the Thomas test is positive (a fixed flexion deformity), a significant problem such as advanced Perthes disease, DDH or SUFE, should be considered.

Limb length discrepancy

- A short leg is typical of DDH.
- Apparent shortening will also be present if there is any fixed flexion deformity.

Palpation

Palpate any painful areas for an associated effusion, any warmth or localized pain. The hip joint cannot be palpated directly because it is a deep joint and so it is important to palpate the groin and greater trochanter for tenderness. Palpation around the knee will reveal joint line tenderness in conditions such as osteochondritis or, in older children, acute soft tissue knee injury, whereas tenderness over the tibial tubercle can be seen in Osgood-Schlatter disease.

Movement

- Restriction of active and passive hip movements indicates underlying pathology.
- DDH results in loss of abduction compared with the other side.
- Perthes disease results in loss of abduction and flexion. Complete loss of abduction is a worrying sign in Perthes as this may indicate subluxation of the joint.
- In septic arthritis, any movement causes extreme pain. The child will hold the joint rigidly still to avoid precipitating pain.

COMMUNICATION

Listening to the child's parents and observing the child at play or rest is a key part of deciding whether a child is unwell. Play may be the only way to examine their painful limb.

INVESTIGATING A CHILD WITH A LIMP

Blood tests

Markedly elevated white cell count (WCC), erythrocyte sedimentation rate (ESR) and C-reactive protein can indicate the presence of infection, but these inflammatory markers can also be mildly increased in transient synovitis or JIA.

Very rare causes of abnormal blood tests include leukaemia. Creatinine kinase is elevated in muscular dystrophy.

X-ray examinations

A plain radiograph is often unremarkable in the younger child, particularly in cases of transient synovitis.

A hip radiograph in a limping child may show:

- an abnormal looking hip with or without subluxation in the case of DDH (Fig. 17.4);
- femoral head changes in Perthes disease (Fig 17.6);
- a slipped upper femoral epiphysis (best seen on frog leg view) (Fig. 17.7);
- evidence of infection including widening of the joint space or a periosteal reaction (remember this is a late sign, X-ray images are initially normal)
- a fracture.

HINTS AND TIPS

If hip pathology is suspected, request a lateral of the hip, and anteroposterior pelvis and frog leg lateral views. If knee pathology is expected, anteroposterior and lateral images should be taken.

Knee radiographs may show:

- Osgood-Schlatter disease (Fig 17.10);
- Osteochondritis dissecans (Fig 17.11);
- a fracture.

Ultrasound examination

Ultrasound examination is very useful for suspected joint problems, particularly of the hip, which is deeply situated, and is also helpful to guide an aspiration.

Effusion will be seen in:

- septic arthritis;
- transient synovitis;
- Perthes disease (early).

Magnetic resonance imaging

Magnetic resonance imaging (MRI) is not a first-line investigation in children; it is difficult for a young child to stay still for the scan. However, if an MRI is necessary, a general anaesthetic can be given to facilitate scanning. MRI is useful in:

- cases where septic arthritis or osteomyelitis is unclear;
- diagnosis of soft knee disorders (see Chapter 17);
- bone and soft-tissue tumours.

Kocher's criteria can be extremely useful clinically for diagnosing septic arthritis. This has been adapted over time, but the original criteria are still widely used.

Kocher's criteria can be used as a tool to help differentiate transient synovitis from septic arthritis in children with hip pain. Four criteria are assessed and a score out of four is then calculated, giving a prediction regarding the likelihood of septic arthritis:

- White cell count >12,000 cells/mm^3
- Inability to bear weight
- Fever >38.5°C
- Erythrocyte sedimentation rate >40 mm/h

Predictive value of Kocher criteria (Kocher et al., 1999).

Score	Chance of septic arthritis as cause for hip pain (%)
1	3
2	40
3	93
4	99

Chapter Summary

- Examine the child thoroughly and assess their gait, carefully assessing whether it is painful or painless.
- Elicit whether the pain is coming from the hip, knee or ankle before investigating further.
- Be sure to rule out any malignant or infective cause and decide whether the child is unwell before considering the more common diagnoses.
- Carefully sort the common diagnoses according to age as shown in Table 7.1. Suspect Perthes disease in those aged 3 to 7 years but think more readily of SUFE in older children.
- An 'irritable hip' is a common problem but should be a diagnosis of exclusion.
- Carry out relevant investigations: blood tests, X-ray examinations and further imaging to rule out serious conditions, in particular, septic arthritis.
- Ultrasound scanning can be useful in these cases. MRI is rarely performed and difficult to achieve in young children.

UKMLA Conditions
Idiopathic arthritis
Nonaccidental injury
Septic arthritis

UKMLA Presentations
Acute joint pain/swelling
Chronic joint pain/stiffness
Fever
Musculoskeletal deformities
Limp

Back pain, or leg pain secondary to pathology in the spine, is extremely common. In fact, as many as 80% of the population will have an episode of significant back pain in their life. Back pain is not uncommonly accompanied by unilateral or bilateral leg pain, and it is important to take a detailed history and perform a thorough examination to try to elicit the true source of the patient's symptoms. There are many potential pitfalls when assessing a patient with back pain, however, the most important thing is to distinguish the common benign musculoskeletal pains from the less frequent, but more sinister pathologies.

DIFFERENTIAL DIAGNOSIS

Musculoskeletal back pain causes:

- muscle strain
- osteoarthritis of the spine
- prolapsed intervertebral disc
- vertebral crush fracture
- osteoporotic wedge fracture
- spinal stenosis
- degenerative spondylolisthesis
- malignancy

Infective and inflammatory back pain causes:

- discitis
- vertebral osteomyelitis
- ankylosing spondylitis

Abdominal causes:

- pancreatitis
- aortic aneurysm rupture
- renal disease

HISTORY FOCUSING ON BACK AND LEG PAIN

- Elicit the timescale of symptoms: were they precipitated by a traumatic event or did they occur spontaneously? Did they come on suddenly or gradually? Has the pain been getting worse?
- Character: what words would the patient use to describe the pain? Sharp/shooting/dull/aching?

- Associated leg pain: is this bilateral or unilateral?
- Associated numbness: what is the distribution?
- Associated weakness: is this bilateral or unilateral?
- Any change in bowel or bladder habits?
- Any weight loss or systemic upset? (For red flags alerting to serious spinal pathology, see Chapter 4.)
- Any previous imaging for back pain, surgical intervention or spinal injections?

EXAMINATION FOCUSING ON BACK AND LEG PAIN

General examination

Look at the patient: do they look well or unwell? Weight loss, anaemia and general ill health may suggest a chronic, concerning cause such as malignancy.

Look

Look at the patient's back, their posture and gait, from the front, from behind and from their sides.

- Look for scars suggesting previous surgery or bruising indicating trauma.
- Posture: look for scoliosis, abnormal kyphosis or lordosis.
    - A stooped posture with flexion of the knee can suggest sciatica as the sciatic nerve is irritated in full stretch.
    - A stooped posture in elderly patient suggests osteoporotic wedge fractures.
    - A very stiff spine may be simple low back pain requiring analgesia to relieve spasm, but may also be, for example, ankylosing spondylitis.
- Look at the iliac crest alignment which may show pelvic tilt suggesting a leg length discrepancy or hip abductor weakness.
- Fixed flexion of the hip with an antalgic or Trendelenburg gait indicates hip pathology. There may be an associated limb-length discrepancy.
- Observe the patient walking away from you and towards you: limping (an antalgic gait) suggests joint pain or weakness surrounding the hip, a Trendelenburg gait suggests unilateral weakness of the hip abductors (remember 'sound side sags' to identify which side is deficient).

If hip pathology is suspected, a full hip examination should be performed as described in Chapter 2.

Feel

- With the patient standing, palpate the spinous processes and sacroiliac joints. Then palpate the paraspinal muscles for tenderness. In simple low back pain, the areas around the posterior superior iliac spines and sacroiliac joints are often tender.

Move

- Assess movements of the spine in the distinct regions separately; cervical, thoracic and lumbar. Diminished movement is likely if pathology is present. It may be impossible for the patient to comply with this part of the examination because of pain.

Special tests

- Schober's test for forward flexion: mark the skin at the level of the dimples of Venus (level of the sacroiliac joints). Next, mark a line 10 cm superior to this and 5 cm inferior to this. The distance between the two lines should increase from 15 to 20 cm in normal forward flexion. If the patient can't achieve this, they have stiffness in their lumbar spine, of which ankylosing spondylitis can be a cause.
- Lasègue's test for lumbar radiculopathy: with the patient supine, lift the leg to flex at the hip, keeping the knee straight. Any limitation with leg or thigh pain (normally patients should be able to achieve 90 degrees flexion) suggests nerve irritation, often at L5.

An examination of the spine must always be accompanied by a neurological examination of the peripheral nerves supplying the upper and lower limbs.

A digital rectal examination is mandatory in all patients with suspected cauda equina syndrome. This should assess for resting anal tone and the ability to distinguish sharp and dull touch.

INVESTIGATION OF A PATIENT WITH BACK PAIN

Blood tests

Blood tests are not always necessary in simple back pain, but should be performed in patients with red flags, to exclude sinister causes. Full blood count and biochemistry may reveal:

- Elevated white cell count, erythrocyte sedimentation rate (ESR) and C-reactive protein (CRP) if infection, such as in discitis or osteomyelitis, or inflammation is present.
- A normocytic anaemia or hypercalcaemia in malignancy.

Blood and urine immunoglobulins (including Bence Jones protein) should be checked to exclude myeloma.

Imaging

Plain radiographs of the spine should only be taken routinely after trauma as normal appearances are seen in simple low back pain, a prolapsed intervertebral disc, and even in malignancy or infection if early in the disease process. However, radiographs can be helpful in identifying:

- Osteoarthritic changes in the spine (if the diagnosis is in doubt)
- Spondylolisthesis
- Destruction of the vertebral body (classically at the pedicle (winking-owl sign; see Chapter 4, Fig. 4.7), indicating malignancy)
- A fracture, which may be secondary to a low-energy injury with underlying osteoporosis (or due to trauma in healthy bone)
- Erosion of a vertebral body around the disc due to infection

Further imaging is needed if there is doubt about the diagnosis or for surgical planning:

- Magnetic resonance imaging (MRI): this is the most common imaging modality for soft-tissue structures, including the identification of disc prolapse and nerve root compression and early detection of malignancy and infection.
- Computed tomography (CT) scanning: useful for looking at bony structures in detail, e.g., spondylolisthesis or fracture in trauma setting.
- Isotope bone scanning: to identify a 'hot spot' of metabolic activity in cases of infection or malignancy.

An algorithm for the suggested investigation of sinister back pain is provided in Fig. 8.1.

MECHANICAL LOW BACK PAIN

Back pain is extremely common and causes a significant burden on the resources of westernized societies in terms of lost working days.

Definition

Mechanical back pain is an overarching term to encompass any kind of musculoskeletal back 'strain' causing pain. The spine (specifically the facet joints), the intervertebral discs and the paraspinal muscles can all be affected.

This diagnosis should only be made after other pathological conditions have been excluded.

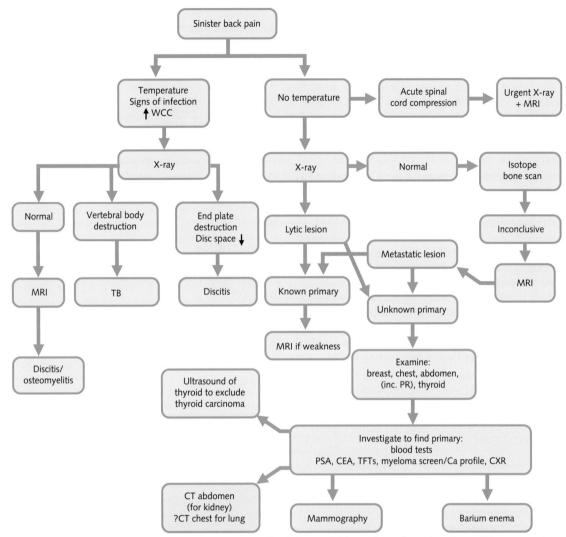

Fig. 8.1 Algorithm for the investigation of sinister back pain. *Ca*, Calcium; *CEA*, carcinoembryonic antigen; *CT*, computed tomography; *CXR*, chest X-ray; *MRI*, magnetic resonance imaging; *PR*, per rectum; *PSA*, prostate-specific antigen; *TB*, tuberculosis; *TFTs*, thyroid function tests; *WCC*, white cell count.

Incidence

Of the population, 80% will have back pain at some stage in their lives.

Aetiology and pathology

As mechanical back pain is so common, it is difficult to define clear aetiological factors for its occurrence. A history of muscle strain during an episode of heavy lifting or vigorous activity may point to an obvious pathology, however, the history may not always be that clear.

A lot of the pathological changes seen on imaging will also be present in the healthy, normal population with no symptoms, so imaging should be used with caution.

Clinical features

There are two typical clinical scenarios: acute back pain over days or weeks and chronic unrelenting back pain for many years.

Acute back pain (<3 months)

Pain is usually solely located in the back, possibly following a precipitating incident. Pain is severe and the patient may have difficulty getting into a comfortable position. Sometimes the patient has pain referred down the back one or both legs, but this differs from true radicular pain in that back pain is still the predominant feature and the pain does not typically radiate beyond the knee. The pain is worse on movement.

Clinical examination will show reduced range of movement in the spine with muscle spasm, paraspinal tenderness and loss of lumbar lordosis.

Sciatic stretch testing and peripheral nerve examination will be negative.

Chronic unrelenting back pain (>3 months)

The patient will be unable to work and often has seen numerous doctors, physiotherapists and other allied health workers, sometimes including alternative medical practitioners, in an attempt to control the pain.

The back pain is usually unrelenting and does not have any relieving factors. Leg pain may or may not be present.

Clinical examination rarely shows any significant features other than reduced movements. Inappropriate signs (Waddell signs) may be present (see Clinical Notes box describing these signs).

CLINICAL NOTES

WADDELL SIGNS FOR NONORGANIC COMPONENT TO LOW BACK PAIN

- Superficial tenderness and tenderness not in keeping with an anatomical source.
- Regional pain not conforming to known neuroanatomy.
- Pain on movements not affecting the lower back, e.g., axial loading and simulated rotation.
- Lack of pain after distraction, e.g., patients being unable to lift a leg straight but able to sit on the examination couch with legs straight and hips flexed to 90 degrees.
- Overreaction to pain (this sign is very subjective and should be used with caution).

Diagnosis and investigation

The majority of patients with a short history (<6 weeks) and mechanical symptoms need no further investigation as symptoms are most commonly self-limiting.

Prolonged symptoms need investigation to exclude sinister causes of back pain.

Blood tests including full blood count, ESR, liver function tests, calcium/phosphate/alkaline phosphatase, myeloma screen and CRP should all be normal in mechanical back pain.

X-ray examination may show:

- normal appearances;
- minor disc narrowing;
- osteoarthritis (Fig. 8.2).

MRI and CT scanning are rarely helpful and may be misleading if they highlight an abnormality that may not be significant.

Treatment

Conservative

Analgesia, nonsteroidal antiinflammatory drugs (NSAIDs) and physiotherapy are used for acute low back pain. Bed rest should be avoided.

Patients with chronic pain require a biopsychosocial approach and need multidisciplinary input to try to manage their pain. Psychological input may be required and the pain management team might have to be consulted. Occasionally, facet joint injections for localized disease can relieve symptoms.

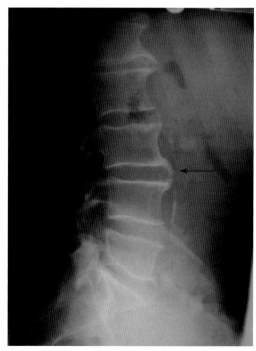

Fig. 8.2 Osteoarthritis of the spine *(black arrow)*.

Surgical

Surgery has no role in the management of mechanical back pain and the patient must be informed of this.

Prognosis

Most acute back pain episodes settle spontaneously and the patient returns to their normal level of activity. Once chronic, back pain becomes very difficult to treat.

PROLAPSED INTERVERTEBRAL DISC

Definition

A disc prolapse occurs when part of the nucleus pulposus herniates through the annulus fibrosus. This can press on a spinal nerve root causing radicular symptoms (Fig. 8.3).

Incidence

Up to 3% of men and 1% of women will suffer with sciatica related to a prolapsed intervertebral disc. Usual presentation is between the ages of 30 and 50 years.

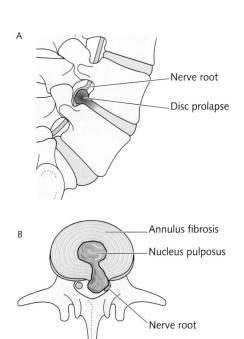

Fig. 8.3 (A and B) Prolapsed intervertebral disc.

Aetiology and pathology

There is good evidence that manual workers involved in repetitive heavy lifting have increased incidence of disc prolapse. As do people who are overweight, and spend prolonged periods sitting at work e.g., taxi or lorry drivers.

The herniation of disc material tends to occur posterolaterally where the posterior longitudinal ligament is weakest, and the disc material can then press on the nearby nerve roots. Central disc prolapse can also occur and the disc can then press on the combined nerve roots, including those supplying the bladder and bowel (sometimes causing cauda equina syndrome). Prolapse can occur without spinal root involvement, in which case the patient will have symptoms of back pain but not sciatica.

Disc prolapse most commonly occurs at L4–L5 or L5–S1 level but can occur at any level (including cervical and rarely thoracic levels). The nerve root crosses its space before exiting the spine beneath the pedicle, i.e., a protruding L4–L5 disc presses on the L5 nerve root as it transits. A protruding L5/S1 disc presses on the L5 nerve root as it exits (Fig. 8.4).

Clinical features

Sciatica is a symptom of lower lumbar or sacral nerve root irritation. The patient complains of severe pain radiating down the leg as far as the toes. There may be numbness and tingling or weakness of the foot. Patients find certain postures (e.g., sitting or standing, depending on their particular pathology) difficult to maintain.

> **RED FLAG**
>
> Symptoms of cauda equina syndrome mandate an immediate MRI:
> - Altered bladder/bowel function: insensate urination, insensate full bladder, difficulty initiating urination, urinary retention or incontinence of either bladder or bowel.
> - Perineal/perianal/genital anaesthesia or 'saddle anaesthesia'. Patients may complain of an odd sensation when wiping themselves after using the toilet.
> - Bilateral sciatica.
> - Progressive bilateral neurological deficit of the legs.
> - Reduced resting anal tone.
> - Sexual dysfunction.

Clinically, a patient will have an abnormal posture, stooping to the affected side and standing with the knee flexed to relieve pressure on the dura (Fig. 8.5).

Nerve root tension signs such as straight-leg raising will be positive.

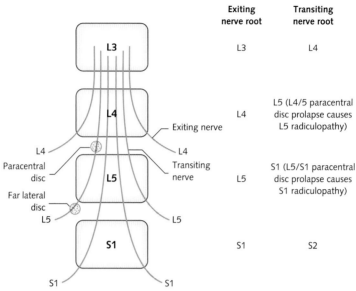

	Exiting nerve root	Transiting nerve root
L3	L3	L4
L4	L4	L5 (L4/5 paracentral disc prolapse causes L5 radiculopathy)
L5	L5	S1 (L5/S1 paracentral disc prolapse causes S1 radiculopathy)
S1	S1	S2

Fig 8.4 Prolapsed intervertebral disc. Radiculopathy in relation to exiting and transiting nerve roots. Paracentral disc lesions compress the transiting nerve. Far lateral disc lesions compress the exiting nerve. (From Delbridge MS, Al-Jundi W. *Basic Science for the MRCS: A Revision Guide for Surgical Trainees*. 4th ed. Elsevier; 2023.)

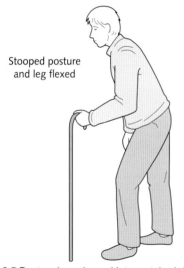

Stooped posture and leg flexed

Fig. 8.5 Posture in prolapsed intervertebral disc.

The crossover sign may be positive (elevation of the opposite or normal leg gives pain shooting down the affected leg).

Numbness in a dermatomal distribution and weakness with loss of reflexes may be present.

Diagnosis and investigation

In older patients, blood tests, described above, should be performed to exclude any sinister causes.

X-ray images are usually normal and are performed to exclude bony pathology such as spondylolisthesis.

MRI scanning is now the investigation of choice in patients with persistent symptoms (Fig. 8.6).

Treatment

Conservative

A short period of bed rest in the acute period, followed by gentle physiotherapy with adequate analgesia (including NSAIDs) is the initial treatment for most disc prolapses.

Surgical

Lumbar nerve root injection can provide a confirmatory diagnosis as well as treatment for nerve root irritation.

The only indications for urgent surgical discectomy are cauda equina syndrome and acutely progressively worsening neurological deficit.

If patients have prolonged intractable back pain (>3 months), elective surgery is considered.

Prognosis

The vast majority of disc prolapses settle spontaneously with conservative treatment. It is important to let your patient know that an acute disc prolapse is usually a self-limiting condition.

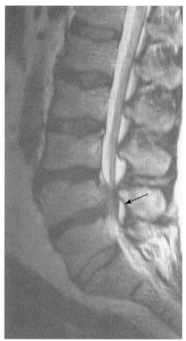

Fig. 8.6 Magnetic resonance imaging scan of prolapsed intervertebral disc at L4–L5 level *(black arrow)*.

SPONDYLOLISTHESIS

Definition

Spondylolisthesis is one vertebral body slipping on another.

> **COMMUNICATION**
>
> It is easy to confuse the terminology. A *spondylolysis* is a defect in the pars interarticularis that may allow the vertebra to slip forward, causing a *spondylolisthesis* (forward slippage of one vertebra on another).

Incidence

The condition occurs in approximately 5% of the population but most are asymptomatic. It is more common in Caucasian males.

Aetiology and pathology

Spondylolisthesis is the most common pathological cause of persistent back pain in children. Certain sports predispose to spondylolysis (gymnasts, ballet dancers and fast bowlers in

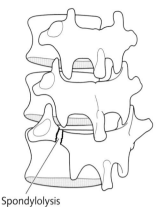

Spondylolysis

Fig. 8.7 Classic 'collar on Scottie dog' defect showing the spondylolysis.

cricket are often affected). Spondylolisthesis usually occurs at the L5–S1 level. The degree of slip is normally assessed as a percentage (0%–25%, 25%–50%, 50%–75% or >75%) and graded 1–4. There can be an associated kyphosis or scoliosis.

Clinical features

Initially, back pain is the sole presentation but if the slip becomes severe, nerve root irritation will occur, causing sciatica. Radicular symptoms are more common in adults.

There may be central spinal tenderness. Movement is usually preserved, but classically hyperextension is painful.

Diagnosis and investigation

Oblique X-rays may show the classic 'collar on Scottie dog' appearance of spondylolysis (Fig. 8.7) and the lateral X-ray image will show the degree and angle of slippage (Fig. 8.8).

CT scans more clearly demonstrate the lesion in 3D.

An MRI should be performed if nerve root irritation or compression is suspected.

Treatment

Conservative

Initial rest and restriction of exacerbating activities may allow a spondylolysis to heal before a slip occurs. In most cases a trial of conservative treatment is advised with physiotherapy, analgesia and activity modification. Unilateral pars defects almost never progress to spondylolisthesis.

Surgical

Persistent pain, radiculopathy and significant deformity are indications for surgery. Fusion with or without bone graft is commonly performed.

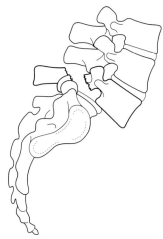

Fig. 8.8 An L5–S1 spondylolisthesis resulting from a pars defect.

Prognosis

The outcome is variable, depending on the type and degree of slip.

SPINAL STENOSIS

Definition

Spinal stenosis has many causes and is the resulting narrowing of the spinal canal causing compression of the nerve roots and therefore nerve root ischaemia.

Incidence

This is a common disorder mainly affecting men over 50 years of age.

Aetiology and pathology

Spinal stenosis can be congenital or acquired. As with many spinal pathologies, acquired spinal stenosis is more common in manual labourers. It is usually secondary to degenerative or posttraumatic changes whereby thickened ligaments, osteophytes and posterior disc bulges encroach into the spinal canal (Figs 8.9 and 8.10). Other causes of acquired spinal stenosis include spondylolisthesis, post-traumatic? spinal stenosis and spinal stenosis secondary to systemic diseases such as Paget's disease, ankylosing spondylitis and acromegaly.

Clinical features

Typically, patients present with discomfort when walking, with pain referred to the buttock, calves and feet due to positional

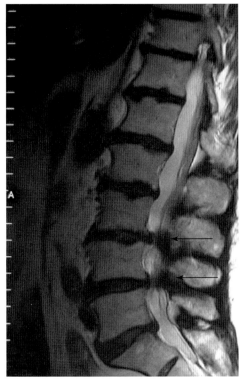

Fig. 8.9 Magnetic resonance imaging scan of spinal stenosis *(arrows)*.

nerve root ischaemia. The pain will be claudicant in nature and therefore relieved by rest. It must be distinguished carefully from vascular claudication. The 'shopping cart sign' may be present, whereby patients who normally suffer severe pain are able to walk greater distances when they have a flexed spine whilst leaning on, for example, their shopping trolley. Flexion is thought to 'open up' the spinal canal, relieving some of the stenosis.

Examination may reveal stiffening of the spine with a reduced range of movement, but sciatic stretch testing should be normal.

It is also important to examine the peripheral vascular system to ascertain whether the cause is spinal or vascular in origin.

Diagnosis and investigation

X-ray examination will usually reveal degenerative changes.

MRI can be used to identify the degree of stenosis and nerve root involvement. If suspected, exclude peripheral vascular insufficiency with ultrasound scanning.

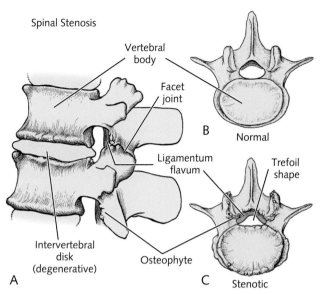

Fig. 8.10 Spinal stenosis. (A) Aging causes loss of disc height and compression of the vertebral body. The ligamentum flavum hypertrophies and osteophytes develop. Degenerative disease occurs at the facet joints. Any or all of these variables can contribute to spinal stenosis. (B) Normal, healthy vertebral body with a widely open vertebral canal. (C) Stenotic spine from a variety of contributing factors. (From Heick JD, Lazaro R. *Goodman and Snyder's Differential Diagnosis for Physical Therapists: Screening for Referral.* 7th ed. Elsevier; 2023.)

Treatment

Conservative
Weight loss, physiotherapy, activity modification and NSAIDs may relieve symptoms sufficiently to avoid surgery.

Surgical
Severe symptoms not responding to conservative measures require surgical decompression.

Prognosis
The condition tends to be progressive.

DISCITIS/VERTEBRAL OSTEOMYELITIS

Definition
Discitis is infection of the disc space and vertebral osteomyelitis is infection of a vertebral body.

Incidence
The incidence is approximately 1/100,000, but the condition is more common in less developed countries.

Aetiology and pathology
Those predisposed to spinal infection include patients with conditions associated with other bone and joint infections (see Chapter 20). Included in this group are intravenous drug users, patients who are immunocompromised or diabetic. Patients with recent sepsis from pneumonia or urinary tract infection can develop discitis by seeding of infection. Discitis can also occur iatrogenically following surgery to the disc.

Common infecting organisms are staphylococci and streptococci in adults and staphylococci and *Haemophilus* in children.

Tuberculosis should also be considered in spinal infection (Pott's disease).

Clinical features
Patients are usually unwell with pyrexia and complain of severe, unrelenting back pain.

Clinical examination may reveal swelling, localized tenderness and, in advanced cases, an angular scoliosis or kyphosis (gibbus). There is pain on palpation, reduced movement and possible abnormal neurology.

Discitis commonly presents late: patients can have weeks of vague symptoms before the correct diagnosis is made.

Diagnosis and investigation
The white cell count, ESR and CRP are elevated.

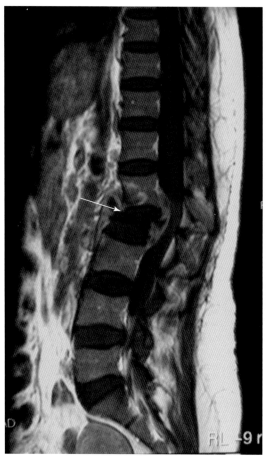

Fig 8.11 Magnetic resonance imaging showing tuberculosis of the spine. There is complete collapse of the vertebra *(white arrow)* with resultant kyphosis.

X-ray examination will not acutely show any changes, but after 10 days to 3 weeks may start to show narrowed disc space (discitis) and bony destruction (osteomyelitis). MRI is the investigation of choice (Fig. 8.11). It is not unusual for the site of infection to be distant from the site of symptoms (i.e., lumbar back pain with a thoracic focus of infection) or for there to be more than one focus of infection and so an MRI of the whole spine is performed. MRI is not 100% sensitive and so should be repeated as an interval scan around 2 weeks later if suspicion of infection remains high.

CT-guided biopsy with samples sent for culture and sensitivity, can be used to guide microbiological therapy.

Treatment

Conservative

After blood cultures and biopsy samples have been taken, antibiotics are given for 6 weeks under advice from microbiology

Table 8.1 Causes of scoliosis

Type	Pathology	Example
Congenital	Abnormal development of spine	Hemivertebra
Idiopathic	Unknown	Adolescent idiopathic scoliosis
Neuromuscular	Abnormal muscle forces acting on the spine	Cerebral palsy
Secondary	Curve develops secondary to another process	Leg-length discrepancy

and pharmacy. This may be a short course (2 weeks) of intravenous antibiotics, followed by oral antibiotics with good bioavailability and bone penetration. Follow-up assessments are made based on clinical assessment and CRP trends.

Surgical

Any abscess should be drained and an unstable spine with significant deformity needs considered for surgical stabilization.

Prognosis

Prognosis is variable: childhood cases respond well and the patient should return to normality; severe adult infections can be life-threatening and surgery carries significant risk.

SCOLIOSIS

Definition

This is a lateral deviation and rotational abnormality of the spine. It is not a painful condition but has been included in this chapter as a common spinal condition.

Incidence

Up to 2.5% of the population are affected by idiopathic scoliosis.

Aetiology and pathology

Causes of scoliosis are listed in Table 8.1. Curves can be thoracic or lumbar (Fig. 8.12).

Clinical features

Pain is not usually a feature; rather the patient or relatives complain of deformity, in the form of an asymmetrical rib hump

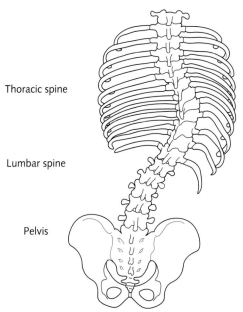

Thoracic spine

Lumbar spine

Pelvis

Fig. 8.12 Thoracolumbar curve in scoliosis.

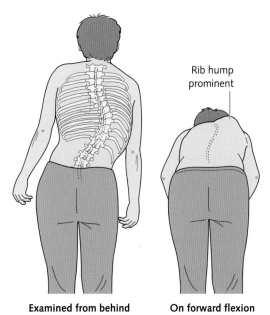

Rib hump prominent

Examined from behind   On forward flexion

Fig. 8.13 Examination of a patient with scoliosis.

(more prominent on forward flexion (Fig. 8.13)), spinal curve, limb length inequality and/or pelvic tilt. Very severe deformity reduces chest expansion.

Diagnosis and investigation

Standing X-ray images show the spinal curve and serial films are important to monitor the progress of the curve.

A significant increase in the severity of the curve is often an indication for surgical stabilization.

MRI scans are performed to exclude any associated spinal cord abnormality.

Treatment

Conservative

The treatment depends on the angle of the curve measured on the X-rays. In idiopathic scoliosis, the initial treatment is bracing for mild to moderate curves.

Surgical

All congenital, most neuromuscular and severe or progressive idiopathic curves will require surgical correction and stabilization.

Prognosis

The majority of curves are minor and require little treatment.

At the other end of the spectrum, in extreme cases, very severe neuromuscular curves can lead to death due to cardiorespiratory compromise.

CLINICAL NOTES

Metastatic cord compression (further discussed in Chapter 21) should be considered in patients with known metastatic disease and back pain. If imaging confirms this, urgent treatment is usually with radiotherapy under the oncology team.

Chapter Summary

- Back pain should be investigated carefully, ruling out any sinister causes first.
- Chronic mechanical back pain has an unpredictable course and can be difficult to treat. It often requires a multidisciplinary team approach.
- Differentials that are cause for concern are primary malignancy, metastases, cauda equina and infection.
- It is essential to ask about red flags to identify patients who need urgent investigation and management.
- Spondylolysis is a defect at the pars interarticularis, whereas spondylolisthesis is one vertebra slipping on another.
- The difference between spinal and vascular claudication can be elicited with a good history spinal claudication is more likely with positional symptoms.
- Discitis and vertebral osteomyelitis should be treated with aggressive antibiotic treatment.
- If in doubt, further imaging of back pain is always indicated in the form of CT or MRI, with MRI being better for analysing discs or nerve roots and CT for bony pathology.

UKMLA Conditions
Ankylosing spondylitis
Osteoarthritis
Osteomyelitis
Osteoporosis
Radiculopathies
Spinal cord compression
Spinal fracture

UKMLA Presentations
Back pain
Chronic joint pain/stiffness
Muscle pain/myalgia
Musculoskeletal deformities

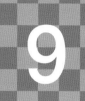
Neurological symptoms such as numbness, 'pins and needles', electric shock-type pain, burning pain, hypersensitivity or weakness, occur when there is irritation or injury to a nerve. This can be due to chronic compression, neuropathic disease or an acute injury. The pattern of these symptoms will help diagnose which nerve is causing the problem. This chapter will show you how to approach someone complaining of symptoms such as these and discuss common upper and lower limb nerve pathologies.

> ### HINTS AND TIPS
>
> Nerves may be injured in different ways giving rise to different sets of symptoms. One way to categorize nerve injury, is by the level of damage sustained (Fig. 9.1):
>
> **Neuropraxia** – the nerve remains in continuity but signalling along the nerve is affected. This can be thought of as a 'bruise' to the nerve which recovers over time.
>
> **Axonotmesis** – there is loss of continuity of the axon and covering myelin but the framework around the nerve is intact and there is recovery potential without need of surgical treatment.
>
> **Neurotmesis** – the nerve is transected, there is no continuity and surgical intervention is necessary.
>
> Wallerian degeneration occurs after a nerve is injured and is the process whereby the axon distal to the injury degenerates. This occurs in axonotmesis and neurotmesis.

DIFFERENTIAL DIAGNOSIS

Peripheral nerve pathology:

- carpal tunnel syndrome (CTS)
- ulnar nerve entrapment (e.g., at the cubital tunnel or in Guyon's canal)
- radial nerve palsy (as in 'Saturday night palsy')
- peroneal nerve palsy
- tarsal tunnel syndrome
- meralgia paraesthetica
- Morton's neuroma
- nerve tumours, e.g., neurofibroma, schwannoma
- postsurgical nerve dysfunction, e.g., superficial radial nerve neuroma
- complex regional pain syndrome (see Chapter 4)

Spinal pathology:

- intervertebral disc prolapse
- spinal stenosis
- osteoarthritis
- cervical rib
- malignancy

Systemic causes:

- medical causes, e.g., multiple sclerosis or stroke
- peripheral neuropathy caused by, for example, alcoholism, diabetes mellitus, drugs, vitamin B_{12} deficiency

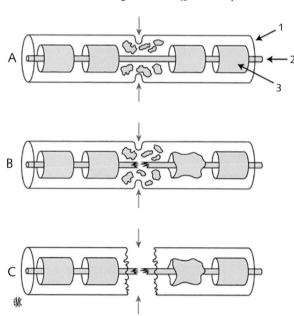

Fig. 9.1 (A) Neuropraxia (1 – epineurium; 2 – axon; 3 – myelin sheath). (B) Axonotmesis. (C) Neurotmesis. (Reproduced from Nollet S, Cosson A, Michel F, Tatu L, Práctica clínica y electroneuromiográfica de las lesiones nerviosas periféricas de los miembros inferiores. EMC - Podología. 2017; 19(1): 1-14. © 2017 Elsevier Masson SAS. All rights reserved.)

HISTORY

The following points should be covered in a systematic manner.

Site

Identifying the site of the neurological problem is key in determining if an individual nerve is affected (Fig. 9.2), a group of nerves are affected, or whether in fact, the underlying problem is due to systemic disease affecting multiple nerves or groups of nerves.

Onset of symptoms

The timing of symptoms can help to establish the pathology affecting the nerve or group of nerves.

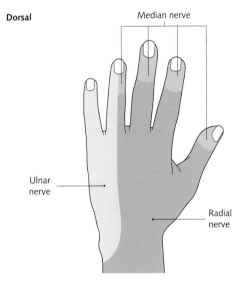

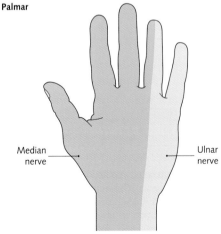

Fig. 9.2 Median, ulnar and radial nerve innervation of the hand.

- Acute onset usually occurs with disc prolapse after for example, lifting a heavy object.
- There is a gradual onset in other compressive neuropathies, e.g., spinal stenosis, CTS, cubital tunnel syndrome and tarsal tunnel syndrome.
- Acute onset of symptoms may also occur after trauma, e.g., CTS after distal radius fracture.
- Accidental laceration to a nerve during surgery can result in immediate postoperative paraesthesia in the distribution of the affected nerve, or a painful neuroma.

Nature of symptoms

Exacerbating features

Sneezing and coughing often exacerbate symptoms of leg pain with disc prolapse. Compressive neuropathies are often worsened in certain positions, e.g., typing at a keyboard with CTS or flexing the elbow at night in cubital tunnel syndrome.

Relieving features

- Patients with CTS often get night pain, which is relieved by hanging their hand down off the bed.
- Patients with lumbar spinal stenosis suffer pain and numbness in their legs after walking short distances (spinal claudication), which is relieved by bending forward.

Associated features

Be aware that the neuropathy may be a sign of underlying disease.

- Patients with undiagnosed diabetes mellitus may have weight loss, polyuria and polydipsia associated with peripheral neuropathy.
- In patients with back pain and radicular symptoms, loss of bowel or bladder function should be treated as cauda equina syndrome until proven otherwise (see Chapter 9).
- Check for constitutional features such as weight loss, malaise and night sweats if malignancy is possible. For example, a Pancoast tumour (an apical lung carcinoma) can present with upper-limb neurological symptoms.

Medical history

The following can predispose to neuropathy and should be asked about in the medical history:

- osteoarthritis and rheumatoid arthritis
- systemic lupus erythematosus
- diabetes
- malignancy
- previous surgery/trauma

A list of causes specific to CTS can be seen later.

Drug history

Some chemotherapy agents can cause peripheral neuropathy, as can some antibiotics such as nitrofurantoin and linezolid. Cardiovascular agents including amiodarone, digoxin and some statins may also be causative.

Social history

Manual jobs may trigger compressive neuropathies such as carpal tunnel or cubital tunnel syndrome. A history of alcohol use is relevant in suspected cases of peripheral neuropathy.

Family history

Examples of important family histories to be aware of include neurofibromatosis (von Recklinghausen disease) or diabetes.

Examination

Examining the specific affected myotomes and dermatomes is key in determining the level of a spinal cord lesion. For peripheral nerve lesions, establish the extent of the sensory and motor deficit present to help you determine which nerve is affected. Some special tests may reproduce nerve symptoms such as tapping a nerve (Tinel's test). Café-au-lait spots are characteristic of neurofibromatosis.

COMMUNICATION

Sleep is affected in severe carpal tunnel syndrome. Patients look tired, unhappy and can even be depressed. When using their hands, the patient may struggle to complete complex fine motor tasks and drop things. Pain might be more severe when using the phone or typing. Simple splints may allow a patient a good night's sleep and to function at work.

Investigation

Dependent on the location of symptoms, different imaging may be useful. Plain radiographs of the spine may show osteophytes causing nerve root compression or the presence of a cervical rib. Magnetic resonance imaging (MRI) provides very detailed soft-tissue images and is commonly used to investigate spinal pathology such as a disc prolapse. Ultrasound scans or MRI can diagnose other compressive neuropathies like a Morton's neuroma. Nerve conduction studies are used in cases of diagnostic doubt to confirm CTS and can be used to diagnose other peripheral nerve lesions. Blood tests may demonstrate the cause of a peripheral neuropathy, e.g., fasting glucose, thyroid function tests, haematinics.

CARPAL TUNNEL SYNDROME

Definition

CTS results from compression of the median nerve as it passes through the carpal tunnel at the wrist. The carpal tunnel is formed by the space between the transverse carpal ligament and the carpal bones. The transverse carpal ligament attaches proximally to the scaphoid tubercle and pisiform and distally to the trapezium and hook of hamate.

Incidence

CTS is the most common compressive neuropathy in the upper limb. It is especially common in middle-aged and elderly women and affects up to 10% of the population.

Aetiology

CTS is usually idiopathic but can be associated with several underlying conditions (see Clinical Notes).

CLINICAL NOTES

CONDITIONS PREDISPOSING TO CARPAL TUNNEL SYNDROME

- Diabetes mellitus
- Hypothyroidism
- Rheumatoid arthritis
- Pregnancy
- Acromegaly
- Obesity
- Chronic renal failure
- Vitamin deficiency
- Alcoholism
- Trauma, e.g., wrist fractures

Clinical features

CTS presents with pain and/or paraesthesia in the median nerve distribution (Fig. 9.2). These symptoms can radiate distally to the fingers but also proximally towards the elbow. They are often worse at night, waking the patient. It is important to try to distinguish this from other types of peripheral neuropathies caused by, for example, alcoholism or diabetes. The presence of bilateral fingertip numbness in all digits should raise doubt about CTS being the cause.

Examination may reveal sensory loss in the median nerve distribution but can be unremarkable at the time of assessment.

The strength of the thenar muscles should be tested; they may be weak and wasted in advanced disease. Carpal tunnel compression testing with Phalen's, Tinel's and Durkan's tests may reproduce the symptoms (Figs 9.3 and 9.4)

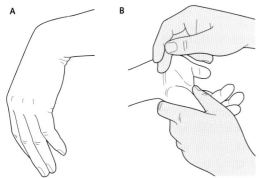

Fig. 9.3 Provocation tests for carpal tunnel syndrome may reproduce the patient's symptoms. (A) Phalen's test: the wrist is held in maximal palmar flexion. (B) Tinel's test: tap over the median nerve proximal to the transverse carpal ligament in the wrist.

Investigations

Nerve conduction studies may be necessary where there is diagnostic doubt and will show reduced nerve conduction velocities across the wrist. This will be helpful in distinguishing entrapment from cervical disc pathology where conduction of nerves distal to the lesion will be unaffected or uniformly reduced. Investigations such as serum glucose and thyroid function tests should be performed to exclude underlying medical conditions.

Management

The most successful treatment is surgical decompression of the carpal tunnel by division of the transverse carpal ligament. This is a very effective procedure and can be performed under local anaesthetic. In less severe cases, wrist splints may help nocturnal symptoms and corticosteroid injection of the carpal tunnel may bring some relief. In cases associated with pregnancy, the patient should be assessed postpartum as symptoms may subsequentially disappear.

ULNAR NERVE ENTRAPMENT

Definition

The ulnar nerve can become compressed at various points in the forearm from where it passes behind the medial epicondyle (cubital tunnel syndrome) down to Guyon's canal in the wrist.

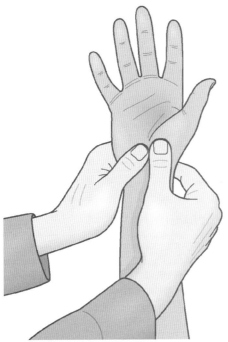

Fig. 9.4 Durkan's test. (From Lowe W. *Suggested variations on standard carpal tunnel syndrome assessment tests*. J Bodyw Mov Ther. 2008;12(2):151–157.)

Incidence

Ulnar nerve compression at the elbow is fairly common due to its superficial position here and is the second most common compression neuropathy of the upper limb.

Aetiology

Ulnar nerve entrapment may be idiopathic like in CTS or due to a precipitating injury.

CLINICAL NOTES

PRECIPITATING FACTORS FOR ULNAR NERVE ENTRAPMENT
- Local trauma, e.g., fractures of the elbow
- Prolonged leaning on the elbow
- Elbow synovitis

Clinical features

Patients develop pain and/or paraesthesia in the medial side of the elbow, which radiates to the medial forearm and the ulnar nerve distribution in the hand (see Fig. 9.2).

Examination usually reveals reduced sensation in the ulnar nerve distribution. Palpation of the nerve behind the medial epicondyle may provoke the symptoms. Motor dysfunction may result in atrophy of the hypothenar eminence and intrinsic muscles, the majority of which are supplied by the ulnar nerve. Due to intrinsic weakness, abduction and adduction of the fingers may be weak and in severe cases there may be clawing of the hand (Fig. 9.5). Observable signs include: Benediction posture, Froment's sign and Wartenberg's sign (Fig. 9.6).

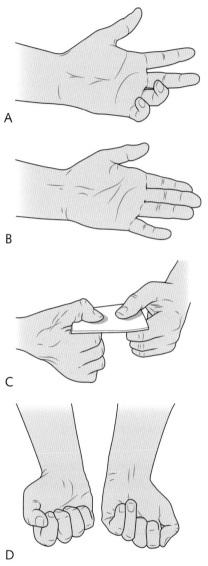

A

B

C

D

Fig. 9.6 (A) Benediction posture, with clawing of the fourth and fifth fingers while the fingers and thumb are held slightly abducted. (B) Wartenberg's sign, abduction of the little finger with the hand at rest. (C) Froment's sign, seen when using the thumb and index finger to pinch an object. (D) Weakness of the ulnar flexor digitorum profundus, inability to completely flex the distal phalanx of the fourth and fifth digits. (From Kasfiki EV, Folwell A, Kelly CWP. *250 Cases in Clinical Medicine*. 5th ed. Elsevier; 2020.)

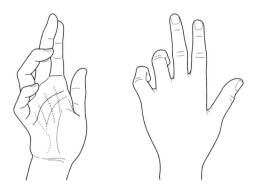

Fig. 9.5 Clawing of the hand due to ulnar nerve palsy.

Investigations

Nerve conduction studies confirm the diagnosis where doubt exists and establish the site of compression.

Management

Conservative management for cubital tunnel syndrome includes using a night splint with the elbow held in extension, with NSAIDs for pain relief and suppression of inflammation. Ulnar nerve compression due to elbow synovitis may respond to corticosteroid injection of the elbow. Surgical decompression should be performed if sensory symptoms cannot be tolerated or if there is muscle weakness or wasting.

RADIAL NERVE INJURIES

Aetiology

Radial nerve compression at the axilla is typically seen in an inebriated person who falls asleep with an arm hanging over the back of a chair ('Saturday night palsy'). The radial nerve may also commonly be injured by fractures of the humeral shaft.

Clinical features

The wrist extensors are paralysed, resulting in wrist drop. Grip strength is dramatically reduced because the finger flexors do not function well with the wrist in a flexed position. Nerve injury in the axilla will also lead to paralysis of the triceps. Due to nerve overlap, sensory loss is best detected in the small area of skin on the dorsum of the hand between the first and second metacarpals where the supply is purely from the radial nerve.

Management

The wrist should be splinted and the cause of the radial nerve palsy should be assessed. Most radial nerve palsies associated with a radial shaft fracture will be a neurapraxia rather than a true radial nerve injury and will heal over time. However, fracture or dislocation reduction is sometimes required for a true nerve entrapment and may sometimes need to be performed surgically. If there is no resolution, tendon transfer or nerve grafting may be indicated.

COMMON PERONEAL NERVE INJURIES

Aetiology

The common peroneal nerve winds around the neck of the fibula and is in a vulnerable position. It may be damaged by a fracture to the neck of the fibula, from the pressure of a tight bandage, or plaster cast or intraoperatively due to patient positioning and prolonged pressure over the head and neck of the fibula.

Clinical features

Common peroneal nerve injury results in paralysis of the ankle and foot extensors. Unopposed action of the foot flexors and inverters causes the foot to be plantar flexed and inverted. This is referred to as 'foot drop'. Patients develop a high-stepping gait, flicking the foot forwards to avoid tripping over it. There is also loss of sensation over the anterior and lateral sides of the leg and the dorsum of the foot and toes.

Management

Pressure on the nerve should be relieved and a splint should be applied. If the foot drop does not resolve, an ankle–foot orthosis can be used to maintain some degree of dorsiflexion. Nerve conduction studies are carried out to assess the integrity of the nerve.

● Chapter Summary

- Nerve injuries can be classified by which part of the nerve is affected. This guides management and can set patient expectations for recovery.
- Entrapments can be differentiated from other patterns of neurological deficit through history and examination.
- Common causes of nerve entrapments include central compressive lesions in the spine and more peripheral nerve entrapments such as carpal or ulnar nerve entrapment.
- Common investigations used to investigate neurological conditions include MRI for the spine and nerve conduction studies for peripheral lesions.
- A thorough drug and past medical history is important. Pregnancy, diabetes and rheumatoid arthritis are common predisposing conditions in carpal tunnel syndrome.
- Release of distal nerve entrapments such as in carpal tunnel syndrome is commonly performed under local anaesthetic.

UKMLA Conditions
Lower limb soft tissue injury
Radiculopathies
Upper limb soft tissue injury

UKMLA Presentations
Soft tissue injury
Trauma

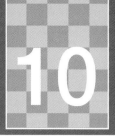
DEFINITION

Osteoarthritis (OA) is a disorder of synovial joints characterized by articular surface damage, formation of new bone and secondary inflammation. It is sometimes known as degenerative joint disease. It causes joint pain, stiffness, swelling and deformity.

INCIDENCE

OA is the most common chronic joint disease, with incidence and prevalence increasing with age. At some point, up to 80% of the population will be affected by OA. However, it is often asymptomatic and the prevalence of true symptoms in the Western world is somewhere around 20%.

PATHOLOGY AND AETIOLOGY

Histologically, repeated microtrauma or abnormal biomechanical forces cause damage to the weight-bearing cartilage surface, which eventually wears away completely exposing the subchondral bone (Fig. 10.1). Chondrocytes attempt repair by releasing degradative enzymes. Cysts occur and new bone is laid down (sclerosis) as a result of microfracturing of the articular surface. Disorganized new bone formation occurs at the joint margins (osteophytes) and the synovial lining becomes thickened and inflamed, producing excess synovial fluid (effusions).

> ### HINTS AND TIPS
>
> These changes explain the four cardinal features found on X-ray examination of osteoarthritis joints:
> - Joint space narrowing
> - Sclerosis
> - Cyst formation
> - Osteophytes

OA is described as primary when no single underlying cause is identified. Risk factors are listed in Table 10.1. They can be classified as modifiable or nonmodifiable risk factors. Secondary OA occurs when a clear cause is identified; it can include trauma, congenital/developmental issues and metabolic diseases.

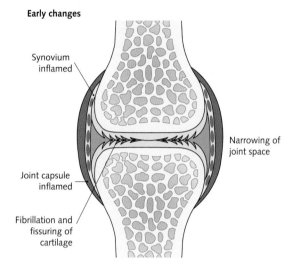

Early changes

- Synovium inflamed
- Joint capsule inflamed
- Fibrillation and fissuring of cartilage
- Narrowing of joint space

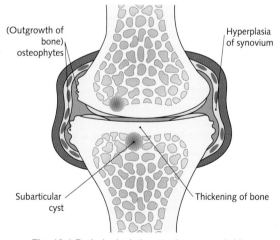

Changes secondary to loss of cartilage

- (Outgrowth of bone) osteophytes
- Subarticular cyst
- Hyperplasia of synovium
- Thickening of bone

Fig. 10.1 Pathological changes in osteoarthritis.

CLINICAL FEATURES

Pain is the predominant symptom of OA. It is usually described as an aching or burning pain within the affected joint but may be referred distally. The onset is gradual and worse on or after activity. As the disease progresses and the joints develop secondary inflammation, night pain can become a feature. Stiffness is often

Table 10.1 Risk factors for osteoarthritis

Modifiable	Nonmodifiable
Occupation	Increasing age
Muscle weakness	Female sex
Obesity	Inflammatory joint disease
Previous trauma	Genetics
High impact activity	Congenital leg length discrepancy
Previous meniscectomy	Lack of osteoporosis
	Oestrogen deficiency

- Do they struggle to use their hands to get undressed?
- Deformity may be obvious but also note previous scars, redness, swelling and wasting of muscles during inspection.
- Palpate effusions and the joint lines for tenderness.
- There may be fixed flexion deformities and movements may be diminished.
- Remember to examine above and below the affected joints.

reported. The pain and stiffness due to OA can reduce daily function and quality of life. The characteristic pain that worsens with activity as experienced with OA, can help differentiate from an inflammatory arthritis which more commonly presents with morning stiffness and pain that improves with activity.

Joints are usually affected in an asymmetrical pattern with single or multiple joints involved.

HINTS AND TIPS

Remember that pain from the hip can be referred to the knee.

Other symptoms can include swelling, deformity and weakness (usually secondary to muscle wasting). Certain activities can become increasingly difficult; for example, a patient with OA in the hip might not be able to put on their own socks.

Almost any synovial joint can become affected by OA, most commonly the knees, hips and hands. Within the hands, the first carpometacarpal joint, distal interphalangeal (DIP) joints and proximal interphalangeal (PIP) joints are usually affected. The wrists, shoulder and elbows are also susceptible (Figs 10.2 and 10.3). Signs of OA can include restricted movements, palpable crepitus, squaring at the base of the thumb due to involvement of the first carpo-metacarpal joint, mild synovitis, and bony swellings. Patients can also suffer from osteoarthritis affecting the spine. The cervical and lumbar spine are most commonly affected and the patient will experience pain localized to these areas. However, pain may radiate to the arms, legs or buttocks, suggesting nerve root compression due to osteophyte formation.

EXAMINATION

Examination should start in the joint where the patient complains of symptoms. Here are some useful general tips:

- Watch as the patient gets out of a chair and comes into the examination room. Do they limp or use a stick? Is their gait antalgic?

DIAGNOSIS AND INVESTIGATION

HINTS AND TIPS

Classical features of osteoarthritis in the hands include Heberden nodes of the distal interphalangeal joints and Bouchard nodes of the proximal interphalangeal joints (Fig. 10.3).

In most cases, the diagnosis is clear from the history and clinical examination. The National Institute for Health and Clinical Excellence (NICE) guidelines state that a patient can be diagnosed with OA without further investigation if they are 45 or over, have activity-related joint pain and have either no morning-related stiffness or morning stiffness that lasts no longer than 30 minutes.

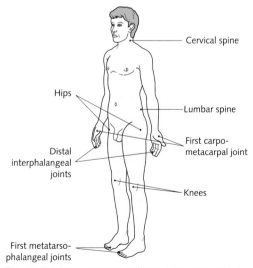

Fig. 10.2 Joints commonly affected by osteoarthritis.

Blood tests and joint aspiration may be undertaken to exclude septic or inflammatory arthritis in uncertain cases.

X-ray is the gold standard imaging technique for OA and will show narrowing of the joint space, sclerosis, osteophyte formation and subchondral cysts (Fig. 10.4). However, it is important to note that X-ray findings may not correlate directly to the severity of symptoms. An MRI should be carried out if nerve root compression due to spinal OA is suspected.

To provide patient-centred care, a holistic assessment of the patient is required. This involves assessing how symptoms impact the patient's life, allowing the clinician to form a management plan that is tailored to the individual patient.

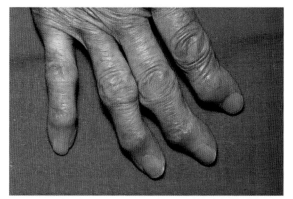

Fig. 10.3 Osteoarthritis of the hand, showing Heberden nodes at the distal interphalangeal joints and Bouchard nodes at the proximal interphalangeal joints. (Reproduced with permission from Ralston SH, McInnes IB, eds. *Davidson's Principles and Practice of Medicine*. 22nd ed. Edinburgh: Churchill Livingstone; 2014.)

HINTS AND TIPS

It is important to look for atypical features that may suggest a diagnosis other than osteoarthritis. These include a history of trauma to the joint, morning stiffness that lasts longer than 30 minutes, presence of an erythematous joint or rapid progression of symptoms. Differential diagnoses would include inflammatory arthritis (e.g., rheumatoid or psoriatic arthritis), crystal arthropathy, bone tumours or septic arthritis.

MANAGEMENT

There is no cure for OA and treatment is aimed at relieving pain and maintaining function. Treatment options are medical or surgical.

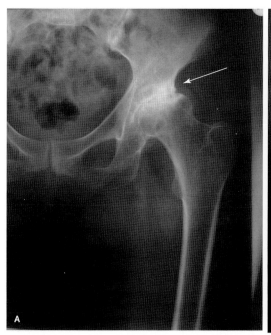
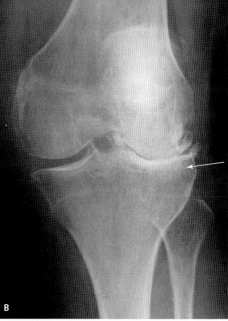

Fig. 10.4 Features of osteoarthritis on X-ray images. (A) Hip joint showing sclerosis, joint space narrowing, cysts and osteophytes. (B) Knee showing OA within the lateral compartment of the femorotibial joint.

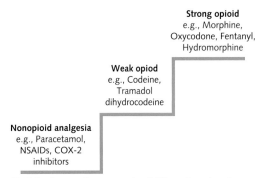

Fig. 10.5 The increasing strength of different analgesic options. *COX-2*, Cyclooxygenase-2; *NSAIDs*, nonsteroidal antiinflammatory drugs.

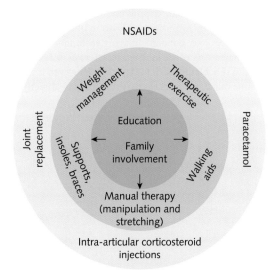

Fig. 10.6 Treatment of osteoarthritis. (Adapted from NG226 Osteoarthritis in over 16s diagnosis and management.)

Medical

- Initial lifestyle advice should be given, with regard to weight loss, regular exercise and the avoidance of impact-loading activities. Input from other healthcare professionals will be of great benefit.
- The first-line pharmacological treatment for osteoarthritis is oral paracetamol. If pain relief is insufficient, addition of an NSAID or COX-2 inhibitor should be considered. These drugs should be used at the lowest effective dose, for the shortest possible time and should be coprescribed with a proton pump inhibitor such as omeprazole. Opioids can be considered, however, it is important to note that opioids have side effects such as dependence and withdrawal and are not always suitable for the treatment of long-term chronic pain. Fig. 10.5 illustrates the increasing strength of different analgesic options.
- Physiotherapy improves gait and function of an affected limb. Simple measures such as the use of a walking stick may improve pain when walking. Orthotic insoles can help with biomechanical off-loading.
- Injections of corticosteroids provide temporary relief from pain and improvement in function. Hyaluronic acid derivative injections may offer relief for those unfit for surgery, but the evidence for this is poor.
- Glucosamine is often tried, but lack of clinical trial data of its benefit means it is not routinely recommended.
- Thermotherapy and transcutaneous electrical nerve stimulation (TENS) should be considered as an adjunct to core treatments.

Fig. 10.6 illustrates the different components in the management of OA.

Surgical

Surgical treatment for OA depends on age, the joint affected, the level of pain and disability experienced. This is dealt with in greater detail in Chapter 24.

There are generally four things a surgeon can do to a joint:

1. Arthroplasty (joint replacement). This is most commonly undertaken for the knee or hip joint. It gives excellent pain relief in 90% of patients for at least 10 years.
2. Arthrodesis (joint fusion). The two sides of the joint are removed and fused together. This is most commonly undertaken in the foot and ankle. When successful, there is good pain relief, but movement is lost.
3. Osteotomy (joint realignment). Increased load through a joint because of a deformity often leads to OA. A surgeon can realign the limb by cutting the bone above or below the joint, removing a wedge of bone and correcting the deformity. The most common site for this is at the knee and is often used to correct a varus deformity (bow legs). The tibia is realigned to redistribute the load more evenly, slowing the progression of OA (Fig. 10.7).
4. Joint excision. This involves removal of the failing joint and is less commonly used. It is still undertaken occasionally when other methods have failed.

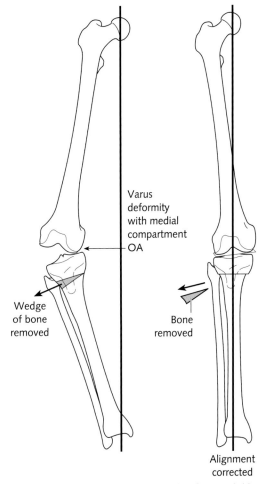

Fig. 10.7 Osteotomy of the knee. *OA*, Osteoarthritis.

Chapter Summary

- Osteoarthritis (OA) is the most common arthritis, with up to 80% of the population affected at some point in their lives.
- It can be primary or secondary, with many alterable lifestyle risk factors.
- The classic X-ray findings of OA are loss of joint space, sclerosis, cyst formation and osteophytes.
- Pain is usually a burning or aching sensation with an asymmetric distribution of joints affected.
- There is no cure for OA and treatment focuses on relieving pain and preserving function either medically or surgically.

UKMLA Conditions
Osteoarthritis
Radiculopathies

UKMLA Presentations
Back pain
Chronic joint pain/stiffness
Musculoskeletal deformities
Trauma

Rheumatoid arthritis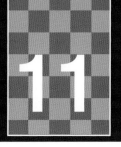

DEFINITION

Rheumatoid arthritis (RA) is a common autoimmune, inflammatory condition characterized by symmetrical swelling in multiple joints. It typically affects the hands and follows a chronic course that results in disability if left untreated. RA is a multisystem disease, the complications of which can cause reduction in life expectancy.

INCIDENCE AND PREVALENCE

RA affects females more commonly than males, with a female-to-male excess of between two and four times. The annual incidence in the UK is 0.1–0.2/1000 for men and 0.2–0.4/1000 for women. RA prevalence in North American and European populations is approximately 1%.

AETIOLOGY

The aetiology of RA remains unclear, but it appears that both genetic and environmental factors have an important influence. It is likely that an environmental trigger (e.g., an infection) triggers an autoimmune response in a genetically susceptible individual.

Genetic factors

The most significant genetic predisposing risk factor for RA is in variations of the human leucocyte antigen (HLA) genes. The most significant appears to be the HLA DR4 gene, therefore, family history is relevant. It is important to note that having one autoimmune condition increases the likelihood of having another.

Environmental factors

Environmental influences on the development of RA are not well understood. The effects of various infections, occupations and lifestyle factors have been examined but no causal links have been found. However, there is an increased risk of the disease in smokers in whom the disease tends to be more aggressive.

COMMUNICATION

Remember to ask about smoking history and give advice about smoking cessation.

IMMUNOLOGICAL ABNORMALITIES

In RA, the normal immunological mechanisms that help fight infections and destroy malignant cells target normal tissue, resulting in joint damage. T-lymphocytes play a key role in initiating inflammation in RA (Fig. 11.1) with B-cells and activated macrophages also playing important roles.

The activated cells produce cytokines (intracellular messenger molecules), e.g., tumour necrosis factor-α (TNF-α) and interleukin 1 (IL-1). These cytokines have many actions, including those listed in the box 'Actions of cytokines'. Understanding these immunological pathways has allowed the production of targeted biological therapies.

ACTIONS OF CYTOKINES

- Stimulation of inflammation
- Attraction of other immune cells (chemotaxis)
- Excess synovial fluid production
- Cartilage destruction
- Bone resorption
- Stimulation of B-lymphocyte differentiation and maturation
- Increased antibody production, including production of rheumatoid factor

Rheumatoid factor and anticitrullinated protein antibodies are produced by activated B-cells in the synovium. They are autoantibodies found in approximately 80% of patients with RA. High levels of antibodies are associated with more aggressive disease and the presence of extraarticular features.

PATHOLOGY

The main pathological abnormality in RA is synovitis. Inflammatory cells and fibroblasts infiltrate the synovium causing

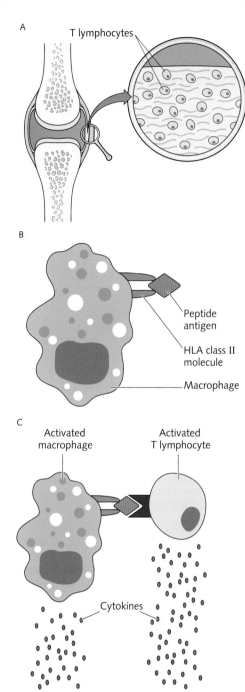

Fig. 11.1 (A) T-lymphocytes (predominantly T-helper cells) accumulate in the synovium. (B) Synovial macrophages (antigen-presenting cells) express peptide antigens on their cell surfaces in association with HLA class II molecules. (C) T-lymphocytes with appropriate receptors interact with the macrophages and both cell types become activated. *HLA,* Human leucocyte antigen.

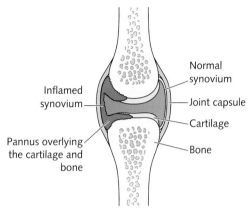

Fig. 11.2 Diagram of a synovial joint. One side is healthy; the other shows the pathological changes of rheumatoid arthritis.

synovial hypertrophy. Macrophages and osteoclasts create a layer of chronically inflamed tissue, pannus, which extends from the joint margins and erodes the articular cartilage (Fig. 11.2). Matrix metalloproteinases (MMPs) released by fibroblasts also cause extensive erosion of cartilage and bone leading to joint deformity. Prostaglandins and nitric acid are released and are accountable for the swelling and pain experienced in RA. Ligament insertions (entheses) are a common site of inflammation and the thickened joint capsule distends due to effusion. Adjacent muscular atrophy is a common feature.

CLINICAL FEATURES

RA can develop at any time of life, but the peak incidence occurs between the ages of 30 and 50 years. Symptoms begin insidiously, developing over weeks and months. Some people may experience a very acute onset. Others can develop monoarthritis or palindromic RA where symptoms are severe but fleeting and affect different joints. Overall, RA follows a clinical course of exacerbation and remission.

The features of RA can be broadly divided into:

- articular features
- extraarticular features

Articular features

Joint pain, stiffness and swelling are the cardinal articular features of RA. Stiffness is typically worse after periods of rest, such as first thing in the morning, and tends to ease on movement. The duration of this stiffness is a useful guide to disease activity. RA affects mainly small- and medium-sized joints in a symmetrical fashion (Fig. 11.3).

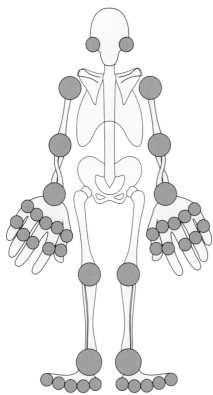

Fig. 11.3 The joints most commonly affected by rheumatoid arthritis.

Pain and stiffness lead to varying degrees of functional loss. Even in early disease, the impact on patients' activities of daily living can be profound. By the late stages of the illness, established bony erosions and joint damage further limit a patient's physical abilities.

> **COMMUNICATION**
>
> Patients can feel extremely frustrated and helpless if they suffer loss of function. It is important to listen sympathetically to their concerns, ideas and expectations. Help patients to find a solution. For example, the secretary who struggles to type because of her wrist pain may benefit from occupational therapy input, corticosteroid injections and wrist splints.

Synovitis causes 'boggy' joint swelling. The skin overlying an affected joint is usually warm and erythematous due to increased local blood flow. Note that infection should first be excluded in a patient that presents with a warm, erythematous joint. On palpation, the swelling is tender and has a similar consistency to that of a grape.

The effects of RA on specific joint regions

Many of the classical deformities of RA are becoming less common in clinical practice due to more effective therapies being used earlier. Some patients still have longstanding classic joint deformities that need recognition.

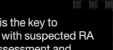

> **RED FLAG**
>
> Urgent recognition and treatment is the key to preventing joint damage. Patients with suspected RA should be referred for specialist assessment and treatment within 6 weeks of symptom onset.

The rheumatoid hand and wrist

The hands and wrists are almost always involved in RA (Fig. 11.4). Synovitis typically occurs in the wrists, the metacarpophalangeal (MCP) and proximal interphalangeal (PIP) joints, sparing the distal interphalangeal (DIP) joints. The inflammation can weaken and damage the tendons and ligaments, producing well-recognized deformities.

Ulnar deviation of the fingers results from MCP joint inflammation (Fig. 11.5). Subluxation of the MCP joints can occur, with the proximal phalanges drifting in an ulnar and palmer direction.

Boutonnière and swan-neck deformities of the digits are due to PIP synovitis and laxity and/or contraction of the extensor and flexor tendon apparatus (Fig. 11.6).

Radial deviation of the wrist occurs partly to compensate for ulnar deviation of the fingers. Subluxation of the wrist joint produces a prominent ulnar styloid.

The foot

The foot is the commonest site of inflammation in RA. The proximal phalanges may sublux dorsally and the metatarsal heads become eroded and displaced towards the floor. They can be easily palpated through the sole of the foot, as the protective fat pad is lost, and can be painful to walk on. Patients often feel as though they are 'walking on marbles'.

Hindfoot involvement can also cause issues with subtalar arthritis. Valgus deformity may develop in patients with longstanding disease. All these deformities are the result of poorly controlled synovitis. The aim of the rheumatologist is to suppress synovitis, limiting bony destruction and reducing disability.

The cervical spine

Inflammation and erosive disease, affecting the first cervical vertebra and the transverse ligament posterior to the odontoid peg, can result in atlantoaxial subluxation. This is a rare and a late

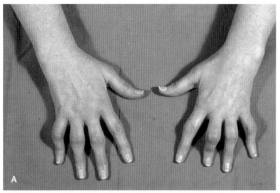

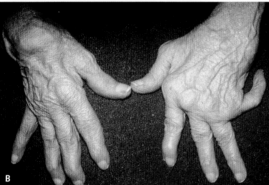

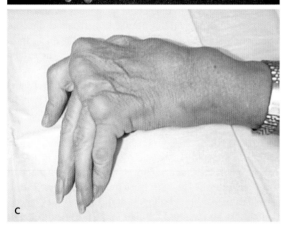

Fig. 11.4 The hands of a patient with rheumatoid arthritis. (A) Polyarticular swelling of the proximal interphalangeal joints along with wrist deformity. (B) Complete subluxation with ulnar deviation at the metacarpophalangeal joints in a patient with advanced disease. (C) 'Zig-zag' deformity of the hand with radial deviation at the wrist and ulnar deviation at the metacarpophalangeal joints. (With permission from Erickson AR, Cannella AC, Mikuls TR. *Clinical Features of Rheumatoid Arthritis, Kelley and Firestein's Textbook of Rheumatology.* 10th ed. Elsevier; 2017. (A and B, Courtesy Dr. Iain McInnes; C, Courtesy Dr. Gerald Moore.))

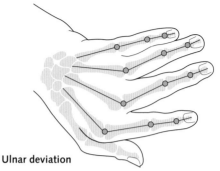

Ulnar deviation

Fig. 11.5 Ulnar deviation.

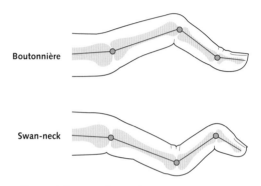

Boutonnière

Swan-neck

Fig. 11.6 Boutonnière and swan-neck deformity.

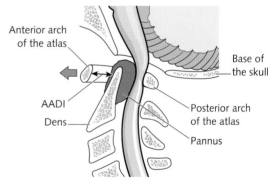

Anterior arch of the atlas

Base of the skull

AADI

Posterior arch of the atlas

Dens

Pannus

Fig. 11.7 In healthy adults, the distance between the anterior arch of the atlas and the dens should not exceed 3 mm. The diagram shows forward subluxation of the atlas on the axis. The spinal cord is compressed between the pannus around the dens and the posterior arch of the atlas. *AADI*, Anterior atlantodental interspace.

complication. The atlas slips forward on the axis, reducing the space around the spinal cord (Fig. 11.7). This produces neck pain, which radiates to the back of the head. Atlantoaxial subluxation should be suspected in an RA patient that presents with a new headache in the occipital region. Upper motor neurone damage resulting in a spastic quadriparesis is a rare complication. Damage to the articulation between the occipital bone and the atlas may allow the odontoid peg to move upwards through the foramen magnum. This can threaten the cord and brainstem, sometimes resulting in sudden death after relatively minor jolts to the head and neck. Subaxial subluxation can also occur (below the first cervical vertebra).

> **HINTS AND TIPS**
>
> It is important to take lateral flexion X-ray images or magnetic resonance imaging of the cervical spine in rheumatoid arthritis patients requiring a general anaesthetic. The anaesthetist must be aware of any neck instability so that precautions can be taken during intubation.

Extraarticular features of RA

Rheumatoid nodules
Rheumatoid nodules are firm subcutaneous nodules found in around 20% of rheumatoid patients. They develop in areas affected by pressure or friction, such as the fingers, elbows and Achilles tendon. They are seen in patients who have positive rheumatoid factor antibodies and are more common in smokers. They tend to accompany more severe disease. Unfortunately, methotrexate, often used to treat RA, has the disadvantage of making nodules worse.

Tenosynovitis and bursitis
Tendon sheaths and bursa are lined with synovium, which can also become inflamed in RA. The flexor tendons of the fingers are commonly affected by tenosynovitis, which can result in tendon rupture. The olecranon and subacromial bursae are common sites of bursitis.

Carpal tunnel syndrome
Synovitis can cause entrapment of peripheral nerves. Medial nerve compression resulting in carpal tunnel syndrome is common (see Chapter 9).

Systemic features of rheumatoid arthritis

As well as causing joint pain and swelling, active RA makes people feel generally unwell. The inflammation can result in systemic symptoms such as low-grade fever, weight loss, muscle aches and lethargy. These symptoms can be prominent, particularly in patients with acute onset RA.

The effects of rheumatoid arthritis on distant organs

RA can affect many different body systems (Fig. 11.8). Extraarticular manifestations can be severe and are associated with an increase in mortality. Some of the more common are explored below.

Anaemia
Anaemia in RA can be due to:

- anaemia of chronic disease (normocytic);
- autoimmune haemolysis;
- Felty syndrome;
- nonsteroidal antiinflammatory drugs (NSAIDs) can cause iron deficiency anaemia through gastrointestinal inflammation and blood loss;
- disease-modifying antirheumatic drugs (DMARDs) sometimes potentiate anaemia through bone marrow suppression. Methotrexate may cause a macrocytic anaemia due to a decrease in folate.

Felty syndrome
Felty syndrome is associated with RA and describes splenomegaly with leukopenia. It usually occurs in patients who are rheumatoid-factor positive. The leukopenia leads to bacterial infections. Lymphadenopathy, anaemia and thrombocytopenia can also occur.

Rheumatoid lung disease
Although pulmonary disease is common in RA, it does not always produce symptoms. Men are more commonly affected than women.

Pneumonitis can cause fibrosis and scarring of the lungs leading to pulmonary fibrosis, with or without the presence of granulomatous lesions. It may also occur as a reaction to DMARDS and is most commonly associated with methotrexate.

Pleural effusions in RA have become less common with more aggressive early disease management. They occasionally precede arthritis and rheumatoid factors can be detected in the fluid, which is a transudate.

Pulmonary nodules can occur in seropositive patients with subcutaneous nodules. They rarely cause symptoms but may produce a chronic dry cough.

Investigations

Blood tests
Full blood count may show anaemia of chronic disease, thrombocytosis due to chronic inflammation or leukopenia due to Felty syndrome.

Erythrocyte sedimentation rate (ESR) and C-reactive protein (CRP) are usually raised in the presence of synovitis and are useful markers of response to treatment.

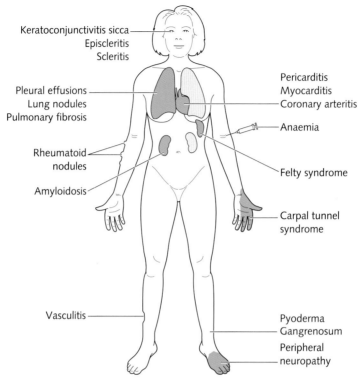

Keratoconjunctivitis sicca
Episcleritis
Scleritis

Pleural effusions
Lung nodules
Pulmonary fibrosis

Rheumatoid
nodules

Amyloidosis

Vasculitis

Pericarditis
Myocarditis
Coronary arteritis

Anaemia

Felty syndrome

Carpal tunnel
syndrome

Pyoderma
Gangrenosum

Peripheral
neuropathy

Fig. 11.8 Extraarticular manifestations of rheumatoid arthritis.

It is important to check serum uric acid levels to help exclude a urate crystal arthropathy.

Rheumatoid factor is found in the serum of 70% to 90% of patients with RA. Patients who lack antibodies are sometimes described as having seronegative rheumatoid arthritis. It is important to remember that rheumatoid factor is found in 5% to 10% of healthy individuals, particularly in the elderly. It may also be raised in conditions such as SLE, Sjogren's, hepatitis and bacterial endocarditis. Patients who are rheumatoid-factor positive have a higher rate of systemic disease and a poorer prognosis than those who are not.

Another serological test is available to help in the diagnosis of RA. Anticyclic citrullinated peptide antibodies can be present in patients who are rheumatoid-factor negative and indicate a worse prognosis. They are not associated with systemic features but have a higher specificity for RA.

HINTS AND TIPS

Rheumatoid factor can be present in healthy people. The diagnosis of rheumatoid arthritis can be made on clinical grounds following history, examination and the application of diagnostic criteria.

Radiological investigations

Plain X-ray images should be obtained to look for radiological evidence of RA (Table 11.1), which tends to be seen first in the small joints of the hands and feet (Fig. 11.9).

X-ray changes are often not present at diagnosis. It may be many months or even years before changes in the joint caused by persistent inflammation can be seen on radiological examination. Ultrasound has now become established in the detection of synovitis in early arthritis and is used to guide treatment to a target of low disease activity. Magnetic resonance imaging (MRI) can also help in the detection of synovitis and early erosions although this technique is expensive and time consuming (Fig. 11.10).

Diagnosis

Diagnosis is aided by the American College of Rheumatology 2010 criteria. This is a points-based criteria based on the number of joints affected, the type of joints affected, the duration of symptoms, rheumatoid factor and anti-CCP levels and the normality of CRP and ESR levels.

Management

Patients with RA should be cared for by a multidisciplinary team. Fig. 11.11 lists the professionals involved in the care of RA patients and explains the roles they play.

Table 11.1 Early and late radiological signs seen in RA

Early changes	Later changes
Soft tissue swelling	Juxta articular erosions
Periarticular osteopenia	Narrowing of joint space
	Subluxation

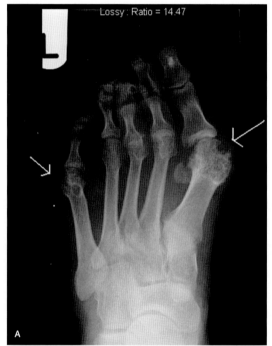

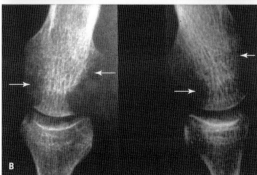

Fig. 11.9 (A) Periarticular osteopenia and erosions of the metatarsophalangeal joints. (B) Large erosions of the two metacarpophalangeal joints.

Drug treatment
There are three main aims of drug treatment in RA:

- Reduction in symptoms.

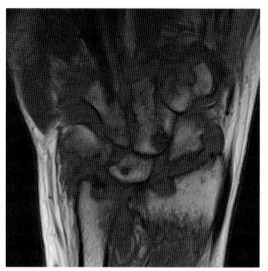

Fig. 11.10 Magnetic resonance imaging of erosions in rheumatoid arthritis.

- Prevention of damage by control of disease, thereby maintaining patient function.
- Nice guidelines (2018) recommend a treat-to-target strategy. This means treating with the aim of disease remission or low disease activity if remission cannot be achieved.

Initial treatment with antiinflammatory drugs
Initial treatment with NSAIDs or COX-2 inhibitors can improve joint pain and stiffness but has no effect on disease progression. Remember that NSAIDs should be coprescribed with a PPI due to the increased risk of gastric ulceration.

Corticosteroids
Corticosteroids can swiftly improve pain and swelling in RA and therefore, are often an initial treatment. Low doses of oral prednisolone can be used to control symptoms early in disease in conjunction with a DMARD, as DMARDs take time to exhibit their antiinflammatory effects. Corticosteroids can be given intraarticularly to treat local synovitis and are sometimes given via the intramuscular route to treat a generalized flare of RA. These would commonly be Kenalog or Depo-Medrone injections.

Disease-modifying antirheumatic drugs
DMARDS suppress inflammation and slow progression of erosive joint disease. They are the mainstay of RA therapy and should be commenced by 6 weeks of disease onset.

DMARDs act slowly and take several weeks to produce a clinical effect. If a patient does not respond adequately to one DMARD, a second one can be added or substituted. In patients

Professional	Role
Rheumatologist	Monitoring of disease activity. Prescription and monitoring of drug therapy. Identification and management of complications. Referral to other specialists when necessary. Coordination of team. Diagnosis.
Specialist nurse	Patient education. DMARD monitoring. Biologic administration and advice. Joint injections.
Orthopaedic surgeon	Replacement of damaged joints. Surgical synovectomy. Tendon repairs.
Physiotherapist	Use of physical therapies to combat inflammation. Prescription of exercises to maintain and improve muscular strength and range of joint movement.
Occupational therapist	Splinting of acutely inflamed joints. Advice on how to function whilst putting as little stress as possible on the joints (joint protection). Provision of aids and appliances to assist with activities of daily living.
Podiatrist	Assessment of footwear and advice on choosing suitable shoes. Provision of insoles to improve the mechanics of deformed feet. Prevention and treatment of skin lesions, such as calluses and ulcers.
Psychologist	RA is a lifelong, chronic condition that will have significant impact on a patient's life. Furthermore, providing psychological support will likely increase the patient's engagement with the treatment plan.

DMARD, Disease-modifying antirheumatic drug.

Fig. 11.11 Professionals involved in the care of rheumatoid arthritis patients and the roles they play.

Table 11.2 DMARDs used in the treatment of RA.

DMARD	Possible side effects
Methotrexate	Gastrointestinal upset Oral ulcers Raised liver enzymes Pneumonitis (methotrexate lung) Bone marrow suppression
Sulphasalazine	Gastrointestinal upset Raised liver enzymes Bone marrow suppression Altered colour of urine, sweat and tears
Hydroxychloroquine	Retinal damage (importance of annual eye tests)
Leflunomide	Hypertension Gastrointestinal upset Bone marrow suppression Peripheral neuropathy

Note: DMARDs used in the treatment of RA.
DMARDs, Disease-modifying antirheumatic drugs.

RED FLAG

Methotrexate is an antiinflammatory drug due to its action as a folate antagonist. It is a teratogen and should not be used during pregnancy. Certolizumab pegol (sold under the brand name Cimzia), sulphasalazine or hydroxychloroquine can be considered in pregnancy. However, remission of RA can occur during pregnancy. The inhibition of folate may also cause a macrocytic anaemia. It is important that patients taking methotrexate receive folate supplementation and have their bloods checked regularly.

ETHICS

Serious side effects to disease-modifying antirheumatic drugs are rare but can cause considerable harm to patients. Ensure patients are given written information about possible side effects and reactions so that they can make informed decisions on their treatment.

with poor prognostic markers, several DMARDs may be commenced at diagnosis.

Like many drugs, DMARDs can cause minor side effects such as nausea, headaches and rashes (Table 11.2). More serious complications, such as bone marrow suppression, abnormal liver function tests and renal impairment are rarer, but well recognized. It is therefore important to closely monitor patients on DMARD therapy both clinically and with regular blood testing.

Biological therapies

Patients who persist with high and moderate disease activity can be eligible for biological therapies. Biological therapies that target inflammatory mediators to treat RA are now widely used.

Table 11.3 Biological drugs used in the treatment of RA and their mechanism of action

Mechanism of action	Drug names
Targeted against TNF-α	Etanercept, infliximab, adalimumab
Targeted against B-cells.	Rituximab
Block IL-6 to suppress the acute phase response of inflammation	Tocilizumab, sarilumab
Inhibition of T cell activation	Abatacept
Inhibition of the JAK family of enzymes that are responsible for phosphorylating cytokine receptors. This blocks the effects of various interleukins	Upadacitinib, filgotinib, tofacitinib, baricitinib (JAK inhibitors).

Note: Biologics used in the treatment of RA.
IL-1, *Interleukin 1; JAK, Janus kinase; TNF-α, tumour necrosis factor-α.*

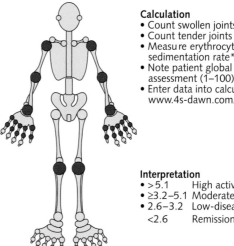

Calculation
- Count swollen joints
- Count tender joints
- Measure erythrocyte sedimentation rate*
- Note patient global health assessment (1–100)
- Enter data into calculator: www.4s-dawn.com/das28

Interpretation
- >5.1 High activity
- ≥3.2–5.1 Moderate activity
- 2.6–3.2 Low-disease activity
-   <2.6   Remission

Fig. 11.12 DAS-28 scoring and interpretation. *Erythrocyte sedimentation rate or C-reactive protein can be used for the calculation. (From Penman ID et al. *Davidson's Principles and Practice of Medicine.* 24th ed. Elsevier; 2023.)

There are many target molecules in the inflammatory cascade that can be the target site of biologics (Table 11.3). These drugs produce excellent clinical effects but remain more expensive than DMARDs and carry an increased risk of infection. In general, they are less toxic than DMARDs as they target a specific immune component. The National Institute for Health and Clinical Excellence (NICE) has issued guidance for their use in the UK. Disease activity scoring systems are employed to select patients for treatment. The development of cheaper generic or biosimilar forms of these drugs is allowing broader access. Janus kinase (JAK) inhibitors have recently been approved by NICE. They are oral agents with rapid onset, but carry an increased risk of shingles. Some uncertainty remains over their use in select patient groups such as those affected by cardiovascular disease.

> **RED FLAG**
>
> Biological therapies suppress the immune system and therefore, there are important steps and considerations that should be taken before starting a patient on these drugs.
> 1. Check HIV, tuberculosis, varicella and hepatitis status.
> 2. Ensure annual vaccination against influenza and pneumococcal illness.
> 3. Do not start these drugs in patients with active infection, tuberculosis, who are pregnant or those who have a malignancy or diverticular disease.
> 4. Be aware of the increased risk of skin and haematological malignancies when using these drugs. Communicate this risk to the patient.

Monitoring disease activity and drug efficacy

Disease activity and the efficacy of treatment can be evaluated using the Disease Activity Score-28 (DAS-28; Fig. 11.12). This score considers the number of swollen and tender joints (out of the 28 assessed), ESR levels and the patient's assessment of their health. This scoring may trigger a step-up in therapy.

The aim is to treat RA with the minimum effective dose. Treatment tends to follow a step-wise pattern:

First line: methotrexate, leflunomide, sulphasalazine or hydroxychloroquine.

Second line: two of the drugs listed above in combination.

Third line: methotrexate plus rituximab.

Fourth line: Any of the drugs mentioned in Table 11.3, selected based on individual patient factors.

Patients should attend a biannual appointment to ensure treatment targets are being met (remission or low disease activity).

Societal impact

A person's engagement with wider society is affected by the diagnosis of RA. Within 3 years of diagnosis, 25% of patients are no longer working. Personal loss of income, government loss of taxation, drug costs and the impact of disability with associated social care costs all contribute to the financial impact of the disease.

● Chapter Summary

- Rheumatoid arthritis is a multisystem disease characterized by symmetrical polyarticular arthritis, usually involving the hands.
- The typical pattern of involvement includes inflammation of the PIP, MCP and wrist joints, although any synovial joint can be affected.
- Classical deformities include boutonnière and swan-neck deformities.
- Extraarticular features include anaemia, respiratory conditions (pleural effusions, lung nodules and pulmonary fibrosis), pericarditis/myocarditis and inflammation of the eyes.
- The classic radiological features of RA are soft-tissue swelling, periarticular osteoporosis, juxta-articular erosions and narrowing of the joint space.
- Methotrexate, sulphasalazine, leflunomide and hydroxychloroquine are the most commonly used synthetic DMARDs.
- Biological DMARDs are extremely effective in reducing inflammation and limiting disease activity.

UKMLA Conditions
Bursitis
Rheumatoid arthritis
Spinal cord compression

UKMLA Presentations
Acute joint pain/swelling
Back pain
Chronic joint pain/stiffness
Musculoskeletal deformities
Neck pain/stiffness
Soft tissue injury

Spondyloarthropathies 12

DEFINITION

The term spondyloarthropathy (SPA) describes a group of related and often overlapping inflammatory joint disorders of the spine or vertebral column (see list in box). Spondyloarthropathy with inflammation is commonly referred to as axial spondyloarthritis. It is characterized by enthesitis (inflammation of the insertions of tendons, ligaments and capsules into bone), as well as synovitis, and occurs in patients who are seronegative for rheumatoid factor. For this reason, these disorders are sometimes referred to as seronegative spondyloarthropathies.

THE SPONDYLOARTHROPATHIES

Ankylosing spondylitis
Psoriatic arthropathy
Reactive arthritis
Enteropathic arthritis
Undifferentiated spondyloar-
thropathy

AETIOLOGY

All types of SPA are genetically associated with the human leucocyte antigen (HLA) B27, a major histocompatibility complex class I antigen. HLA B27 is more closely linked with some forms of SPA than others. Around 10% of the world's Caucasian population is positive for HLA B27.

The true aetiology of SPAs is unknown. Infection is thought to be important; bacterial infections may trigger an immune reaction in genetically susceptible people. This is particularly true for reactive arthritis. In other forms of SPA, a combination of genetic and environmental factors might trigger inflammation.

PATHOLOGY

The entheses are the key sites of inflammation in SPA. Initial inflammation and erosions are followed by fibrosis and ossification (bone formation), which can result in ankylosis of the joints. In ankylosing spondylitis (AS), the outer fibres of the vertebral discs become inflamed where they attach to the corners of the vertebral bodies. The characteristic squaring of the anterior contour of the vertebra results from destructive osteitis and repair. Ossification leads to formation of syndesmophytes (bony bridges). The sacroiliac joints are commonly affected and become fused. Synovitis is another feature of SPA. Peripheral joints tend to be more commonly affected in psoriatic arthritis and reactive arthritis than in enteropathic arthritis and AS.

Pathological changes are not always confined to the musculoskeletal system (discussed in more detail later). The four main seronegative spondyloarthropathies (that will be discussed in this chapter), and their genetic association and clinical features are illustrated in Fig. 12.1.

ANKYLOSING SPONDYLITIS

Clinical features

The prevalence of AS amongst the Caucasian population is 0.5% to 1%. It is three times more common in men than women and tends to be more severe in men. It usually develops in the teenage years and early adulthood, with a peak age of onset in the mid-20s. Presentations over the age of 45 years are rare.

Clinical features fall into two groups:

- musculoskeletal
- extraskeletal

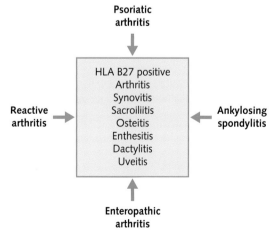

Fig. 12.1 The genetic association and clinical features seen in the seronegative spondyloarthropathies.

It is important to note that AS lies on a spectrum of axial spondyloarthritis. The condition can be classified as AS when it has progressed to show radiological damage. Not all patients go on to develop ankylosing spondylitis, however, risk factors for the progression to radiological damage include the presence of existing damage, being male and being a smoker.

Musculoskeletal features

Most symptoms in AS are due to spinal and sacroiliac disease. The typical patient presents with gradual onset of lower back or gluteal region pain and stiffness. As symptoms progress, there is loss of anterior flexion, lateral flexion and extension of the spine. The time of onset to diagnosis remains unacceptably high, with many patients having had symptoms for a number of years before referral. Early identification allows for prompt treatment to preserve spinal mobility, limit functional loss and reduce pain and stiffness. Symptoms are worse in the morning and generally improve with exercise. Involvement of the thoracic spine and enthesitis of the costovertebral joints can cause chest pain, breathlessness and reduce chest expansion. Features of AS are described in the NICE (2019) guidelines shown in the following box.

ANKYLOSING SPONDYLITIS: HOW DO I MAKE A WORKING DIAGNOSIS OF ANKYLOSING SPONDYLITIS? (NICE GUIDELINES (2019))

Suspect AS in anyone with chronic or recurrent low back pain, fatigue and stiffness, especially if:
- They are 45 years old or younger.
- The back pain has been present for more than 3 months.
- The back pain is worse in the morning, lasts for over 30 minutes and improves with movement.
- They have current or previous: buttock pain, pain in the thoracic or cervical spine, arthritis, enthesitis, anterior uveitis or have psoriasis/inflammatory bowel disease/genitourinary infection.
- Symptoms wake them during the night.
- Symptoms respond to nonsteroidal antiinflammatory drugs (NSAIDs) within 48 hours of use.
- There is a positive family history for spondyloarthritis.

COMMUNICATION

Lower back pain is common and usually due to mechanical or degenerative issues. When assessing a younger person with back pain, always ask about morning stiffness.

In the early stages of disease, patients may have few clinical signs. In addition to Regional Examination of the Musculoskeletal System (REMS), the following examinations may be useful:

- The sacroiliac joints are often tender and pain can be reproduced by applying pressure to the joints. The sacroiliac squeeze test is achieved by applying pressure on the anterior iliac spines whilst the patient is supine.
- Mobility of the lumbar spine is reduced. The Schober test is used to assess anterior flexion of the lumbar spine (Fig. 12.2). With a pen, a mark is made on the skin at the lumbosacral joint, level with the dimples of Venus. A second mark is made 10 cm above. The patient bends forward with the legs straight and attempts to touch the floor. The distance between the marks should increase by at least 5 cm.
- Lateral flexion of the spine (see Chapter 2) is even more sensitive at identifying AS.

Later in the disease process and in those with severe disease, the spine becomes progressively stiff and immobile and posture deteriorates (Fig. 12.3). The normal lumbar lordosis is lost and the thoracic and cervical spines become increasingly kyphotic. The resulting stooped posture restricts chest expansion and causes the abdomen to protrude. It is sometimes referred to as the question mark posture. The Bath AS Functional Index (BASFI), Bath AS Disease Activity Index (BASDAI) and the Bath AS Metrology Index (BASMI) are three scoring systems commonly used to objectify functional capacity and disease activity.

RED FLAG

Spinal disease can be complicated by atlantoaxial subluxation and fractures. Be sure to perform a full neurological examination in AS patients presenting with acute pain.

The peripheral joints are less commonly involved than the axial skeleton in AS. Inflammation tends to target the medium and large joints such as the shoulders, knees and hips. Pain and tenderness due to enthesitis may occur in multiple sites. Achilles tendonitis and plantar fasciitis are common examples of this.

Extraskeletal features

Extraskeletal features are commonly referred to as the four-As:

- *A*cute anterior uveitis: also called iritis, this occurs in approximately one-third of AS patients. The eye becomes red and painful and vision is blurred. It requires urgent assessment by an ophthalmologist as blindness may occur if left untreated. Steroid eye drops are the usual treatment.

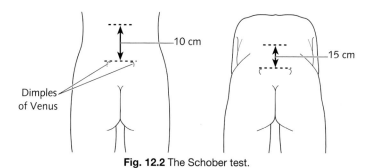

Fig. 12.2 The Schober test.

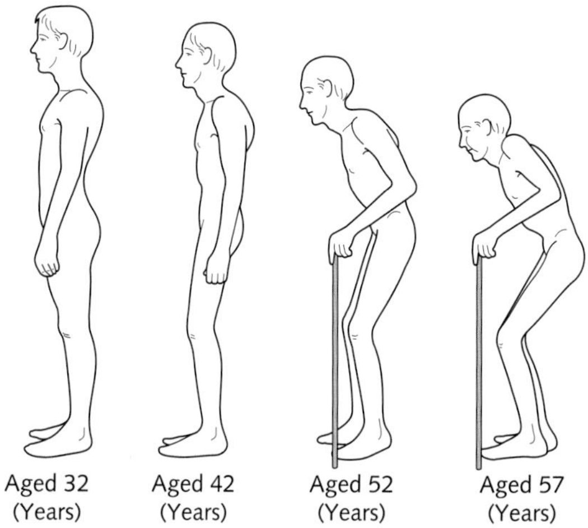

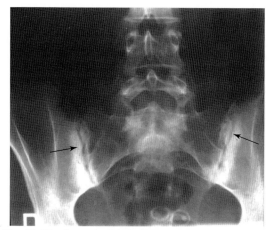

Fig. 12.4 Radiograph showing bilateral sacroiliitis (*arrows*).

Aged 32 (Years)   Aged 42 (Years)   Aged 52 (Years)   Aged 57 (Years)

Fig. 12.3 Deterioration in posture in ankylosing spondylitis patients over time.

- Aortic incompetence/ascending aortitis.
- Apical lung fibrosis.
- Amyloidosis.

In addition, constitutional features such as anorexia, fever, weight loss and fatigue may occur.

Investigations

Blood tests
- A full blood count may show anaemia of chronic disease.
- Erythrocyte sedimentation rate (ESR) and C-reactive protein (CRP) are often elevated during the active phases of the disease.
- Serological tests for rheumatoid factor are negative.
- Genotyping for HLA B27 is not required for diagnosis but may be useful where doubt exists.
- A raised faecal calprotectin will suggest clinical features are instead due to enteropathic arthritis.

Radiological investigation
The investigation of choice is magnetic resonance imaging (MRI). This technique is able to detect inflammatory back disease in cases where X-ray images may be normal in appearance. MRI also prevents X-ray exposure in the pelvis, which is particularly important in young patients. Sacroiliitis (Figs 12.4 and 12.5) and bone oedema highlight ongoing inflammation, amenable to therapy. Note that sacroiliac joint inflammation may be a normal finding in pregnant and post-partum women and in those that do a lot of recreational running. X-ray images have a role in assessing established damage where substantial mechanical change has occurred. Views of the lumbar spine may show squaring of the vertebrae and formation of syndesmophytes (Fig. 12.6). These are due to ossification of the longitudinal ligaments and produce a 'bamboo spine' appearance. The incidence of osteoporosis is also more common in these patients and X-rays should be assessed for vertebral fractures. Radiographs taken at other sites of enthesitis may show erosions, for example at the insertion of the plantar fascia of Achilles tendon.

Management

Patients with AS require a multidisciplinary approach to care.

Physiotherapy

This is an important element in the management of AS. Each patient should follow a long-term exercise programme with the aim of maintaining normal posture and exercise activity. Hydrotherapy is also beneficial.

Drug treatment

NSAIDs are the mainstay of initial treatment and provide benefit in the majority of patients. Continuous therapy should occur in patients with ongoing evidence of inflammation. Both NSAID types, cyclooxygenase-1 (COX-1) and COX-2 inhibitors, have shown benefit to patients and may even suppress radiological progression. Local glucocorticoid injections have also shown to be effective.

Immunosuppressive drugs, such as methotrexate and sulphasalazine, are of less benefit in AS, except where a concomitant peripheral arthritis occurs.

The tumour necrosis factor (TNF) inhibitors, however, have excellent efficacy in treating active axial disease and preventing AS progression. Patients who respond well include those who are young, those who have elevated inflammatory markers and those with a shorter disease progression. Fig. 12.7 shows the general pathophysiology of inflammation in spondyloarthropathies with biological targets of treatment. In AS, anti-IL17 biologics such as secukinumab are licensed for use, as well as some JAK inhibitors.

PSORIATIC ARTHRITIS

Clinical features

Psoriatic arthropathy is an inflammatory arthritis associated with psoriasis and HLA B27. Psoriasis occurs in 1% to 3% of the population and approximately 10% of those are affected by psoriatic arthritis. The PEST questionnaire should be completed annually by patients with psoriasis as a screening tool to detect for psoriatic arthritis. Psoriatic arthritis is particularly common in patients with psoriatic nail involvement (Fig. 12.8). Nail features to look out for include:

- Onycholysis. This describes detachment of the nail from the nail bed due to enthesitis.
- Nail pitting.
- Subungual hyperkeratosis.

Psoriatic arthritis affects men and women with a similar frequency.

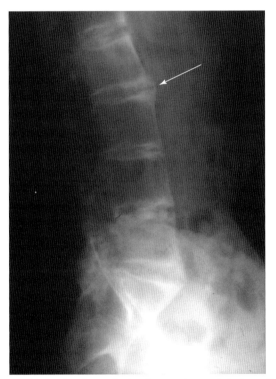

Fig. 12.6 Lateral radiograph showing syndesmophyte formation (*arrow*) in the lumbar spine of a patient with advanced ankylosing spondylitis.

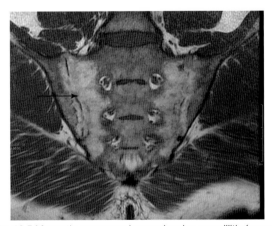

Fig. 12.5 Magnetic resonance image showing sacroiliitis (*arrow*).

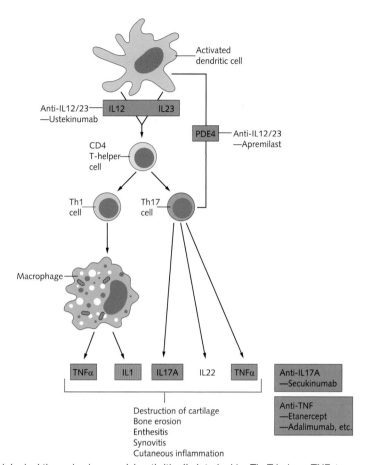

Fig. 12.7 Target sites of biological therapies in spondyloarthritis. *IL,* Interleukin; *Th,* T helper; *TNF,* tumour necrosis factor.

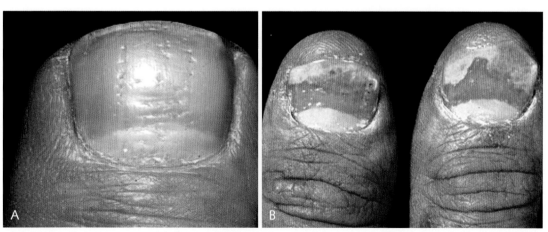

Fig. 12.8 Psoriatic nail changes. Image (A) shows nail pitting while image (B) shows onycholysis. (From Firestone GS et al. *Kelley's Textbook of Rheumatology.* 9th ed. Philadelphia. Elsevier Saunders; 2013, p 1234, Fig. 77-2 A, B.)

Psoriatic arthritis may precede the diagnosis of psoriatic skin disease and does not correlate with the severity of the skin involvement. Differing patterns of joint involvement are listed in the box.

PATTERNS OF JOINT DISEASE IN PSORIATIC ARTHRITIS

- Distal arthritis involving the distal interphalangeal joints
- Asymmetrical oligoarthritis
- Symmetrical polyarthritis indistinguishable from rheumatoid arthritis
- Spondylitis
- Arthritis mutilans

Examination for synovitis is important because patients present with joint pain, stiffness and sometimes swelling. The disease normally follows a relapsing and remitting course. Dactylitis and enthesitis are common features. Involvement of the distal interphalangeal (DIP) joints may be associated with pitting or onycholysis of the nail. Arthritis mutilans is an extremely destructive pattern of joint destruction mainly seen in the hands and feet. Thankfully, it is rare.

Resorption of bone at the metacarpals and phalanges causes telescoping of the digits. They appear shortened but can be passively extended to their original lengths. Psoriatic spondylitis tends to cause milder symptoms than classic AS and sacroiliitis is often asymmetrical and asymptomatic.

The diagnosis is clinical but can be facilitated by using the CASPAR criteria.

HINTS AND TIPS

Some patients present with articular features of psoriatic arthritis but no features of skin involvement. Careful inspection of the scalp, naval and natal cleft may reveal small patches of psoriasis. A family history of psoriasis is also clinically important.

Metabolic syndrome is a collection of risk factors including hypertension, hyperlipidaemia and insulin resistance that is becoming more prevalent with increased rates of obesity within the population. It has been shown that there is a close association between metabolic syndrome, psoriasis and psoriatic arthritis. It is therefore important to screen for these risk factors and encourage weight loss where appropriate in patients presenting with psoriatic arthritis and metabolic syndrome. This may play a role in limiting the clinical impact of the disease. The risk factors that are described in metabolic syndrome are shown in Fig. 12.9.

Investigations

Blood tests
Full blood count, ESR and CRP show a similar picture to that of AS. Rheumatoid factor is usually absent.

Radiological investigations
The radiological changes of psoriatic arthritis are asymmetrical and target the small joints of the hands and feet, particularly

THE CLASSIFICATION CRITERIA FOR PSORIATIC ARTHRITIS (CASPAR)

Inflammatory articular disease (joint, spine or entheseal) with ≥3 points from the following:

• Evidence of current psoriasis, a personal history of psoriasis or a family history of psoriasis	2 points
• Typical psoriatic nail dystrophy, including onycholysis, pitting and hyperkeratosis observed on current physical examination	1 point
• A negative test result for the presence of rheumatoid factor by any method except latex	1 point
• Either current dactylitis, defined as swelling of an entire digit, or a history of dactylitis recorded by a rheumatologist	1 point
• Radiographic evidence of juxta-articular new bone formation appearing as ill-defined ossification near joint margins (but excluding osteophyte formation) on plain radiographs of the hand or foot	1 point

Definitions: Current psoriasis is skin or scalp disease present today as judged by a rheumatologist or dermatologist. A personal history of psoriasis is a history of psoriasis that may be obtained from a patient, family physician, dermatologist, rheumatologist or other qualified healthcare provider. A family history of psoriasis is a history of psoriasis in a first- or second-degree relative according to patient report.

(Adapted from Taylor W, Gladman D, Helliwell P, et al. Classification criteria for psoriatic arthritis: development of new criteria from a large international study. Arthritis and Rheumatism 2006;54:2665–2673.)

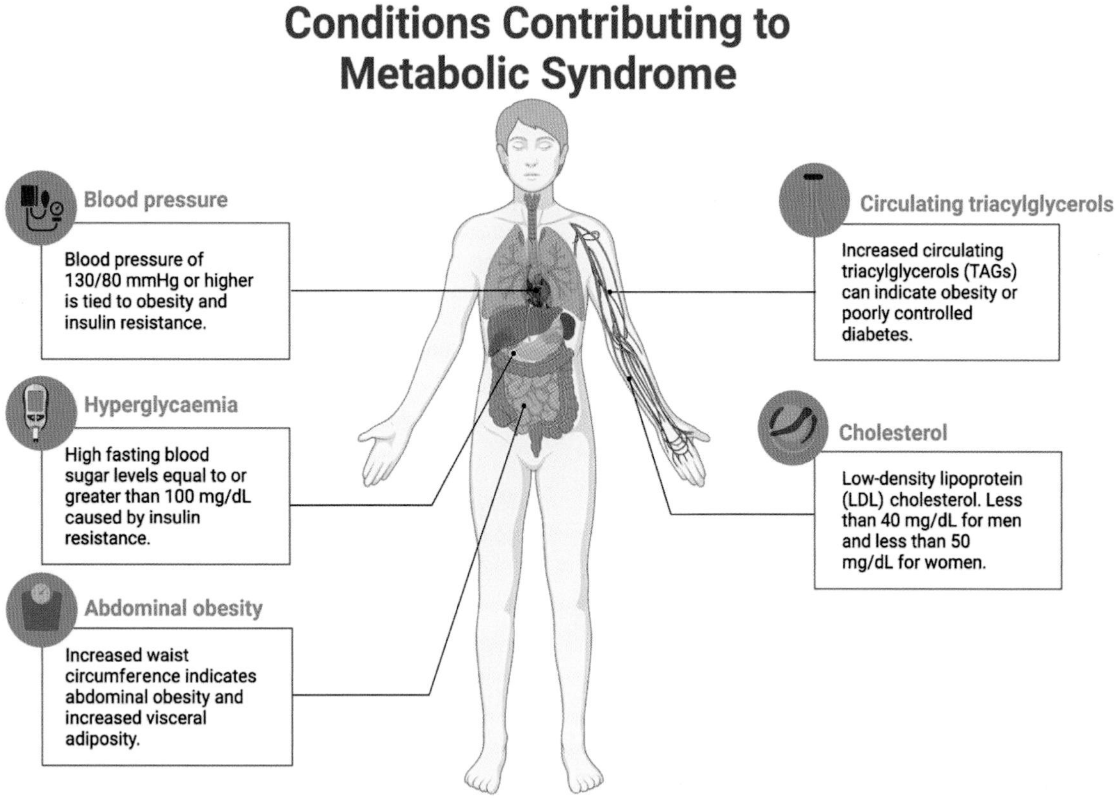

Conditions Contributing to Metabolic Syndrome

Blood pressure

Blood pressure of 130/80 mmHg or higher is tied to obesity and insulin resistance.

Circulating triacylglycerols

Increased circulating triacylglycerols (TAGs) can indicate obesity or poorly controlled diabetes.

Hyperglycaemia

High fasting blood sugar levels equal to or greater than 100 mg/dL caused by insulin resistance.

Cholesterol

Low-density lipoprotein (LDL) cholesterol. Less than 40 mg/dL for men and less than 50 mg/dL for women.

Abdominal obesity

Increased waist circumference indicates abdominal obesity and increased visceral adiposity.

Fig. 12.9 Metabolic syndrome. (From Lamb H. *Visceral and Ectopic Fat.* Elsevier; 2023.)

the DIP joints (Fig. 12.10). Changes that can be seen on X-ray images include:

- erosions with proliferation of the adjacent bone
- resorption of the terminal phalanges
- pencil-in-cup deformities, seen in arthritis mutilans
- periostitis
- ankylosis
- new bone formation at entheses
- sacroiliitis is found in up to 30% of cases and is usually asymmetrical (Fig. 12.5)

Management

Treatment depends on the pattern of joint disease:

- Peripheral joint disease is treated with NSAIDS, methotrexate, leflunomide and sulphasalazine. In the case of isolated synovitis, intraarticular glucocorticoid injections should be considered. Anti-TNF therapies work well in selected patients where conventional synthetic

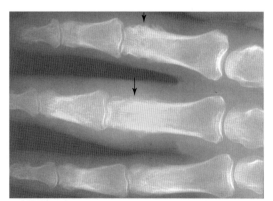

Fig. 12.10 Radiograph showing fluffy periosteal reaction and erosive changes (*arrows*) in the digits in a patient with psoriatic arthritis.

disease-modifying antirheumatic drugs (DMARDs) have failed.
- Axial disease is treated in a similar way to AS with physiotherapy, NSAIDs and biologic therapy as the

mainstay. Anti-IL12/23 and anti-IL17A are particularly effective in psoriatic arthritis with axial involvement and are licensed for first-line use alongside anti-TNF treatment. Ustekinumab is an anti-IL23 biological therapy that has shown efficacy as a last-line treatment for psoriatic arthritis. PDE4 inhibitors and JAK inhibitors are small molecules that are given orally which have demonstrated effectiveness in peripheral joint disease.

- All patients benefit from a multidisciplinary team approach. There should be efficient communication between the rheumatology and dermatology teams.

Prognosis

The prognosis for psoriatic arthritis is generally good, with joint function being preserved in most cases. Chronic, destructive and deforming arthritis may occasionally develop.

REACTIVE ARTHRITIS

Clinical features

Reactive arthritis is an aseptic arthritis that occurs after an anatomically distant infection. It mainly affects young adults and the triggering infection is usually of the gastrointestinal or genitourinary tract. Occasionally the incidental infection is not found and other triggers such as drug treatment have been rarely found.

Symptoms start to develop a few days to weeks after the infection. The onset is sometimes acute, with stiffness, fatigue and occasionally fever.

> **RED FLAG**
>
> Remember that *Salmonella* and *Neisseria* can cause septic arthritis. Always ensure joint aspirate cultures are negative!

Musculoskeletal features

The arthritis is typically asymmetrical and oligoarticular. It targets the larger weight-bearing joints, fingers and toes. Dactylitis and enthesitis occur and some patients experience pain and stiffness in the sacroiliac region.

Conjunctivitis

This is sterile and can be unilateral or bilateral.

Urethritis

Sterile inflammation of the urogenital tract can cause symptoms of frequency, dysuria and urethral discharge. It is important patients are screened for sexually transmitted infections if at risk, as these can also trigger reactive arthritis.

Skin and mucosal lesions

Circinate balanitis can accompany uveitis. Some patients develop a sterile pustulosis on the palms of the hands and soles of the feet. This looks similar to pustular psoriasis and is called keratoderma blennorrhagica (see Fig. 12.11). Mouth ulcers and erythema nodosum are another recognized associations.

> **HINTS AND TIPS**
>
> The presence of arthritis, conjunctivitis and uveitis following infection is a key triad to look out for that suggests reactive arthritis.

> **ETHICS**
>
> It is important to ask about sexual history in patients with reactive arthritis. Although this discussion can be difficult or embarrassing for the patient, you should explain it is necessary to ensure correct diagnosis. In patients who test positive for sexually transmitted infections, contact testing and partner tracing are important.

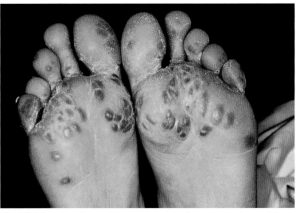

Fig.12.11 Keratoderma blennorrhagica. (Image courtesy of the CDC.)

Investigations

- Full blood count, ESR and CRP show a similar picture to that of AS. CRP and ESR may be significantly elevated.
- Serological tests, including antibodies against *Salmonella, Campylobacter, Chlamydia*, gonorrhoea and *Neisseria,* may help identify the causative organism.
- Synovial fluid from the affected joints should be examined for Gram stain and cultures performed. Cultures are negative in reactive arthritis, but it is important to exclude a septic arthritis or crystal arthropathy.
- A cervical/penile swab, midstream specimen of urine and stool sample should all be obtained for culture and to exclude ongoing infection. Partners should be offered advice where possible. Consider testing the patient for HIV.
- X-ray images are initially normal. Later, fluffy periostitis may be seen in the calcaneus, digits or pelvis. Plantar spurs are common, but erosions are rare. Sacroiliitis and typical AS changes develop in some patients.
- HLA B27 is often associated with the risk of developing reactive arthritis and patients who are HLA B27 positive are more likely to have subsequent episodes.

Management

Reactive arthritis varies in severity from mild symptoms that do not require treatment, to relapsing inflammation requiring steroid/DMARD treatment. The course of treatment is generally as follows:

- Treat any underlying infection with antibiotics.
- NSAIDs.
- Corticosteroid joint injections +/− systemic steroids.
- Rarely, DMARDs may be required.

Prognosis

The vast majority of cases are mild and self-limiting. Relapses following a further infective trigger can occur. At least 60% of those affected will experience a further episode. Permanent joint damage can occur but is rare.

ENTEROPATHIC ARTHRITIS

Clinical features

Arthritis occurring with inflammatory bowel disease (IBD) is known as enteropathic arthritis. It occurs in approximately 10% to 20% of patients with Crohn disease or ulcerative colitis.

Peripheral arthritis

A peripheral arthritis that is a mono- or oligoarthritis may develop. It worsens with flaring of the bowel disease and improves if the affected bowel is surgically removed. It is important to note that many patients with IBD get arthralgia but not arthritis; this is an important distinction to make.

Spondylitis and sacroiliitis

These are not related to the activity of the bowel disease and often predate the onset of Crohn disease or ulcerative colitis.

Enthesopathy

This can accompany peripheral or axial joint disease.

Investigations

Most X-ray images are normal. Spinal imaging may show changes similar to AS. In the case of active spinal inflammation, MRI is the imaging modality of choice. Blood tests are generally unhelpful, unless inflammatory markers correlate with active bowel disease activity. If IBD is suspected, faecal calprotectin and inflammatory markers should be tested and the patient referred to a gastroenterologist.

Management

Treatment of the IBD is the priority and will help with active peripheral arthritis. Drugs, such as corticosteroids and sulphasalazine, should improve both bowel and joint disease. Anti-TNF biologics are licensed for IBD and are extremely effective in managing axial disease.

HINTS AND TIPS

Nonsteroidal antiinflammatory drugs often aggravate gastrointestinal symptoms in inflammatory bowel disease. They risk causing upper gastrointestinal (GI) bleeding, particularly in patients with Crohn disease, where inflammation/ulceration can occur at any point in the GI tract.

● Chapter Summary

- Spondyloarthropathies are a group of overlapping conditions associated with HLA B27.
- The general aetiology of spondyloarthritis is of inflammatory axial enthesitis with or without associated synovitis.
- Back pain is common; inflammatory back pain is recognized as being worse on rest and better on movement, often with associated stiffness.
- Ankylosing spondylitis is more common in men, typically does not involve the peripheral joints and is associated with the 'four-As': acute anterior uveitis, aortic incompetence, apical lung fibrosis and amyloidosis.
- Psoriatic arthritis occurs in around 10% of patients with psoriasis, although it is more common in those with nail involvement. There are differing axial and peripheral patterns of disease.
- Reactive arthritis is commonly seen after a bacterial infection; always consider STIs in sexually active patients.
- Treatment for axial disease typically involves the use of biologic therapies: anti-TNF, anti-IL12/23 and anti-IL17.
- Enteropathic arthritis occurs in approximately 10% to 20% of patients with Crohn disease or ulcerative colitis.

UKMLA Conditions
Ankylosing spondylitis
Inflammatory bowel disease
Psoriasis
Reactive arthritis
Septic arthritis

UKMLA Presentations
Acute joint pain/swelling
Back pain
Chronic joint pain/stiffness
Eye pain/discomfort
Musculoskeletal deformity
Neck pain/stiffness
Red eye
Soft tissue injury

Connective tissue diseases 13

Connective tissue disease (CTD) is a broad term used to describe conditions where the connective tissues of the body are targeted. There is no strict unifying definition, but generally these diseases are multisystem inflammatory disorders associated with immunological abnormalities. There are overlaps between many of the disorders, which share many clinical features.

SYSTEMIC LUPUS ERYTHEMATOSUS

Definition

Systemic lupus erythematosus (SLE) is an autoimmune inflammatory disease characterized by autoantibodies to nuclear material, which can involve almost any organ or system of the body.

Prevalence

SLE has an average worldwide prevalence of 10 to 50 per 100,000. However, this varies significantly according to ethnicity. It is more common in Indian and Afro-Caribbean people, than in Caucasians and affects women at least 10 times more frequently than men.

Aetiology

There are genetic, environmental and hormonal factors thought to be important to the aetiology. SLE can be induced by drugs, notably, the oral contraceptive pill. Oestrogen is thought to play a role in producing autoreactive B cells. Environmental triggers include viruses and ultraviolet B light. Drug-induced lupus tends to be mild and does not affect the kidneys.

Pathology

Immune function in SLE is abnormal, with T- and B-cell dysfunction causing B-cell hyperactivity and impaired immune complex clearance from tissues. Dysfunction of the complement system and aberrant programmed cell death means that intracellular material is not disposed of correctly, allowing autoantibody production to develop against nuclear material. A wide variety of autoantibodies have been described, some of which are directly pathogenic (anti-double-stranded DNA, anti-Ro). The coagulation system may be abnormal and vasculopathy

is common, resulting from clotting cascade antibodies. The pathogenesis of SLE is illustrated in Fig. 13.1.

Clinical features

SLE usually develops between the ages of 15 and 40 years. The clinical features are diverse and vary in severity over time. Initial symptoms may be mild and vague, but it is the exacerbations of SLE and resultant tissue damage that cause significant ill health. Severe lupus flares can result in life-threatening complications including renal failure and cerebral vasculitis. Factors that may trigger a flare of SLE are listed in the box.

FACTORS CAPABLE OF TRIGGERING FLARES OF SYSTEMIC LUPUS ERYTHEMATOSUS

- Overexposure to sunlight: ultraviolet light B > A
- Oestrogen-containing contraceptive therapy
- Drugs: hydralazine, minocycline, etc.
- Infection
- Stress

Constitutional features

Fatigue, malaise, lymphadenopathy and weight loss are common features of SLE. Fatigue, in particular, can be extremely debilitating and difficult to manage.

Musculoskeletal features

Approximately 90% of patients with SLE experience arthralgia, usually polyarticular. Nonerosive arthritis occurs in approximately 25% of patients and symptoms are usually more dramatic than clinical signs. Deformity is due to tenosynovitis and fibrosis, rather than cartilage or bone erosions. Jaccoud arthropathy is the term used to describe tendon laxity causing twisting and deformity of the joints.

Myalgia is a common feature in SLE and myositis (inflamed muscle) can occur (see later section on myositis). Avascular necrosis of bone and osteoporosis are recognized but are usually a consequence of corticosteroid treatment or vasculopathy.

Dermatological features

There are many cutaneous manifestations of lupus. Photosensitivity is common (approximately 60%). The characteristic 'butterfly' malar rash develops over the nose and cheeks and can

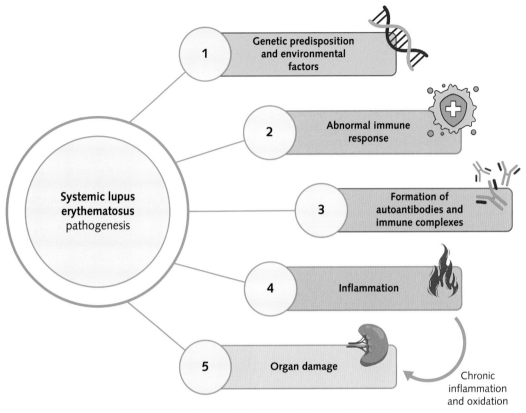

Fig. 13.1 The pathogenesis of Systemic lupus erythematosus.

be painful (Fig. 13.2). Discoid lupus (demarcated, pigmented or atrophic plaques) can develop with no systemic features (Fig. 13.3).

Hair loss reflects disease activity and patients may develop alopecia. Mucosal ulceration may affect the nose, mouth and vagina. Cutaneous vasculitis can present with urticarial lesions and splinter haemorrhages.

Cardiovascular features

Serositis is common in SLE and pericarditis is the most common manifestation. It tends to cause a sharp pain in the chest, alleviated by sitting forward and associated with diffuse saddle-shaped ST-segment elevation on an electrocardiogram.

Myocarditis may accompany myositis and can present with arrhythmias or heart failure. Myocarditis will cause a rise in blood troponin. Libman–Sacks endocarditis is due to noninfective vegetations and seldom causes clinical problems.

At least a third of patients with SLE suffer from Raynaud phenomenon (vasospasm, typically precipitated by the cold, causing peripheral ischaemia). This can be seen in the digits, tip of the nose, earlobes and occasionally the tongue, which become pale and numb before turning blue. The final phase is redness

and flushing due to eventual vasodilation. Raynaud phenomenon may predate other symptoms by many months or years.

Vasculitis may present with digital infarcts, skin rashes or ulcers that can occasionally affect internal organs such as the lungs and brain.

There is an increased risk of atherosclerosis, myocardial infarction and stroke in patients with SLE due to antiphospholipid syndrome. This will be discussed in full later in this chapter.

Pulmonary features

Amongst the pulmonary features of SLE, inflammation of the pleura and pleural effusions are the most common. Acute pneumonitis can mimic pneumonia. Chronic pneumonitis causes fibrosis, alveolar haemorrhage and a decrease in lung volume. Pulmonary hypertension is rare.

Renal features

Glomerulonephritis is the most common cause of lupus-related deaths in patients with SLE. Nephritis does not cause clinical symptoms until there is significant renal damage. It can show signs of nephrotic syndrome (heavy proteinuria,

Issues such as anxiety, depression and psychosis are well recognized effects of lupus.

Haematological features

Lymphopenia is very common in SLE but neutropenia is also found. When patients are taking immunosuppressants, it can be difficult to differentiate between drug effects and disease-related aetiology. Anaemia can be due to chronic inflammation or auto-immune haemolysis, which affects up to 5% of lupus sufferers. Antiphospholipid antibodies and coagulopathies are discussed later in this chapter.

Gastrointestinal features

Gastrointestinal (GI) features tend to be rarer than other systemic involvement. Aseptic peritonitis can present with abdominal pain and nausea, with or without ascites. Other manifestations include lupus hepatitis, mild hepatosplenomegaly from haemolysis or vasculitis affecting the mesenteric vessels.

Investigations

Serological tests

SLE is characterized by the presence of serum autoantibodies against nuclear components (Table 13.1).

Other tests

- Urine should be tested with a dipstick to look for blood and protein. These are signs of nephritis.
- Full blood count should be performed regularly to look for anaemia, leukopenia and thrombocytopenia. Urea, creatinine and electrolyte levels should also be monitored.
- The erythrocyte sedimentation rate (ESR) will increase during a flare of SLE (see box) but may also be high even when the patient feels well. C-reactive protein tends to be normal or mildly elevated unless infection, synovitis or serositis is present.
- SLE is a disease of compliment consumption so low C3 and C4 levels may occur in a SLE flare.
- Coombs test will be positive in patients with autoimmune haemolytic anaemia. A direct Coombs test checks for antibodies bound to RBCs and an indirect Coombs test looks for free antibodies in the serum.
- Skin biopsy shows deposition of immunoglobulin G (IgG) and complement at the dermal–epidermal junction in patients with rashes (lupus band test).
- Renal biopsy is sometimes performed to aid diagnosis or to establish prognosis in patients with abnormal renal function.

The SLICC criteria is used in the diagnosis of SLE. It considers clinical features of the disease and immunological markers.

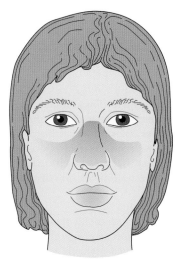

Fig. 13.2 The classic butterfly rash of systemic lupus erythematosus.

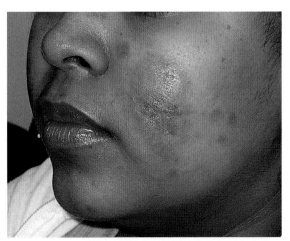

Fig. 13.3 Lesions of discoid lupus. (With permission from Aranow C, Diamond B, Mackay M. Systemic lupus erythematosus. In: Rich RR et al., eds. *Clinical Immunology: Principles and Practice*. 5th ed. Elsevier; 2019.)

decreased serum albumin levels and oedema) or nephritic syndrome (hypertension and haematuria). It is important to monitor patients closely, checking their blood pressure and urine for blood and protein, so that renal disease can be acted upon early.

Neurological features

SLE can involve the central nervous system, cranial and peripheral nerves, producing a wide range of clinical features. These include headaches, neuropsychiatric problems, seizures, neuropathies and chorea.

Table 13.1 Autoantibodies associated with systemic lupus erythematosus

Autoantibodies found in SLE	Comments
Antinuclear antibodies	Detected in >95% of patients
Anti-Ro and anti-La antibodies	Associated with secondary Sjögren syndrome and pulmonary fibrosis. Mothers are at risk of having babies with neonatal SLE and congenital heart block. Sensitivity = 25%
Anti-double-stranded DNA antibodies	Present in 50% of SLE patients. Very specific indicator of disease when present.
Antihistone antibodies	Often positive in drug-induced SLE; sensitivity = 90%
Antiphospholipid and anticardiollpin antibodies	May be positive in around 10%–20% of SLE patients

SLE, *Systemic lupus erythematosus.*

INDICATORS OF HIGH DISEASE ACTIVITY IN SYSTEMIC LUPUS ERYTHEMATOSUS

- Raised ESR
- High anti-DsDNA titres
- Low C3 and C4 complement levels

HINTS AND TIPS

Consider lupus in patients who present with multisystem symptoms, particularly mouth ulcers, rashes, arthralgia, Raynaud, lymphopenia and positive antinuclear antibody titre with a raised ESR.

Management

General measures

Education about SLE is essential. Patients are advised to avoid factors that can precipitate lupus flares (see earlier box). They should wear long-sleeved clothes and use complete sunblock in sunny weather. Infections should be treated promptly.

Pharmacological treatment

The choice of drug treatment depends on the severity of the disease and the organs involved.

Mild SLE

Patients with symptoms such as arthralgia, lethargy or a faint rash may respond to nonsteroidal antiinflammatory drugs and/or antimalarials such as hydroxychloroquine.

Moderate SLE

Patients with more severe clinical features, such as serositis, severe arthritis, nephritis autoimmune haemolysis, thrombocytopenia and neurological or psychiatric disorders, often require treatment with corticosteroids. Once disease remission is achieved, steroid-sparing agents such as azathioprine, methotrexate and mycophenolate mofetil are often used.

Severe SLE

An SLE flare may cause severe life-threatening complications such as acute renal failure, neurological or haematology problems and must be treated promptly with cytotoxic medication and corticosteroids. Cyclophosphamide is very effective. Tacrolimus and mycophenolate are alternatives. Ciclosporin is often also used. Newer, biologic agents have been used in treatment of refractory disease and include anifrolumab (interferon blocker), rituximab (CD20 B-cell inhibitor) and belimumab (a B-cell-activating factor blocker) (see Fig. 13.4). Renal replacement would need to be considered in end-stage kidney disease.

Adjunctive treatment

Hypertension due to nephritis should be managed aggressively. Intravenous immunoglobulin infusions may help thrombocytopenia or neutropenia. Antiplatelet medication or warfarin are required for patients with antiphospholipid syndrome (see later section). Anticonvulsants may be required for epilepsy associated with a disease of the central nervous system.

Prognosis

The outlook for patients with SLE is improving. Ten-year survival is over 90%. It is widely recognized that patients have a higher cardiovascular mortality and risks are managed aggressively. Malignancy and infection rates are higher.

THE ANTIPHOSPHOLIPID SYNDROME

Definition

The antiphospholipid syndrome (APS) is a systemic autoimmune condition characterized by arterial and venous thrombosis, fetal loss and thrombocytopenia associated with persistent levels of antiphospholipid antibodies.

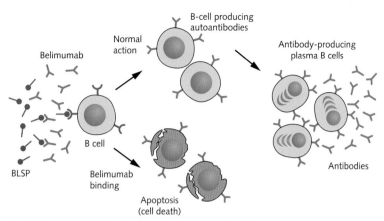

Fig. 13.4 B-lymphocyte stimulating protein is blocked by the monoclonal antibody, belimumab, thus inhibiting B cells from producing pathogenic autoantibody.

Antiphospholipid antibodies often complicate other CTDs, such as lupus. In these cases, the patient is said to have secondary APS.

Incidence

Overall incidence of APS is unclear; it was first described in patients with SLE, but it has become apparent that it has its own clinical entity.

Pathology

The three main antiphospholipid antibodies are anticardiolipin, beta-2 glycoprotein I and lupus anticoagulant. They have a pro-coagulant effect in susceptible individuals, associated impaired fibrinolysis and increased vascular tone, all contributing to clot formation and infarction.

Clinical features

The major features and additional clinical features of APS are shown in the boxes.

The Major Features of Antiphospholipid Syndrome

Venous thrombosis	Deep vein thrombosis and pulmonary emboli are the most common Other veins can be affected (e.g., inferior vena cava, pelvic, renal, portal and hepatic veins)
Arterial thrombosis	Cerebral ischaemia (stroke, transient ischaemic attacks) Peripheral ischaemia
Fetal complications	Spontaneous abortion, premature births
Thrombocytopenia	Not severe enough to cause haemorrhage

> **ASSOCIATED CLINICAL FEATURES OF ANTIPHOSPHOLIPID SYNDROME**
>
> - Livedo reticularis
> - Leg ulcers
> - Cardiac valve abnormalities (e.g., aortic and mitral regurgitation)
> - Chorea
> - Epilepsy
> - Migraine
> - Haemolytic anaemia

Investigations

Diagnosis is based on the detection of at least one of the three antiphospholipid antibodies on at least two occasions separated by at least a 12-week interval. The interval is necessary because the antibodies can sometimes develop transiently in relation to other events (such as infection) and exist harmlessly in the body.

An APTT 50:50 mixing study can be conducted to assess the intrinsic and common coagulation pathways. In this test, patient blood is added to plasma sufficient in coagulation factors in a 50:50 ratio. If the prolonged APTT value is then corrected, this suggests the patient's blood was coagulation factor deficient (e.g., due to vitamin K deficiency). If the APTT is prolonged despite addition of normal plasma, this suggests that there was an inhibitor present in the patient's blood (e.g., lupus anticoagulant).

Management

General advice

The following steps are advisable:

- Avoidance of the oral contraceptive pill.
- Avoidance of smoking.
- Treatment of hypertension, diabetes and hyperlipidaemia.

Asymptomatic patients

Current recommendations are that asymptomatic patients should be monitored closely, but those with no clinical features should not be treated. Those with high cardiovascular risk factors or with a concurrent separate autoimmune disease should receive low-dose aspirin prophylaxis. During high-risk periods, such as after elective surgery, patient should receive thrombosis prophylaxis with low-molecular-weight heparin.

Venous or arterial thrombosis

Patients who experience thrombosis should be managed with conventional anticoagulation. However, anticoagulation should be lifelong, because there is an ongoing risk of repeated thrombosis. Warfarin is the typical anticoagulant used in patients with a confirmed arterial or venous thrombus.

Recurrent fetal loss

Warfarin should be stopped before conception, when attempting another pregnancy, because it is teratogenic. Subcutaneous heparin and aspirin should be given throughout pregnancy to reduce the risk of fetal loss.

SJÖGREN SYNDROME

Definition

Sjögren syndrome is a chronic autoimmune disease, characterized by inflammation of exocrine glands. The salivary and lacrimal glands are the most commonly involved, resulting in dryness of the mouth and eyes. Sjögren syndrome can be primary or secondary (associated with another autoimmune disease). Causes of secondary Sjögren syndrome are shown in the box.

DISEASES ASSOCIATED WITH SECONDARY SJÖGREN SYNDROME

- Rheumatoid arthritis
- Systemic lupus erythematosus
- Systemic sclerosis
- Polymyositis
- Primary biliary cirrhosis
- Chronic active hepatitis

Sicca syndrome is the presence of dry eyes or mouth as a result of nonautoimmune disease, such as smoking or drugs.

Prevalence

In terms of prevalence, Sjogrens syndrome is thought to affect 1-3% of the population. It is nine times more common in women than in men.

Aetiology

The exact aetiology is unknown. The primary disease has a strong association with human leukocyte antigen (HLA class II DR and DQ) haplotypes and the signal transducer and activator of transcription 4 (*STAT4*) gene. It is thought that a viral infection might trigger an immune response in susceptible individuals.

Pathology

All organs affected by Sjögren syndrome are infiltrated by lymphocytes. In the salivary glands, this results in duct dilatation, acinar atrophy and interstitial fibrosis. There is marked activation of B cells, resulting in increased immunoglobulin production.

Clinical features

Sjögren syndrome predominantly affects people aged between 40 and 50 years. The main symptoms are ocular and oral.

Ocular symptoms

Reduced tear secretion results in the destruction of the corneal and conjunctival epithelium. Patients complain of dry, gritty, sore eyes that might be reddened. Bacterial conjunctivitis is common and corneal ulcers can occur.

Oral symptoms

Xerostomia (dryness of the mouth) leads to difficulties in swallowing dry food or talking for extended periods of time. On examination of the oral cavity, the mucosa is dry, there is very little saliva and the tongue may be fissured. Dental caries and gingivitis are common and oral candidiasis often occurs. Intermittent parotid swelling affects at least half of patients with primary Sjögren syndrome but is less common in secondary disease.

Other symptoms of exocrine dysfunction

Secretions from other exocrine glands can also be affected. Patients may experience vaginal dryness which can cause painful intercourse and candidiasis. Lack of secretions in the GI tract can result in oesophagitis and gastritis. Lymphadenopathy can also be found.

Systemic features

Primary Sjögren syndrome is a systemic disease and many patients develop extraglandular manifestations that mimic SLE:

- Constitutional features such as fatigue, weight loss and fever.
- Arthritis is episodic, nonerosive and very similar to the joint disease seen in SLE.
- Circulation: Raynaud phenomenon affects up to 50% of patients. Vasculitis affects approximately 5% of patients and usually causes cutaneous lesions, purpura and urticaria.
- Respiratory: interstitial lung disease is mild and often subclinical.
- Renal: interstitial nephritis can lead to renal tubular acidosis or nephrogenic diabetes insipidus.
- Neurological features vary widely. Peripheral neuropathies result from small vessel vasculitis. Cranial neuropathies, hemiparesis, seizures and movement disorders can also occur.
- Malignancy: There is a 40-fold increased lifetime risk of lymphomas (usually B cell) in patients with Sjögren syndrome when compared to the general population. They develop in the salivary glands, reticuloendothelial system, GI tract, lungs or kidneys. In cases of progressive lymphadenopathy, it is important to take a lymph node biopsy to exclude lymphoma.

Investigations

Schirmer test

Schirmer test is used to demonstrate a reduction in tear production from the lacrimal glands. One end of a strip of filter paper is placed beneath the lower eyelid. Wetting the paper by less than 5 mm in 5 minutes suggests reduced tear secretion.

Labial gland biopsy and histology

Biopsy and histology of the buccal surface of the lower lip is very useful. Lymphocytic infiltration can be seen.

Blood tests

- ESR is usually elevated.
- Immunoglobulin levels can be very high.
- Anti-Ro/La antibodies are a diagnostic aid but rheumatoid factor and antinuclear antibodies (ANA) are often also found.

HINTS AND TIPS

Do not assume every patient with arthralgia and a positive rheumatoid factor has rheumatoid arthritis (RA). Titres of rheumatoid factor can be very high in Sjögren syndrome and patients with primary Sjögren syndrome are often misdiagnosed as having RA.

Management

Treatment of Sjögren syndrome is mainly topical and symptomatic. Tear substitutes such as hypromellose eye drops can help to lubricate the eyes. Occlusion of the canaliculi can help block the drainage of tears and keep the conjunctiva moist.

Xerostomia can be treated with saliva substitutes. Pilocarpine tablets can help but might cause cholinergic side effects such as sweating, flushing and abdominal cramps. Careful attention to dental hygiene is essential.

Vaginal lubricants can be prescribed to treat vaginal dryness.

Hydroxychloroquine can help the arthritis. Corticosteroids and other immunosuppressants are prescribed for serious complications such as vasculitis and renal disease.

POLYMYOSITIS AND DERMATOMYOSITIS

Definition

Polymyositis (PM) and dermatomyositis (DM) are autoimmune, inflammatory muscle diseases. DM affects the skin as well as the muscles.

Incidence

Both muscle diseases are rare, with a combined annual incidence of between 2 and 10 cases per million. There is a female predominance of 2:1.

Aetiology

The aetiology is unknown in both diseases. Family studies support a genetic predisposition. Associations with various HLA types have been reported but are weak.

Pathology

In both conditions, muscle fibres are infiltrated by inflammatory cells and there is subsequent degeneration, necrosis and phagocytosis. In PM, the main driver of damage is thought to be predominantly via cytotoxic T-cell damage. In DM, muscle damage is driven by complement-mediated damage of the intramuscular microvasculature. Skin biopsies in DM show the same histological features as in lupus.

Clinical features

Inflammatory muscle disease can affect people of any age, but the peak onset is between 40 and 60 years of age.

Myositis

PM and DM are characterized by an insidious, symmetrical and progressive proximal muscle weakness that develops over weeks and months. Patients describe difficulty in rising from a chair or walking up stairs. It can be difficult to reach things above head height.

Involvement of the intercostal muscles and diaphragm can affect ventilation and lead to a type 2 respiratory failure. Involvement of the muscles of the head, neck and oesophagus can result in dysphagia and regurgitation.

Patients may complain of muscle pain and tenderness. Muscle bulk and reflexes appear normal, except in advanced cases.

Cutaneous manifestations

The skin rashes of DM usually precede the weakness. Typical lesions are:

- Gottron papules: erythematous, scaly papules or plaques over the metacarpophalangeal and proximal interphalangeal joints and also over the extensor surfaces of the hands and elbows (Fig. 13.5).
- A heliotrope rash develops over the eyelids; lilac discolouration is often accompanied by periorbital oedema (Fig. 13.6).
- A macular erythematous rash may develop on the face, neck, chest, shoulders and hands. This rash is photosensitive and has been described as the 'shawl sign' (Fig. 13.7).
- Cutaneous vasculitis can cause ulceration.
- Periungal telangiectasia may be seen and the cuticles are often thickened and irregular.
- Mechanic's hands: Erythema and hyperkeratotic changes on the hands associated with Jo-1 autoantibody-positive myositis (Fig. 13.8).

Extramuscular features of polymyositis and dermatomyositis

Constitutional features

Fatigue, malaise, fever and weight loss are common.

Skeletal features

Many patients develop polyarthralgia as well as myalgia.

Pulmonary features

Interstitial lung disease occurs in up to 30% of patients. Ventilatory failure can result from weakness of the intercostal muscles and diaphragm. Patients with dysphagia and regurgitation may develop aspiration pneumonia.

Cardiovascular features

Myocarditis can occur with heart failure and arrhythmias, but most cases are asymptomatic. Raynaud phenomenon and vasculitis can accompany myositis.

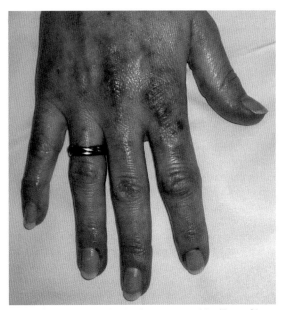

Fig. 13.5 Gottron's papules in dermatomyositis. (From Glynn M, Drake W. *Hutchison's Clinical Methods*. 25th ed. Elsevier; 2023.)

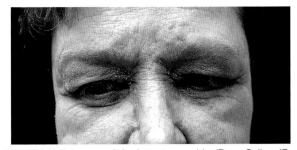

Fig. 13.6 Heliotrope rash in dermatomyositis. (From Callen JP, Jorisso JL, Bolognia JL, Piette WW, Zone JZ. *Dermatological signs of internal disease*., 4th ed. Elsevier; 2009.)

Gastrointestinal features

Vasculitis can result in intestinal haemorrhage or perforation. It is more common in juvenile DM.

> **RED FLAG**
>
> Approximately 10% to 15% of adults with inflammatory muscle disease have an underlying malignancy. The association is thought to be much stronger with DM than PM. It is important to assess for a possible underlying cancer in patients presenting with inflammatory muscle disease.

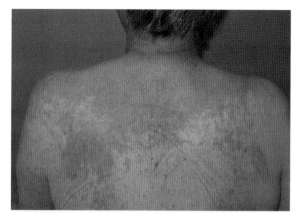

Fig. 13.7 'Shawl sign' in dermatomyositis. (From Hochberg M, et al. *Rheumatology*. 8th ed. Elsevier; 2023.)

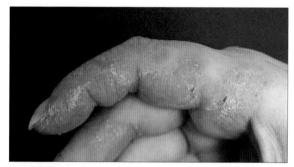

Fig. 13.8 Mechanic's hands. (From Hochberg M, et al. *Rheumatology*. 8th ed. Elsevier; 2023.)

Investigations

Serum levels of muscle enzymes

Serum levels of muscle enzymes (such as creatine kinase) are elevated due to myositis.

Erythrocyte sedimentation rate

The ESR is usually raised but does not closely correlate with disease activity.

Autoantibodies

A positive autoantibody test is found in around 60% of patients with inflammatory myositis. Anti-Jo-1 antibodies are more common in patients with PM than those with DM and are associated with Raynaud phenomenon and interstitial lung disease (the antisynthetase syndrome). Anti-Mi-2 antibodies are specific for DM but are only found in around 25% of patients.

Muscle biopsy

This is the most definitive diagnostic test. Histology shows the typical inflammatory infiltrate pattern of PM or DM.

Electromyography and nerve conduction studies

Electromyography and nerve conduction studies can show that the weakness is due to a myopathic process but do not provide a specific diagnosis.

Magnetic resonance imaging

Magnetic resonance imaging (MRI) can identify areas of anatomical muscle oedema and then be used to target a biopsy.

Management

Although the muscle enzymes respond quickly to treatment, muscle strength is usually much slower to recover. Physiotherapy plays a key role in the rehabilitation of patients with inflammatory muscle disease.

Most patients with PM and DM require immunosuppressive therapy. Corticosteroids are used to control myositis. They are initially prescribed at high doses. Serum creatine kinase is monitored and, as it falls, the corticosteroid dose is gradually reduced. Methotrexate and azathioprine are used as steroid sparing agents. Cyclophosphamide may be prescribed for patients with severe interstitial lung disease. If an underlying malignancy is found, it should be promptly treated.

> **HINTS AND TIPS**
>
> Steroid myopathy is a common complication of treatment. It may be difficult to distinguish from active myositis, but it should be considered in patients with normal creatine kinase levels whose muscle strength is deteriorating. Biopsy may help differentiate.

Prognosis

The 5-year survival for PM and DM has improved and is currently over 80%. Despite this, many patients are still left with persisting symptoms, or side effects due to their treatments.

SYSTEMIC SCLEROSIS

Definition

Scleroderma means hardening of the skin and describes a spectrum of disorders, which may be confined to the skin

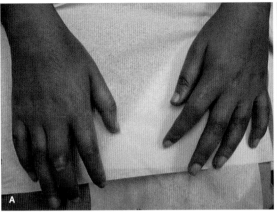
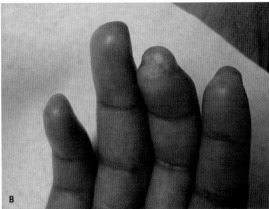

Fig. 13.9 (A) Sclerodactyly and (B) digital pitting and ulceration. (With permission from Torok KS. Pediatric scleroderma: systemic or localized forms. *Pediatric Clinics of North America* 2012;59(2):381–405.)

(cutaneous) or involve other organs (systemic sclerosis). Both terms (scleroderma and systemic sclerosis) are often used interchangeably. Most patients with skin changes will also have involvement of other organs. The systemic form is further subdivided into a limited and diffuse disease, the latter having more extensive skin involvement than the former.

Incidence and prevalence

These are rare conditions. The annual incidence of scleroderma is 0.6 to 1.9 per million. The UK prevalence is approximately 100 per million. Women are affected four times more often as men.

Aetiology

In most patients the aetiology is unknown.

Pathology

The two main pathological processes in systemic sclerosis are fibrosis and microvascular occlusion. Overactive fibroblasts produce excessive extracellular matrix in the dermis. Perivascular inflammatory infiltrates and intimal proliferation lead to narrowing of arteries and arterioles and obliteration of the capillary bed. There is immune activation and release of cytokines.

Clinical manifestations

Skin manifestations

Scleroderma begins with an inflammatory phase. The skin becomes puffy and tight and sometimes feels itchy. These symptoms typically affect the forearms, hands and feet initially. Over several months, skin thickening and induration develop. Common features found on examination are:

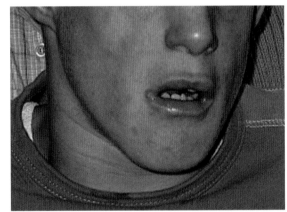

Fig. 13.10 Microstomia: note the tightness of the skin around the mouth. (With permission from de Ravel TJ, Balikova I, Thiry P et al. Another patient with a de novo deletion further delineates the 2q33.1 microdeletion syndrome. *European Journal of Medical Genetics* 2009;52(2):120–122.)

- Sclerodactyly (Fig. 13.9). This causes the skin to tighten, and functional capacity to be reduced. Protective fat pads are lost and the skin can ulcerate.
- Microstomia (Fig. 13.10). Microstomia describes tightening of the skin around the mouth, causing difficulty in opening the mouth fully. This leads to difficulties in eating, speaking and brushing teeth.
- Loss of normal skin creases.
- Tethering of skin to underlying structures.
- Skin hypo- and hyperpigmentation.
- Flexion contractures at joints.
- Thinning and atrophy (late stage).

The skin changes can differ between the limited and diffuse forms of systemic sclerosis. They are outlined in Table 13.2.

Table 13.2 A comparison of skin disease between limited and diffuse systemic sclerosis

	Limited systemic sclerosis	Diffuse systemic sclerosis
Distribution of skin fibrosis	Hands[a] and feet Over the face and neck	Limbs, face, neck and trunk
Skin tethering to underlying structures	Common	Less common
Inflammatory features	Mild	Swelling and pruritus prominent
Telangiectasia	Commonly occurs on the face and digits	Less common
Calcinosis	Cutaneous and subcutaneous calcification common	Less common

[a]*Scleroderma affecting the fingers is often referred to as sclerodactyly.*

Effects of systemic sclerosis on other body systems

In addition to causing disfiguring skin changes, systemic sclerosis can have profound effects on other organs. Limited disease is sometimes referred to as CREST syndrome (CREST = *c*alcinosis, *R*aynaud phenomenon, *o*esophageal disease, *s*clerodactyly and *t*elangiectasia). Symptoms develop most commonly between 40 and 50 years of age.

Involvement of internal organs is more frequent in diffuse than in limited disease. Limited disease makes up around 70% of cases.

Cardiovascular manifestations

Raynaud phenomenon

This occurs in nearly every patient with systemic sclerosis. Severe disease may cause ischaemic changes in the fingertips and possibly gangrene. Unlike in benign primary Raynaud phenomenon, there is destruction of the capillary structures at the peripheries, which can be seen using nail-fold capillaroscopy techniques.

Cardiac disease

Myocardial fibrosis can cause cardiac failure and arrhythmias. Pericarditis can be silent.

Pulmonary manifestations

Pulmonary disease is the most common cause of death in systemic sclerosis.

Interstitial lung disease

This affects around 25% of patients with limited disease and up to 40% of those with diffuse systemic sclerosis.

Pulmonary hypertension

This affects around 10% to 15% of patients and now represents a major cause of death in scleroderma patients.

Primary pulmonary hypertension is more common in limited disease and is not associated with additional lung pathology. Secondary pulmonary hypertension is more common in diffuse disease and is caused by interstitial lung disease and fibrosis.

Renal manifestations

Scleroderma renal crisis

This is a cause of rapidly progressive renal failure associated with severe hypertension. It tends to occur in patients with diffuse cutaneous disease within 5 years of diagnosis and is often preceded by a deterioration in skin disease. Mortality is high and poor outcomes are common. Aggressive but cautious blood pressure control is the mainstay of treatment. Patients often present with headaches, blurred vision and sometimes seizures. Acute left ventricular failure can occur and death from renal failure is common without urgent intervention.

> **RED FLAG**
>
> Scleroderma renal crisis is a life-threatening medical emergency that requires urgent treatment.

Gastrointestinal manifestations

Scleroderma can affect any part of the GI tract but commonly involves the oesophagus. Reflux oesophagitis and dysmotility are common and are a significant source of distress and worry to patients. Hypomotility can lead to bacterial overgrowth, with constipation or diarrhoea. Many patients complain of worsening dysphagia to solids, which warrants a barium swallow study.

Musculoskeletal manifestations

Most patients suffer from a degree of arthralgia and joint stiffness, but overt synovitis is uncommon. Flexion contractors of the interphalangeal joints due to skin changes are common.

Neurological manifestations

Both central and peripheral neuropathies can develop and overlap myopathy/myositis is a recognized feature.

Investigations

The diagnostic criteria are based on clinical findings and serological status (see box). It is important to establish whether patients have limited or diffuse disease, as this impacts upon prognosis.

DIAGNOSTIC CRITERIA FOR SYSTEMIC SCLEROSIS

Item	Subitem	Score
Skin thickening of the fingers of both hands extending proximal to the MCP joints		9
Skin thickening of the fingers (only count the highest score)	Puffy fingers	2
	Sclerodactyly (distal to the MCP joints but proximal to the PIP joints	4
Fingertip lesions (only count the highest score)	Digital tip ulcers	2
	Fingertip pitting scars	3
Telangiectasia		2
Abnormal nail-fold capillaries (visualized through nail-fold capillaroscopy)		2
Lung disease (max score is 2)	Pulmonary artery hypertension	2
	Interstitial lung disease	2
Raynaud phenomenon		3
Related antibodies (max score is 3)	Anticentromere	3
	Antitopoisomerase I (Scl-70) Anti-RNA polymerase III	

The highest score for each criterion is counted.
Patients with a score of 9 or above are classified as having definite scleroderma (sensitivity 91%, specificity 92%).
MCP, Metacarpophalangeal; PIP, proximal interphalangeal.
Adapted from 2013 ACR/EULAR criteria for the classification of systemic sclerosis.

Serological tests

ANA are found in most patients. The presence or absence of other autoantibodies can help predict complications and prognosis, for example:

- Anticentromere antibodies are associated with limited disease and a relatively good prognosis. They signify a risk of pulmonary hypertension, but not pulmonary fibrosis.
- Antitopoisomerase-I (Scl-70) antibodies are associated with diffuse disease, a higher risk of pulmonary fibrosis, renal involvement and mortality.

Management

Treatment

To date, no definitive treatment exists. Symptoms and complications should be treated on an organ-by-organ basis (see Table 13.3).

Table 13.3 Treatment of end-organ disease in systemic sclerosis

Complication	Intervention
• Raynaud phenomenon	Hand warmers Vasodilators • Calcium-channel blockers • Angiotensin-receptor blockers • Intravenous prostacyclin (iloprost) for severe ischaemia. Digital sympathectomy is useful for ischaemia of one or two digits
Pulmonary fibrosis	Prednisolone, with or without cyclophosphamide
Pulmonary hypertension	Anticoagulation Vasodilators • Calcium-channel blockers • Bosentan • Sildenafil • Prostacyclins Diuretics for right ventricular failure, if present
Gastrointestinal problems	Proton pump inhibitor for gastro-oesophageal reflux Antibiotics for small-bowel overgrowth Bulk-forming agents for constipation
Renal crisis	Antihypertensives (give immediately): • ACE inhibitors • Calcium-channel blockers • Temporary dialysis may be required
Cardiac problems	Diuretics and ACE inhibitors for cardiac failure Antiarrhythmics if necessary Corticosteroids for myocarditis

ACE, Angiotensin-converting enzyme.

Screening for complications

Monitoring pulmonary function tests, echocardiography, blood pressure and renal function help to detect complications early in systemic sclerosis.

Prognosis

The 5-year survival rate for scleroderma is about 85%, with 10-year survival less than 70%. Markers that suggest a poorer prognosis include diffuse disease, older age, high ESR and proteinuria. Improving survival rates reflect better disease management, but many patients still suffer a significant burden of morbidity.

SARCOIDOSIS

Sarcoidosis is a multisystem inflammatory disease that mainly affects the lungs and intrathoracic lymph nodes. It is normally dealt with by respiratory physicians, however, it is still important to consider it as a CTD with systemic manifestations.

The cause of sarcoidosis is unclear. It predominantly affects women and onset is usually between 20 and 30 years of age.

It is a granulomatous inflammatory condition. A granuloma describes a collection of macrophages surrounded by epithelioid cells (that fuse to form multinucleate giant cells) and lymphocytes. Granuloma formation is a key feature of sarcoidosis, and the site of granuloma deposition dictates the organs involved.

Approximately 30% to 50% of patients are asymptomatic. For others, the onset of symptoms may be insidious or acute. The main clinical manifestations of sarcoidosis are listed in Table 13.4.

> **HINTS AND TIPS**
>
> A key triad named Löfgren syndrome should be noted in sarcoidosis. This is an acute manifestation of erythema nodosum, arthritis and bilateral lymphadenopathy.

To diagnose sarcoidosis a combination of clinical features, radiological findings, biopsy and blood results should be used. A chest X-ray will show hilar lymphadenopathy (see Fig. 13.12) and a CT scan will show hilar lymphadenopathy with pulmonary fibrosis in more advanced disease. The gold standard for diagnosing sarcoidosis is a lung biopsy obtained through ultrasound-guided bronchoscopy. This will show characteristic granuloma formation. Serum calcium should be measured as

Table 13.4 Clinical features of sarcoidosis

System	Clinical features
Respiratory	Dyspnoea on exertion, cough, vague chest pain, wheeze
Skin	Erythema nodosum (see Fig. 13.11)
Gastrointestinal	Liver nodules and liver cirrhosis
Cardiac	Heart block
Eyes and nose	Uveitis, conjunctivitis, anosmia, nasal deformity
Neurological	Optic neuritis, facial nerve palsy, pituitary gland involvement (mainly affecting gonadotrophin secretion)
Renal	Kidney stone formation
Musculoskeletal	Arthralgia, arthritis
Systemic features	Fatigue, weight loss, lymphadenopathy, night sweats

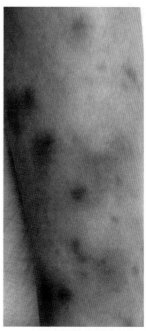

Fig. 13.11 Erythema nodosum. (From Micheletti R, James W, et al. *Andrews' Diseases of the Skin Clinical Atlas*. 2nd ed. Elsevier; 2023.)

macrophage activity leads to an increase in active vitamin D, thereby causing hypercalcemia. This is the mechanism behind the formation of kidney stones in sarcoidosis. In 60% of patients there is an increase in serum angiotensin-converting enzyme (ACE). ESR and CRP will likely be raised. An ECG should be

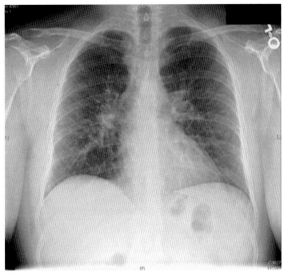

Fig. 13.12 Hilar lymphadenopathy seen in sarcoidosis. (From Mason RJ et al. (eds). *Murray and Nadel's Textbook of Respiratory Medicine*. 5th ed. Philadelphia: Saunders; 2010.)

Table 13.5 Connective tissue diseases with corresponding associated autoantibody summary table

Associated disease(s)	Autoantibody
Many connective tissue diseases	ANA
SLE	Anti-dsDNA
Drug-induced lupus	Anti-histone
Antiphospholipid syndrome & SLE	Antiphospholipid and anticardiolipin
Sjögren syndrome	Anti-Ro/La
Polymyositis > dermatomyositis	Anti-Jo-1
Dermatomyositis	Anti-Mi-2
Systemic sclerosis – limited pattern	Anti-centromere
Systemic sclerosis – diffuse pattern	Antitopoisomerase-1 (Scl-70)
Granulomatosis with polyangiitis	c-ANCA (PR3)
Eosinophilic granulomatosis with polyangiitis	p-ANCA (MPO)

ANA, *Antinuclear antibodies*; ANCA, *antineutrophil cytoplasmic antibodies*; SLE, *systemic lupus erythematosus*.

conducted on admission due to the cardiovascular complications of sarcoidosis.

Treatment of sarcoidosis is dependent on severity. In asymptomatic patients, treatment should not be given. In symptomatic cases glucocorticoids should be used followed by methotrexate or azathioprine. In severe cases of pulmonary fibrosis due to sarcoidosis, a lung transplant may be required.

Chapter Summary

- Connective tissue diseases (CTDs) are a broad spectrum of inflammatory disorders affecting the connective tissues.
- SLE is a common CTD that presents with multisystemic symptoms. It is much more common in women than in men. Anti-dsDNA antibodies are commonly found.
- Antiphospholipid syndrome causes venous and arterial thrombosis and is associated with recurrent fetal loss. It may require lifelong treatment with anticoagulants.
- Sjögren syndrome causes inflammation of the exocrine glands, resulting in dry eyes and a dry mouth.
- Inflammatory myositis (polymyositis and dermatomyositis) is rare but causes significant disability. Many patients require aggressive immunosuppression.
- Scleroderma/systemic sclerosis is a rare multisystem disorder characterized by fibrosis and vascular occlusion. Ulcerating Raynaud phenomenon is usually the presenting feature.
- Sarcoidosis is a multisystem inflammatory disease that mainly affects the lungs and intrathoracic lymph nodes.
- Table 13.5 contains a summary of the autoantibodies associated with various connective tissue diseases.

UKMLA Conditions
Systemic lupus erythematous
Sarcoidosis

UKMLA Presentations
Acute joint pain/swelling
Chronic joint pain/stiffness
Eye pain/discomfort
Muscle pain/myalgia
Musculoskeletal deformity
Red eye

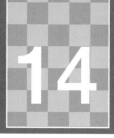
Vasculitis is inflammation of blood vessels. It is a feature of many illnesses and can be primary or secondary. The primary vasculitides are uncommon diseases in which vasculitis is the predominant feature. Secondary vasculitis complicates other established diseases, such as rheumatoid arthritis and systemic lupus erythematosus (SLE). Although these are rare diseases, they should be considered in any patients presenting with lethargy, fever, weight loss, rashes (see Fig. 14.1) and signs of kidney disease (proteinuria seen on urinalysis).

In addition, vasculitis can be caused by infections, drugs and malignancy. Only primary vasculitis is discussed below.

PATHOLOGY

Vasculitis is characterized by idiopathic autoimmune-driven inflammation caused by inflammatory cell infiltration of the blood vessel wall, resulting in fibrinoid necrosis. For this reason, the term necrotizing vasculitis is sometimes used. There is often associated granuloma formation. Vascular inflammation can have severe consequences:

- Vessel stenosis leading to occlusion and distal infarction.
- Aneurysm formation can lead to rupture of vessels and haemorrhage.

Antineutrophil cytoplasmic antibodies (ANCA) are particularly specific for vasculitis and helpful for diagnosis and classification. These antibodies bind to enzymes in the cytoplasm of neutrophils. There are two associated antigen/antibody subtypes:

- Proteinase-3 (PR3) is an enzyme found throughout the neutrophil cytoplasm and anti-PR3 antibodies are sometimes called c-ANCA (cytoplasm ANCA). This enzyme is found in patients with granulomatosis with polyangiitis (GPA, formerly Wegener granulomatosis) and is highly specific.
- Myeloperoxidase (MPO) is an enzyme found in a perinuclear distribution in neutrophils and anti-MPO antibodies are called perinuclear-ANCA (p-ANCA). This enzyme is found in eosinophilic granulomatosis with polyangiitis (EGPA, formerly Churg-Strauss syndrome), polyarteritis nodosa and microscopic polyangiitis.

CLASSIFICATION OF PRIMARY VASCULITIS

The vasculitides are commonly classified by the size of the vessels they affect (see Fig. 14.2).

CLINICAL FEATURES

Although vasculitis is rare, it can affect any system of the body and has the potential to be life-threatening. It is important to be aware of the general effects it can cause (Table 14.1), but detailed knowledge of specific diseases is beyond the scope of this textbook.

Giant cell arteritis and polymyalgia rheumatica

Giant cell arteritis (GCA) is a large vessel vasculitis. It often coexists with polymyalgia rheumatica (PMR), a nonvasculitic illness, which is why they are discussed together here. Both conditions are thought to be manifestations of the same underlying disorder. They have an incidence of approximately 1 to 5 in 10,000. They both affect people over the age of 60 years and are twice as common in women than in men. About 50% of patients with GCA have symptoms of PMR and approximately 25% to 50% of patients with PMR may experience GCA symptoms.

Giant cell arteritis

Most symptoms are due to inflammation of the carotid arteries and their branches, although any large artery can be involved.

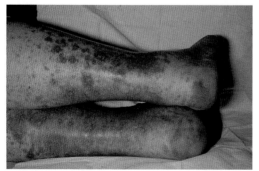

Fig. 14.1 Severe vasculitic rash. (From Herrick AL et al. *Orthopaedics and Rheumatology in Focus*. Churchill Livingstone; 2010.)

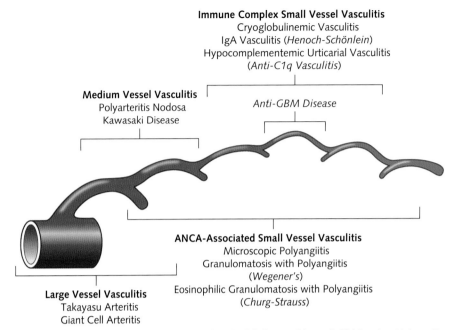

Immune Complex Small Vessel Vasculitis
Cryoglobulinemic Vasculitis
IgA Vasculitis (*Henoch-Schönlein*)
Hypocomplementemic Urticarial Vasculitis
(*Anti-C1q Vasculitis*)

Medium Vessel Vasculitis
Polyarteritis Nodosa
Kawasaki Disease

Anti-GBM Disease

ANCA-Associated Small Vessel Vasculitis
Microscopic Polyangiitis
Granulomatosis with Polyangiitis
(*Wegener's*)
Eosinophilic Granulomatosis with Polyangiitis
(*Churg-Strauss*)

Large Vessel Vasculitis
Takayasu Arteritis
Giant Cell Arteritis

Fig. 14.2 Classification of the vasculitides. (From Jennette JC, Falk RJ, Bacon PA, et al. 2012 revised International Chapel Hill Consensus Conference Nomenclature of Vasculitides. *Arthritis Rheum.* 2013;65:1-11.)

Table 14.1 The effects vasculitis can have on specific body systems

Body system or organ	Manifestations of vasculitis
Constitutional	Fatigue, anorexia, weight loss, fever
Skin	Rashes Nonblanching palpable purpura Ulceration Ischaemia (Fig. 14.3)
Joints	Arthralgia Arthritis
Kidneys	Glomerulonephritis
Gastrointestinal tract	Ischaemia
Nervous system	Neuropathies Stroke
Lungs	Pulmonary haemorrhage

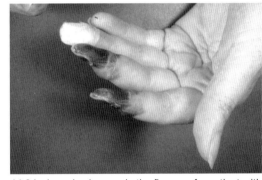

Fig. 14.3 Ischaemic changes in the fingers of a patient with vasculitis.

The onset of GCA can be insidious or abrupt with symptoms appearing overnight. Patients complain of:

- Severe unilateral headache that does not improve with analgesia and scalp tenderness from skin ischaemia.
- Pain on chewing food (jaw claudication from masseter muscle ischaemia).

- The temporal artery is thickened and beaded on palpation and may be pulseless.
- Visual change: optic artery ischaemia, which may be preceded by temporary vision loss known as amaurosis fugax.

Blindness can occur. This is due to ischaemic optic neuropathy, caused by arteritis of the posterior ciliary artery and branches of the ophthalmic arteries. Patients may experience transient visual disturbance at first. A stroke is another serious complication.

RED FLAG

Corticosteroids must be prescribed urgently in GCA to reduce the risk of blindness and stroke. In patients with rapid onset or progressive symptoms, it might be necessary to admit them for pulsed intravenous steroids to preserve vision. Other treatments are as per PMR, described below.

Polymyalgia rheumatica

PMR is the most commonly diagnosed rheumatic disease in older people in the UK. The cause of PMR is unknown but genetic and environmental factors are thought to play a role. Patients present with symmetrical pain and stiffness in the shoulder, pelvic girdle and neck, often without synovitis (see Fig. 14.4). Shoulder pain may radiate to the elbow and is often worse in the morning. Proximal muscles are often tender. A medium-sized joint synovitis can occasionally occur. Systemic features such as lethargy and loss of appetite are common. Pitting oedema may also occur. PMR is not associated with increased mortality but carries a definite increase in morbidity.

Investigations

The diagnosis of PMR is through clinical features of the disease and a positive response to steroid treatment after 1 week. ESR and CRP are commonly raised. If both are normal, it is not PMR. It is important to exclude mimics such as malignancy (e.g., myeloma) and other connective tissue diseases such as rheumatoid arthritis, osteoarthritis, thyroid disease and SLE.

Temporal artery biopsy is the investigation of choice in GCA, but it does not always achieve a diagnosis. Arterial wall thickening may occur as skip lesions and the biopsy may fail to target one. Inflammatory cell infiltrates, giant cells and granulomas should be detected. Increasingly, ultrasound is used as an alternative to biopsy.

The ESR is almost always raised in both conditions.

Management

Both GCA and PMR should be treated with corticosteroids. Prednisolone at a dose of 15–20 mg/day is usually prescribed for PMR. A higher dose of 1 mg/kg/day is used initially in GCA. Guidelines suggest blood tests should be monitored and clinical symptoms assessed regularly and when the patient has clinically improved, the steroid dose should be reduced.

There is usually a dramatic response to initiating steroids, provided an appropriate dose has been used. Failure to respond to steroids should challenge the diagnosis.

PMR is one of the most common indications for long-term steroid treatment. Most patients should be no longer receiving treatment after 2 years. Symptoms may occasionally flare at lower doses and if recurrent, a steroid-sparing agent such as methotrexate or azathioprine should be prescribed to avoid longer-term high-dose steroid use. A biologic drug, tocilizumab (IL-6 blocker) has proven effective to treat GCA and can be considered as an alternative for induction or when steroid dose remains high after induction treatment. A small but significant number of patients remain on long-term low-dose steroids.

RED FLAG

Most patients with GCA and PMR will be on steroids for more than a year. Over time, the body will stop endogenous steroid production and the patient will become dependent on prescribed corticosteroids. Therefore, the patient's steroid dosage should be reduced slowly to reactivate endogenous steroid production. Patients must be warned against immediately stopping steroid treatment. Immediate cessation of treatment may result in adrenal crisis, a life-threatening condition characterized by dehydration and hypotension. Patients should carry a steroid emergency card and should be taught how to inject emergency hydrocortisone in the event of an adrenal crisis. Long-term corticosteroid use also leads to systemic complications. Prescribing bone-protective drugs such as bisphosphonates and calcium and vitamin D supplements is suggested for the prevention of osteoporosis.

Takayasu arteritis

This is a rare disease that predominantly affects young women. The arteritis affects the aortic arch and its branches. Symptoms are due to vascular ischaemia and include claudication, visual disturbance, dizziness and stroke. Differences in blood pressure between limbs may occur, as well as subclavian bruits. Imaging with computed tomography (CT), MRI, Doppler ultrasound or positron emission tomography (PET) may help confirm the diagnosis. Steroids are the mainstay of treatment, but vascular complications are not uncommon and surgery, such as vascular bypass surgery, may be needed.

Polyarteritis nodosa

Polyarteritis nodosa is a necrotizing arteritis that leads to aneurysm formation. It affects men more commonly than women. Clinical features include skin ulceration and rashes (such as livedo reticularis), peripheral neuropathy, renal disease and gut infarction, which presents as bleeding with abdominal pain.

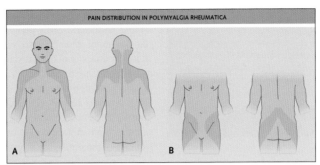

Fig. 14.4 Distribution of pain in polymyalgia rheumatica. (From Hochberg MC. *Rheumatology*. 7th ed. Philadelphia. Elsevier; 2019.)

Angiography may show microaneurysms, which are usually found in the renal arteries and the coeliac axis. Renal, rectal and sural nerve biopsies can be helpful in achieving a diagnosis.

Polyarteritis nodosa is occasionally seen secondary to hepatitis B infection.

Treatment is with corticosteroids and, in severe cases, cyclophosphamide.

Kawasaki disease (mucocutaneous lymph node syndrome)

This vasculitis predominantly affects children under the age of 5 years but may rarely occur in adults. Patients will first present with a persistent high fever and an erythematous rash. Characteristic features include desquamation of the skin of the hands and feet, conjunctival congestion, cervical lymphadenopathy, arteritis and coronary artery aneurysms, which can lead to myocardial infarction and heart failure. The key finding in children is of a strawberry tongue (see Fig. 14.5). Treatment is with intravenous immunoglobulin and low-dose aspirin.

Granulomatosis with polyangiitis

Granulomatosis with polyangiitis (GPA, formerly Wegener granulomatosis) is a granulomatous disorder associated with necrotizing vasculitis. It is strongly linked to the presence of PR3 ANCA. The peak age of onset is between 30 and 40 years of age. Many systems can be affected (Table 14.2), but it is the respiratory and renal complications that are often the most serious, including pulmonary haemorrhage and renal failure.

Survival in cases of GPA has improved significantly since the introduction of cyclophosphamide, which is given in conjunction with corticosteroids. Rituximab (B-cell depletion therapy) has been shown to have equivalence to cyclophosphamide and is licensed for treatment. Some patients with a more limited, non–life-threatening GPA are prescribed immunosuppressants such as mycophenolate, azathioprine and methotrexate.

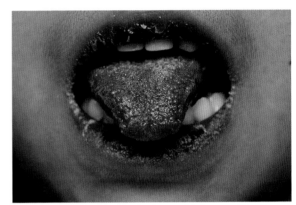

Fig. 14.5 Strawberry tongue in Kawasaki disease. (Courtesy: Kawasaki Disease Foundation.)

Other forms of vasculitis

Eosinophilic granulomatosis with polyangiitis

Eosinophilic granulomatosis with polyangiitis (EGPA, formerly Churg-Strauss syndrome) usually has three stages. The atopic phase is characterized by atopy with allergic rhinitis and adult-onset asthma, often requiring frequent steroids. The eosinophilic stage is marked by abnormally high eosinophils in peripheral blood samples. Weight loss, night sweats, cough, diarrhoea and wheeze may be present due to the effects of eosinophils on the body's systems. The third phase, the vasculitis stage, is the hallmark of EGPA. Inflammation and damage to blood vessels results in rashes, a mononeuritis multiplex, renal failure and abdominal pains.

Treatment is as for GPA. MPO ANCA is commonly detected in affected patients.

Microscopic polyarteritis

Microscopic polyarteritis (MPA) shares many features with GPA and presents with a rash, rapidly progressive glomerulonephritis and occasional alveolar haemorrhage.

Table 14.2 Clinical features of granulomatosis with polyangiitis

Body system or organ affected	Clinical features
Upper and lower respiratory tracts	Subglottic stenosis Lung nodules with or without cavitation Pulmonary haemorrhage Pulmonary infiltrates
Kidneys	Glomerulonephritis (often rapidly progressive)
Ear, nose and throat	Sensorineural deafness Nasal discharge, crusting and epistaxis Saddling of the nose due to destruction of the septal cartilage (Fig. 14.6) Ulceration of oral mucosa, chronic otitis media, loss of colour vision
Joints	Arthralgia Arthritis
Skin	Rashes Palpable purpura Livedo reticularis
Nervous system	Cranial nerve palsies Peripheral neuropathy Granulomatous meningitis

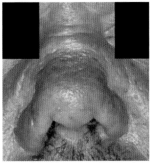
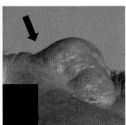

Fig. 14.6 Saddle nose deformity of granulomatosis with polyangiitis (late complication). (With permission from Comarmond C, Cacoub P. Granulomatosis with polyangiitis (Wegener): Clinical aspects and treatment. *Autoimmunity Reviews* 2014;13(11):1121–1125.)

Henoch-Schönlein purpura

Henoch-Schönlein purpura (HSP) typically presents with a palpable purpuric rash on the legs and buttocks in children and adolescents but it can occur at any age. It is an immune complex, small vessel vasculitis most commonly associated with IgA deposition. It is normally precipitated by a strep throat infection (e.g., tonsilitis). GI involvement results in abdominal pains and there may be associated asymmetric arthritis. Around 40% of patients develop a glomerulonephritis, which is usually self-limiting. Treatment is usually supportive with analgesia, rest and rehydration, but in rare cases, immunosuppression may be required.

Behçet disease

This is a rare systemic inflammatory disorder that has features of vasculitis in a number of patients. The classical symptoms are of oral and genital ulceration, anterior and posterior uveitis or retinal vascular lesions, cutaneous lesions (erythema nodosum and cutaneous pustular vasculitis), arthralgia, neurological features (memory impairment and aseptic meningitis) and GI features of anorexia and diarrhoea. It is a condition that follows a relapsing and remitting course. Treatment involves topical and systemic corticosteroid treatment, lidocaine ointment for ulcers and azathioprine or biologics (e.g., infliximab) in more severe cases.

● Chapter Summary

- Vasculitides cover a broad range of inflammatory conditions affecting the arteries. GCA and PMR are relatively common, with urgent high doses of steroids indicated in the former to reduce the risk of blindness.
- Table 13.5 contains a summary of the autoantibodies associated with various connective tissue diseases.

UKMLA Conditions
Kawasaki disease
Polymyalgia rheumatica

UKMLA Presentations
Back pain
Muscle pain/myalgia
Neck pain/stiffness

Metabolic bone disease 15

OSTEOPOROSIS

Because of the ageing population, fractures resulting from osteoporosis can put pressure on medical services incurring costs at both personal and societal levels.

Definition

Osteoporosis is a condition characterized by weakness of the bones, due to lower-than-normal bone mass or greater-than-normal bone loss. It results in increased bone fragility, which translates into an increased risk of fractures. Note that mineralization of bone in osteoporosis is normal. Bone mineral density (BMD) is used to measure bone strength and is expressed as a T-score. This is the number of standard deviations by which the BMD varies in relation to the mean density of young adults. The World Health Organization defines osteoporosis as a T-score of less than –2.5. Osteopenia is defined as a T-score of between –1 and –2.5. Normal bone density is expressed as a T-score greater than or equal to –1. A Z-score may also be used, and this is the number of standard deviations by which BMD varies in relation to the mean bone density of someone of the same age and sex.

Aetiology and pathology

Peak bone mass is usually achieved around the age of 30 years and declines thereafter (Fig. 15.1). Healthy bone structure is maintained through a balance of osteoclastic resorption and osteoblastic proliferation. In osteoporosis, this balance is lost, and osteoclastic resorption outweighs osteoblastic proliferation (Fig. 15.2). Risk factors for osteoporosis can be modifiable or nonmodifiable (see box: Risk factors for osteoporosis). Female sex is a risk factor for osteoporosis as oestrogen is essential for normal bone maturation and mineral acquisition. In the 8 to 10 years following the menopause, this reduction in oestrogen leads to 2% to 3% of bone lost per year (see Fig. 15.3).

RISK FACTORS FOR OSTEOPOROSIS

Nonmodifiable	Modifiable
Age	Poor calcium and vitamin
Race (Caucasian, Asian)	D intake
Female sex	Lack of exercise
Early menopause	Smoking
Small size	Alcohol excess
Positive family history	

Osteoporosis is divided into primary (idiopathic and age related) and secondary (resulting from another disease process). The causes of secondary osteoporosis are outlined in the following box.

CAUSES OF SECONDARY OSTEOPOROSIS

- Hyperthyroidism
- Hyperparathyroidism
- Hypogonadism
- Cushing syndrome
- Rheumatoid arthritis
- Inflammatory bowel disease
- Coeliac disease and malabsorption states
- Renal failure
- Multiple myeloma
- Anorexia nervosa
- Medications:
  - Corticosteroids
  - Anticonvulsants
  - Heparin

Clinical features

Patients present with pain, deformity and immobility due to fractures or they are detected by screening measurements of their BMD. Many areas now have automatic screening programmes for patients presenting with fragility fractures: these

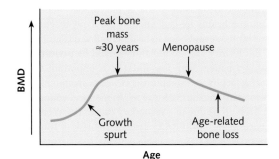

Fig. 15.1 Lifeline of bone mineral density. *BMD,* Bone mineral density.

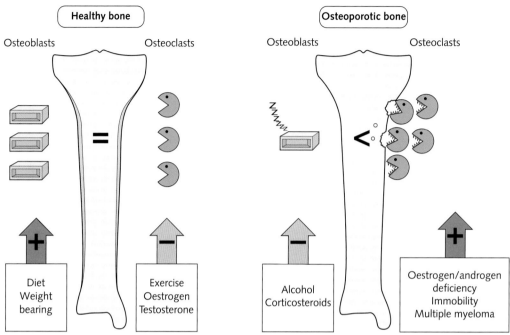

Fig. 15.2 Cell interactions in normal and osteoporotic bone.

are fractures that occur during normal activities, such as a fall from standing height or less. The skeleton should be able to withstand this without injury.

The three typical fragility fractures are a Colles fracture of the wrist, a fractured neck of the femur and a vertebral body fracture.

RED FLAG

Due to the anatomy of the vascular supply to the femoral head, a fractured femoral neck is susceptible to avascular necrosis. Physicians should be aware of this complication as it can progress to degenerative arthritis. Fifty per cent of patients that suffer a hip fracture due to osteoporosis will not regain full independence.

COMMUNICATION

Osteoporosis is often asymptomatic and therefore the importance of treatment to prevent fractures must be emphasized to patients.

Vertebral fractures

Vertebral compression (or wedge) fractures (Fig. 15.4) usually present with severe and sudden thoracic or lumbar back pain after a minor fall. They are frequently multiple and result in a loss of height and kyphotic deformity of the spine. Some patients do not experience pain but complain that they are shrinking or becoming round-shouldered.

These fractures are stable and treatment is aimed at controlling symptoms with analgesia.

Other common fractures include hip and wrist fractures and these are discussed in more detail in Chapter 18.

Diagnosis and investigation

Plain X-ray images cannot be used to diagnose osteoporosis, but osteopenia appearances may indicate the need for further investigation. The usual diagnostic test for osteoporosis is dual-energy X-ray absorptiometry (DEXA). DEXA is used in most departments to measure BMD at the lumbar spine and hip. Two photon beams are generated by the X-ray machine, which allows soft tissue and bone to be differentiated (Fig. 15.5).

A full history and examination should be performed when assessing a patient with low BMD. It is important to enquire about risk factors for osteoporosis as well as symptoms of potential secondary causes. Osteoporosis in men and young people is more likely to be due to a secondary cause. The WHO fracture risk assessment tool (FRAX) assesses the risk of fragility fracture over the next 10 years using patients' risk factors.

Investigations to exclude secondary causes will be necessary in some patients. Full blood count, alkaline phosphatase, renal function, serum electrophoresis, thyroid function, parathyroid

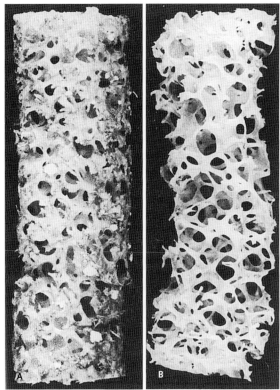

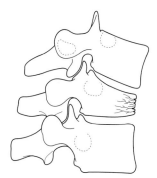

Fig. 15.4 Compression fracture of a thoracic vertebra.

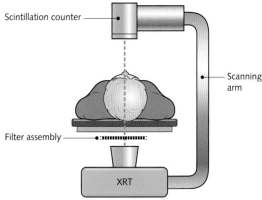

Fig. 15.3 (A) Normal bone in a premenopausal woman. (B) Osteoporotic bone in a postmenopausal woman. (Reproduced from Klippel J, Silman A, Dieppe P. *Rheumatology*. 2nd ed. Metabolic Bone Disease. London. Mosby; 1998.)

Fig. 15.5 Dual X-ray absorptiometry (DEXA) apparatus. The patient lies with the X-ray tube below. The filter allows two different beams to be produced, which are narrow to reduce scatter radiation. The beams are detected by the scintillation counter, which then generates an image. *XRT*, X-ray tube.

hormone (PTH) levels and vitamin D levels are commonly tested. Serum testosterone should be measured in men.

Management

The aim is to reduce the risk of fractures. This can be achieved by the following methods:

Modification of risk factors

Patients should try and change their modifiable risk factors (see box: Risk factors for osteoporosis), for example by stopping smoking or by increasing weight-bearing exercise.

Drug therapies to increase bone mass

Bisphosphonates

These are first-line therapeutic drugs usually used in combination with calcium supplements and vitamin D. Bisphosphonates are antiresorptive and work by inhibiting osteoclast activity.

Daily, weekly, monthly and yearly preparations are available and have good efficacy. These drugs should be taken on an empty stomach with the patient sitting upright for 30 minutes after administration due to the risk of reflux and oesophageal erosions.

Denosumab

This is a second-line monoclonal antibody directed against RANK-L. RANK-L is a ligand produced by osteoblasts that upregulates osteoclast formation, activity and survival, which in turn causes loss of BMD. It is useful in patients who are intolerant to bisphosphonates.

Teriparatide

This is a PTH analogue. It is very expensive but useful in patients intolerant to other treatments. Intermittent PTH exposure causes an increase in osteoblast activation (above that of osteoclasts) and therefore results in a net BMD increase.

Other drugs

Raloxifene, a selective oestrogen receptor modulator, is sometimes used in postmenopausal women but its popularity has significantly decreased. Calcitonin is an antagonistic hormone to PTH, reducing osteoclast activity and therefore increasing BMD. Strontium ranelate works by decreasing osteoclast activity and increasing osteoblast activity. Another drug that can be used is romosozumab. Romosozumab is a humanized monoclonal antibody which inhibits sclerostin, thus, increasing bone formation and reducing bone resorption.

Prevention of falls

As the majority of osteoporotic fractures are caused by falls, a significant amount of time and resource is spent on falls clinics to try to reduce the risk of falling. There are a number of factors that predispose patients to falls:

Intrinsic factors

- The ageing process: this leads to slower reaction times and sarcopenia (muscle loss).
- Poor mobility: patients often have other conditions such as osteoarthritis and neurological issues.
- Poor eyesight.
- Medical comorbidities: Parkinson's disease, pre-syncope and syncope, etc.

Extrinsic factors

- Lack of social support.
- Inadequate/unsafe housing environment.

Falls can be reduced through various interventions and often involve a multidisciplinary approach. Physiotherapists, occupational therapists, specialist nurses and social workers often have a key role to play. Home modifications such as improved lighting and railings can prevent falls.

> **HINTS AND TIPS**
>
> When looking at why patients fall, make sure to review a patient's drugs. Many drugs have mild sedative effects that might increase the risk of falling.

OSTEOGENESIS IMPERFECTA

Osteogenesis imperfecta (sometimes referred to as brittle bone disease) is another example of a disease characterized by low bone mass. This is a rare genetic disorder of collagen type 1 deficiency. It presents in a paediatric population as recurrent childhood fractures (without predisposing trauma), low muscle tone,

bowing of the legs and blue discolouration of the sclerae. It is treated with bisphosphonate therapy.

PAGET'S DISEASE

Definition

Paget's disease is a disorder of bone metabolism characterized by focal increases in bone remodelling, resulting in abnormal bone production. This leads to mechanical weakness of the bone and increased fracture risk.

Incidence

The incidence varies greatly across the world. It is very rare within the Asian population, whereas the UK has the highest incidence in the world at approximately 2% to 3% of people over the age of 40 years.

Aetiology

The cause of Paget's disease is unknown. However, clustering in families has been observed suggesting a strong genetic contribution. Another hypothesis suggests that the disease process may be triggered by a virus.

Pathology

There is a dramatic focal increase in bone metabolism with increased bone resorption, mediated by large multinucleated osteoclasts. Osteoblasts then respond by producing weak, disorganized bone. Repeated cycles of this result in abnormal hypertrophied areas of bone with increased vascularity (Fig. 15.6).

Clinical features

Less than a third of patients are symptomatic and many patients are diagnosed incidentally due to abnormal blood test results (raised alkaline phosphatase) and X-ray examination findings.

Symptomatic patients present with bone pain, deformity and fractures. Bone pain is most common in the spine, pelvis, femurs, skull and tibia. Deformity may lead to compression of other structures, such as the 8th cranial nerve, resulting in unilateral deafness. Spinal stenosis with spinal cord compression may also occur and present as claudication in the calves while walking. Fractures are often atypical such as low-energy femoral shaft fractures.

Fig. 15.7 shows some possible complications from Paget's disease.

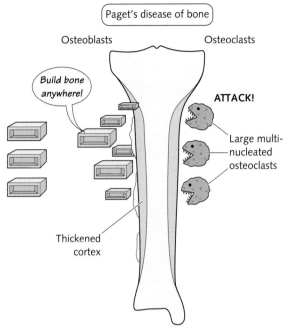

Fig. 15.6 Cell interactions in Paget's disease of bone.

Diagnosis and investigation

- Serum alkaline phosphatase is elevated and correlated to the amount of skeletal involvement. Serum alkaline phosphatase is a measure of bone turnover.
- Plain radiographs show patchy areas of disorganized bone with areas of lysis and sclerosis. The cortex is usually thickened.
- Isotope bone scans often show multiple areas of focal increased uptake and are the most sensitive test for detecting pagetic lesions.

Treatment

Bisphosphonates are very effective in inhibiting bone resorption and reducing the symptoms of Paget's disease. Calcitonin is sometimes also used but is less tolerated. NSAIDs will be used to treat bone pain.

Asymptomatic disease may not require treatment and should simply be observed; the key is to determine whether lesions are active or inactive. Pain is often the main reason for commencing pharmacological therapies.

Surgical treatment is needed to manage complications:

- Fractures: need for surgical stabilization.
- Deformity: osteotomy is rarely performed.
- Osteosarcoma: this is a rare tumour seen in Paget's disease. It is discussed further in Chapter 21.

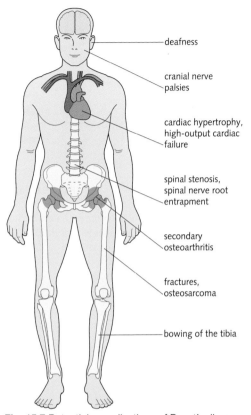

Fig. 15.7 Potential complications of Paget's disease.

> **RED FLAG**
>
> Pagetic bone is highly vascular and bleeds a lot during surgery. Ensure patients are cross matched for blood in advance of planned surgery and make blood available for emergency situations.

RICKETS AND OSTEOMALACIA

Both of these conditions are the result of failure of mineralization of bone. Rickets affects the growing skeleton in children and is a disorder of effective mineralization of cartilage in the epiphyseal growth plates of children. Osteomalacia occurs in adults. Osteomalacia literally translates as 'soft bone'.

Aetiology

Long standing and severe vitamin D deficiency is the most common cause of both conditions. Hypophosphataemia is a

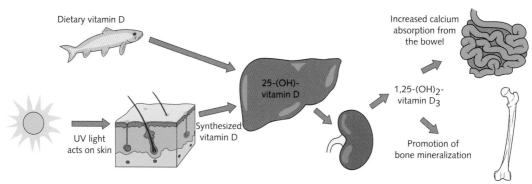

Fig. 15.8 Pathways of vitamin D metabolism.

much rarer cause. Fig. 15.8 illustrates the pathways of vitamin D metabolism. Low vitamin D describes as serum 25-hydroxyvitamin D <25 nmol/L. The causes of vitamin D deficiency are shown in the box.

CAUSES OF VITAMIN D DEFICIENCY

- Low dietary intake plus inadequate sunlight exposure
- Intestinal malabsorption (coeliac disease, gastric surgery)
- Liver disease
- Renal disease
- Drugs that affect vitamin D metabolism (anticonvulsants)

Pathology

Histological examination of bone biopsies in both conditions shows increased amounts of osteoid with deficient mineralization.

Clinical features

The main features of rickets and osteomalacia are:

- bone pain
- skeletal deformity
- muscle weakness
- fracturing

Lethargy, tetany and convulsions due to hypocalcaemia can occur.

Rickets

Growth is impaired in children with rickets. The clinical manifestations depend on the age of the child. Those under 12 months of age may have softening and frontal bossing of the skull. There may be swelling of the epiphyses of the wrists and at the costochondral junctions (the rickety rosary). Older children develop bowing of the long bones and valgus or varus deformities of the knee.

The following radiological changes are seen in rickets:

- delayed opacification of the epiphyses
- widened growth plates
- thin cortices

Osteomalacia

Osteomalacia tends to present with vague bone pain, especially in the long bone and pelvis. Severe localized pain may be due to a fracture. Patients can develop proximal myopathy and often complain of lethargy.

Diagnosis and investigation

The following laboratory abnormalities are usually found:

- low or low/normal calcium
- low or low/normal phosphate
- raised serum alkaline phosphatase
- low serum vitamin D
- raised PTH levels
- low urinary calcium excretion

Low vitamin D causes hypocalcaemia. This low level of calcium in the blood triggers secondary hyperparathyroidism, explaining the increase in PTH seen in the blood.

In osteomalacia, the characteristic appearance on X-ray images is Looser zones, which are spontaneous incomplete fractures.

Treatment

Both rickets and osteomalacia can be treated with vitamin D replacement. The underlying cause of vitamin D deficiency should be addressed.

Chapter Summary

- Osteoporosis results in increased risk of fractures in susceptible individuals.
- A DEXA scan is the diagnostic test of choice with a T-score of between –1 and –2.5 indicating osteopenia and a T-score less than –2.5 indicating osteoporosis.
- Treatment is with bisphosphonates, denosumab or teriparatide with calcium and vitamin D supplementation. Modifiable risk factors such as smoking should also be addressed.
- Osteogenesis Imperfecta is a rare genetic disease of low bone mass seen in paediatric patients.
- Paget's disease is relatively common (2%–3% in the UK over 40 years of age), but many patients are asymptomatic. It causes abnormal bone metabolism resulting in areas of weakened and structurally abnormal bone.
- Vitamin D deficiency causes rickets in children and osteomalacia in adults. Treatment is with vitamin D replacement.

UKMLA Conditions
Lower limb fractures
Osteomalacia
Osteoporosis
Pathological fracture
Spinal cord compression
Spinal fracture
Upper limb fractures

UKMLA Presentations
Bone pain
Musculoskeletal deformities

Gout and pseudogout 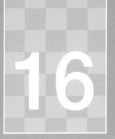 16

GOUT

Definition

Gout is the consequence of hyperuricaemia and uric acid crystal formation. Clinical features include:

- joint inflammation
- crystal deposition in soft tissues (tophi)
- renal disease
- uric acid renal stones

Prevalence

Gout affects 2.5% of people in the UK. It is more common in men with a current 5:1 male predominance. However, the incidence in women is increasing.

Aetiology

Gout is caused by a sustained increase in serum uric acid levels leading to the formation of monosodium urate crystals. Uric acid is a breakdown product of purine bases, which are components of nucleic acids.

Uric acid can arise from dietary sources, however, the majority of uric acid in the body comes from endogenous purine metabolism. The kidneys are responsible for the majority of uric acid excretion, however, the gut also plays a small role. Many factors influence uric acid excretion by the kidneys; age, sex, body mass, diet and genetic factors all contribute.

Hyperuricaemia is usually due to reduced renal excretion of uric acid, rather than increased production. A summary of risk factors for gout can be seen in the following box.

> **RISK FACTORS FOR GOUT**
>
> - Alcohol: especially beer
> - Diet: high protein, shellfish, red meats, high fructose content
> - Obesity
> - Thiazide diuretic use
> - Drugs: ciclosporin, aspirin
> - Male gender
> - Hypertension and renal disease
> - Cancer, especially myeloproliferative and lymphoproliferative disorders
> - Psoriasis (metabolic syndrome)

Pathology

Prolonged hyperuricaemia leads to the formation of monosodium urate crystals. These crystals can reside in the joint for extended periods of time without causing any symptoms, however, when they are released, inflammation occurs. A triggering event such as illness or surgery may cause the release of these crystals. Inflammation occurs due to the physical shape and negative charge of the crystals triggering phagocytosis by macrophages. The mechanism of crystal formation causing inflammation is illustrated in Fig. 16.1. Uric acid crystal deposition in the kidneys can cause interstitial nephritis, renal stones and acute tubular damage.

Clinical features

Acute gout

Acute gout is extremely painful. Joint swelling develops rapidly and can reach its peak severity in 2 to 6 hours. Swelling is often associated with shiny skin, skin redness, warmth and excruciating pain. Systemic symptoms such as fever and delirium may also occur. Gout most commonly occurs as a monoarthropathy but might involve several joints at the same time in severe cases. The first metatarsophalangeal joint is the most commonly affected (also known as a podagra, see Fig. 16.2), but the ankles, knees, elbows, wrists and hands can also be involved. Attacks often subside spontaneously after days or weeks but may require treatment for symptom control.

The bursa can also be affected and gout is a common cause of acute olecranon bursitis.

Acute attacks usually resolve themselves, leaving the patients free of pain. Some people only suffer a single attack, although many have recurrent flares within a year. Without treatment, acute attacks become more frequent and bony erosive damage occurs.

Chronic gout

Chronic gout occurs in patients with longstanding hyperuricaemia who have had many gouty flares. Within the skeleton and soft tissues, bony erosions form and tophi are deposited into the soft tissues; these can rupture, leading to discharge of chalky-white material, and can become infected. Tophi tend to form on the extensor surfaces of fingers, the hands, the elbows and the Achilles tendon. They can be differentiated from

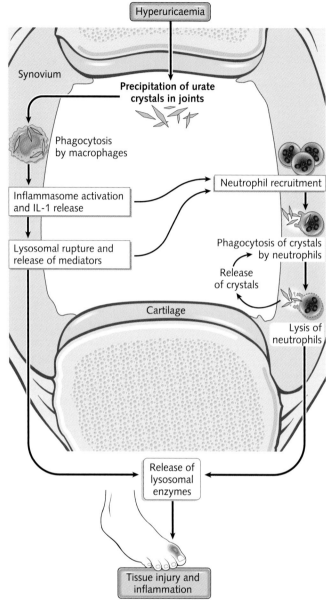

Fig. 16.1 Monosodium urate crystals causing inflammation of the joint in gout. (From Kumar V, et al. *Robbins & Kumar Basic Pathology*. 11th ed. Elsevier; 2023.)

rheumatoid nodules due to their characteristic white colour. Progressive damage to bones, ligaments and tendons leads to deformity (Fig. 16.3).

Within the kidneys, longstanding urate deposition may lead to progressive nephropathy. Uric acid stones may also form in the urinary tract.

Investigations

Synovial fluid analysis

This is the most important test for suspected gout. Synovial fluid should be obtained by needle aspiration from symptomatic joints and examined with a microscope under polarized light.

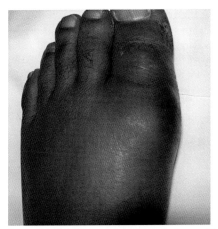

Fig. 16.2 Gout affecting the first metatarsophalangeal joint (a podagra). (From Goldman L, Shafer AI. *Goldman-Cecil Medicine*. 26th ed. Philadelphia. Elsevier; 2020.)

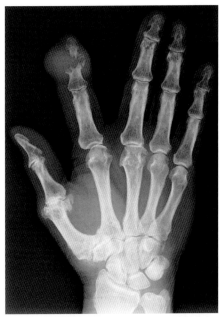

Fig. 16.3 Image of the right hand showing extensive bone erosive destruction of the 2nd digit with soft tissue calcified tophi on X-ray.

Monosodium urate crystals are needle shaped and show strong negative birefringence (Fig. 16.4). This means crystals parallel to the plane of light appear yellow and those perpendicular appear blue. Synovial fluid will likely appear turbid in an acute attack due to the presence of neutrophils phagocytosing crystals. Importantly, no bacterial growth will occur. Material aspirated from tophi can be examined in a similar way. Fluid should be examined soon after aspiration to increase the chance of seeing crystals.

> **RED FLAG**
>
> Septic arthritis is another common cause of an acute monoarthropathy. All acute monoarthritis is septic until proven otherwise. Gram stain and culture should be performed on samples to exclude infection. Look for other features of systemic upset or shock in keeping with sepsis (high temperature, tachycardia, a high respiratory rate and low blood pressure). If in doubt, treat the patient with antibiotics. Septic arthritis can be life-threatening!

Blood tests

Serum uric acid is usually elevated, but one-third of patients have normal serum uric acids during an acute flare as hyperuricaemia sometimes occurs between gout flares. Markers of inflammation (erythrocyte sedimentation rate (ESR) and C-reactive protein (CRP)) are often elevated in an acute flare, as is white blood cell count. It is important to assess renal function by checking U&Es and eGFR due to the association between gout and kidney damage. There is also an increased incidence of gout in those with metabolic syndrome so checking glucose and a lipid profile may be appropriate.

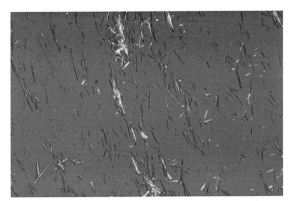

Fig. 16.4 Monosodium urate crystals under polarized light. (With permission from Klatt EC. Bones, joints, and soft-tissue tumors. In *Robbins and Cotran Atlas of Pathology*. 3rd ed. Saunders; 2015.)

Radiology

Radiological appearances are not normally visible until years of recurrent gouty flares have occurred. X-ray images show erosions in the juxta-articular regions with surrounded sclerosis of the bone, which helps differentiate between gouty erosions and erosions from inflammatory joint disease such as rheumatoid arthritis (RA).

Management

Acute Gout

Acute gout treatment should be initiated promptly after diagnosis during an acute flare. The aim of acute treatment is to improve pain and inflammation.

- Nonsteroidal antiinflammatory drugs (NSAIDs) are most commonly used first. They should be continued until pain and inflammation subside.
- Colchicine is a suitable alternative in those with contraindications to NSAIDs (asthma, previous peptic ulcers, renal impairment, etc.).
- Corticosteroids are useful in patients who are unable to tolerate NSAIDs or colchicine. They are not suitable for long-term use. Steroid injections into affected joints are very successful in relieving symptoms.
- Applying ice packs to the area of inflammation should be carried out in conjunction with prescribed medication. This will improve pain and inflammation.

Patients that have a single, acute attack of gout may not need to be prescribed further urate-lowering therapy.

Prophylactic therapy

Drugs that lower serum uric acid levels can be used to prevent gout attacks. Indications for the use of serum uric acid-lowering drugs are:

- The patient is suffering from recurrent gout attacks.
- Tophi are present.
- Renal.
- Presence of uric acid renal stones.
- Evidence of bone or joint damage.

Allopurinol should be used first. It reduces uric acid production by inhibiting the enzyme xanthine oxidase, a key enzyme in the uric acid synthesis pathway. The dose should be increased until the patient's uric acid level is <360 μg/mL. Caution is needed in the elderly and those with renal disease.

Febuxostat is another xanthine oxidase inhibitor that can be used as an alternative to allopurinol.

> **HINTS AND TIPS**
>
> Changes in serum uric acid levels can precipitate acute flares. Urate-lowering drugs should not be prescribed until an acute flare has completely settled. Time limited co-prescription of NSAID/colchicine/steroid should occur in parallel to initiation of urate lowering therapy.

Lifestyle factors

It is important to identify and reduce the patients alterable risk factors, encourage good dietary practices and reduce alcohol intake (especially beer). Review medication and try to find alternatives for medications that are known to increase the likelihood of developing gout.

> **COMMUNICATION**
>
> It is important to take a detailed drug and alcohol history from patients.

> **HINTS AND TIPS**
>
> Do not stop allopurinol in acute flares unless indicated for another reason, i.e., acute renal impairment.

CALCIUM PYROPHOSPHATE DIHYDRATE DISEASE

Definition

Calcium pyrophosphate dihydrate (CPPD) disease is an arthropathy associated with the deposition of CPPD crystals.

Prevalence

CPPD disease is much less common than gout, but much more common in the elderly. There is a slight female preponderance to the condition.

Aetiology

The absolute cause is unknown but the condition is associated with osteoarthritis and other metabolic bone diseases. Attacks are often preceded by intercurrent illness, episodes of physical stress and dehydration.

> **METABOLIC DISEASES THAT PREDISPOSE TO CPPD DISEASE**
>
> - Hypothyroidism
> - Hyperparathyroidism
> - Haemochromatosis
> - Acromegaly
> - Gout

Clinical features

There are two main clinical presentations of CPPD disease:

1. Acute synovitis (pseudogout): This is the most common cause of acute monoarthritis in the elderly. Wrists and knees are most commonly affected. Patients experience pain, swelling, stiffness and occasionally fever. The clinical appearance of affected joints is very similar to gout.
2. Chronic pyrophosphate arthropathy: This is very similar to osteoarthritis with a gradual onset of pain, swelling and loss of joint function. Again, the knees and wrists are most commonly affected, along with the hips, shoulders, elbows and metacarpophalangeal joints. Some patients experience acute attacks of synovitis. Examination reveals changes in keeping with osteoarthritis.

Investigations

Synovial fluid examination

Synovial fluid examination with polarized light microscopy is key to the diagnosis. The CPPD crystals are small rhomboid or rod-shaped crystals that show weak positive birefringence. As with gout, fluid examination should include Gram stain and culture to exclude infection.

Radiology

CPPD causes changes in osteoarthritis that are visible on radiographs, with associated chondrocalcinosis. This calcification is often seen in the menisci of the knee, triangular cartilage of the wrist and symphysis pubis.

Other investigations

Serum calcium should be checked in younger patients. CPPD is very unusual in those <50 years old and if found, prompt screening should be performed for other metabolic diseases.

Management

Attacks of pseudogout are treated with analgesia. Joint aspiration, joint injection with steroids and the use of colchicine can also help. Unlike gout, there is no prophylactic medication that can be given. Other lifestyle factors include losing weight, physiotherapy, pain control and occasionally joint replacement. In very severe cases, a joint washout may be carried out.

● Chapter Summary

- Gout is one of the most common causes of an acute monoarthropathy. It is associated with hyperuricaemia and the deposition of monosodium urate crystals in the joint.
- Clinical features of acute gout include a hot, extremely tender, swollen joint, often with red shiny skin over it. The 1st metatarsal-phalangeal joint is often the first site affected.
- In chronic gout, erosive changes appear on X-ray images, the joints affected may be deformed and there are often hard, chalky deposits (tophi) within the soft tissues.
- Acute gout is managed with nonsteroidal antiinflammatory drugs, colchicine and occasionally corticosteroids. Urate-lowering therapies, such as allopurinol, help prevent against future attacks.
- Calcium pyrophosphate dihydrate disease (pseudogout) is another crystal-arthropathy more common in the elderly and is associated with osteoarthritis and other metabolic bone diseases. It predominantly affects different joints from those affected by gout (wrists and knees). Acute flares of pseudogout are managed similarly to gout attacks.
- Joint aspiration and fluid microscopy is the gold standard test to differentiate between the two conditions.
- All acute monoarthritis is septic until proven otherwise.

UKMLA Conditions
Bursitis
Crystal arthropathy
Septic arthritis

UKMLA Presentations
Acute joint pain/swelling
Musculoskeletal deformity
Soft tissue injury

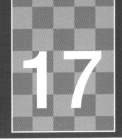
NORMAL VARIANTS

Many referrals to paediatric orthopaedic surgeons are for normal variations in growth of a healthy child noticed by concerned parents. The single most reassuring feature is the symmetrical appearance of the limbs. If the child has only one side affected, the condition is much more likely to be pathological.

Examples of normal conditions commonly referred include the following.

Flat feet

This condition is usually physiological, painless and may be associated with laxity of ligaments. Simple advice should be given as even the use of insoles is questionable and most children develop normally regardless. Pain or fixed deformity suggests an underlying pathological condition.

Toe walkers

Children often take their first steps on tiptoes. Usually the child grows out of this, but examination is required to exclude a tight Achilles tendon or an underlying condition such as cerebral palsy.

In-toeing gait

Causes of in-toeing are found at three levels: the hip, the tibia and the foot.

Persistent femoral torsion leaves the patient with an excessive internal rotation and the child often sits in a W position rather than cross-legged (Fig. 17.1). This condition usually resolves spontaneously as the child grows, but a small number require surgical correction with a femoral osteotomy.

Internal tibial torsion also leads to in-toeing but almost always resolves with no treatment.

In the foot, metatarsus adductus (inwardly pointing forefoot) is a cause of in-toeing and again, this usually resolves over time.

Bow legs (genu varum)

It is normal for toddlers to have bow legs and they almost always grow out of this. Very rarely, pathological conditions such as rickets can cause bowing.

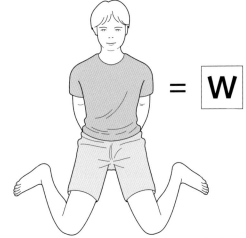

Fig. 17.1 Child sitting in the W position in excessive femoral anteversion.

Knock knees (genu valgum)

Older children (3–8 years old) gradually become more valgus as they grow and the majority straighten spontaneously. Pathological genu valgum is rare, usually asymmetrical, severe and progressive.

PAEDIATRIC HIP DISORDERS

Of all the joint disorders affecting children, the most important are those affecting the hip. Many children with hip disorders will require hip replacement surgery in adult life, with the most severely affected having such surgery aged in their 20s or 30s, and some even in teenage years.

Developmental dysplasia of the hip

Introduction
Previously called congenital dislocation of the hip (CDH), developmental dysplasia of the hip (DDH) describes an abnormal relationship between the femoral head and the acetabulum. This disorder encompasses the spectrum of disease from a frankly dislocated hip to acetabular dysplasia (in which the angle of slope of the acetabular roof is too steep).

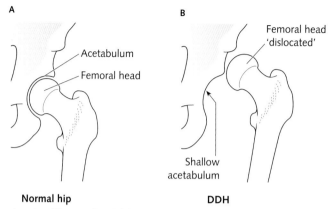

Fig. 17.2 Anatomy of the hip showing (A) normal and (B) pathological hip development. DDH, *Development dysplasia of the hip*.

Incidence

The UK incidence is approximately 1 per 100 live births; however, most of these settle, stabilize and develop normally without treatment.

Aetiology and pathology

The condition is six times more common in females. It is also more common in certain races (northern Italy and North American indigenous population).

DDH is associated with:

- breech presentation
- firstborn children
- family history
- other congenital deformities

The left side is more commonly affected but the condition is bilateral in 20% of cases.

The acetabulum relies on the presence of the femoral head for normal development. In DDH there is excessive laxity of the joint with a shallow acetabulum (Fig. 17.2). This allows the femoral head to develop out of the socket, in severe cases forming a false acetabulum (located superiorly to the normal one).

Clinical features

The majority are picked up on routine baby checks and referred appropriately.

Late-presenting DDH can occur as the child begins to walk. The child will have a limp and shortness of one leg (if unilateral).

The clinical findings of DDH include:

- loss of abduction
- leg length discrepancy
- asymmetrical posterior skin crease

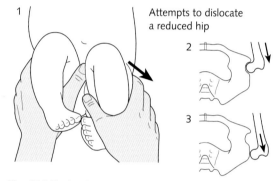

Fig. 17.3 Barlow test: attempts to dislocate a reduced hip.

The special tests for dysplastic hips are called Barlow and Ortolani tests.

Barlow test

This is an attempt to dislocate a dislocatable reduced hip.

The examiner holds the child's thigh so that the thumb is on the medial aspect of the thigh with the middle finger on the trochanter. Then with the child's hip and knee flexed to 90 degrees, the hip is slightly adducted and a gentle downward force applied to try to dislocate the hip. A clunk is felt if positive (Fig. 17.3).

Ortolani test

This is an attempt to reduce a dislocated hip.

Both hips are examined together. The hand is placed in a similar position and the hip is flexed to 90 degrees and then gently abducted. The test is positive if the hip reduces with a clunk.

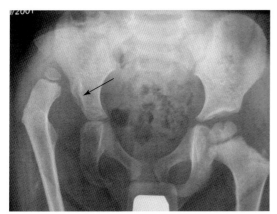

Fig. 17.4 X-ray image showing developmental dysplasia of the hip (*arrow*).

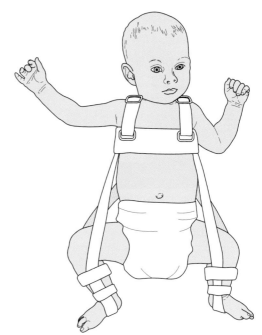

Fig. 17.5 Pavlik harness.

Diagnosis and investigation

All babies are screened clinically by examination at birth but unfortunately this is unreliable. At-risk babies with the factors listed above are also screened with ultrasound. If there is doubt, this investigation can be repeated.

Once the femoral head has ossified, older children should be investigated using X-ray images, which should clearly show if there is a dislocation (Fig. 17.4).

Management

This depends on whether the hip is dislocated and, if so, whether the hip is easily reducible.

Conservative

Conservative treatment can be used in young children who have reducible hips. An abduction splint can be employed to hold the hip in an abducted and stable position, keeping the hip in the joint. The Pavlik harness is an example of such splintage (Fig. 17.5).

Surgical

If the hip cannot be reduced closed, open reduction is performed.

A variety of surgical osteotomies to the pelvis or femur can be used to correct anatomy and maintain reduction.

Prognosis

The outcome depends upon the degree of dysplasia, duration of dislocation and whether or not complications such as osteonecrosis develop. Secondary osteoarthritis is common in this group of patients.

Perthes disease

Introduction

This is a rare disease of unknown aetiology, in which blood supply to the femoral head is interrupted, causing segmental avascular necrosis and collapse of the femoral head. It is often referred to as Legg-Calvé-Perthes disease.

Epidemiology

Approximately 5 to 12 in 100,000 are affected. Perthes disease is four times more common in boys and is bilateral in 12%. It usually presents between the ages of 4 and 8 years but can affect children from the age of 2 to 12 years. It is more common in Whites than in other ethnic groups.

The condition is associated with:

- family history
- lower socioeconomic groups
- low birth weight children
- second-hand smoking
- delayed bone age
- northerly latitude regardless of race

Variable amounts of the femoral head are involved and this affects the outcome. In severe cases of collapse, the proximal femur migrates out of the joint (subluxation).

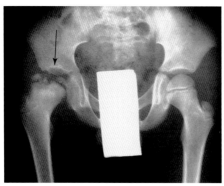

Fig. 17.6 X-ray image of Perthes disease *(arrow)*.

Clinical features

The child (usually a boy) presents with a gradual history of hip or knee pain associated with a limp or Trendelenburg gait. Clinical features will show loss of hip motion, particularly abduction and internal rotation, and there may be fixed deformity. Complete loss of abduction is a worrying sign and may signify subluxation of the hip.

Diagnosis and investigation

Acute Perthes disease in a child could be confused with septic arthritis and therefore inflammatory markers should be checked. These markers are normal in Perthes disease.

A plain X-ray image (Fig. 17.6) is the mainstay of diagnosis. The features of Perthes on X-ray images are:

- Medial joint space widening (earliest)
- Loss of epiphyseal height
- Increased density of the femoral epiphysis
- Subchondral fracture, partial collapse and fragmentation of the head.
- Abnormal shape and size of femoral head
- Subluxation

Magnetic resonance imaging (MRI) is very sensitive for diagnosis and staging and is especially in the early stages of the disease.

Treatment

This depends upon the age of the patient and the extent of the disease. Overall, 75% of children require no treatment and will have a good long-term outcome. Young patients with less than 50% involvement of the femoral head have a good prognosis.

Conservative

Conservative management includes activity restriction and protected weight-bearing, with guided physiotherapy to preserve range of motion and abductor function. This is used in young children with femoral head necrosis of less than 50%.

Surgical

Older patients, female patients (closer to skeletal maturity) and patients with greater than 50% involvement of the epiphysis have a poor prognosis and significant early osteoarthritis is likely. These children may require containment of the femoral head with surgery, e.g., a pelvic or femoral osteotomy.

Slipped capital femoral epiphysis (SCFE)

This condition, previously known as slipped upper femoral epiphysis, is a disorder in which there is structural failure through the growth plate of an immature hip.

Incidence

Approximately 10 per 100,000 children are affected.

It is more common in boys than in girls, usually occurring during the early adolescence growth spurt between 11 and 14 years of age. Approximately 17% to 50% of cases are bilateral.

Aetiology and pathology

Two groups are typically affected: athletic children of either sex or overweight boys with delayed puberty.

The exact cause is not known but may relate to failure of the epiphyseal cartilage to mature as the child grows. Rotational forces acting through the physis then cause the epiphysis to slip.

Obesity is the single greatest risk factor, along with position of femoral head and previous radiation to femoral head. Some hormonal conditions are associated, e.g., hypothyroidism, diabetes mellitus and growth hormone deficiency.

The slip results in the epiphysis lying posterior and inferior to the femoral neck.

Clinical features

The child presents with usually atraumatic groin or knee pain (or both) and a limp. The history can be acute or gradual.

Examination findings reveal an abnormal gait and an external rotation deformity with limitation of most movements. There might be a slight discrepancy in leg length. Check for evidence of hypogonadism, hypopituitarism and hypothyroidism.

Diagnosis and investigation

Diagnosis is based on changes seen in X-ray images. An anteroposterior (AP) X-ray image is taken, but the frog lateral view demonstrates the pathology most clearly (Fig. 17.7).

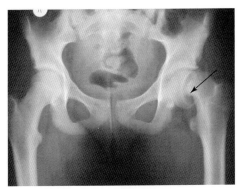

Fig. 17.7 X-ray image of slipped upper femoral epiphysis *(arrow)*.

Management

Surgical

Once diagnosed, the epiphysis should be pinned in situ to prevent further displacement as soon as possible. Consideration should be given to fixing the other hip prophylactically.

Attempts to reduce severe slips are associated with avascular necrosis and these cases are approached cautiously.

Prognosis

There is a high incidence of secondary degenerative osteoarthritis.

CONGENITAL TALIPES EQUINOVARUS (CLUBFOOT)

Congenital talipes equinovarus encompasses a deformity of the lower limb with calf wasting and the classic inwardly pointing foot.

Incidence

The incidence is approximately 1 per 1000 live births. Boys are affected twice as often as girls and half of cases are bilateral.

Aetiology and pathology

The exact aetiology is not known, but arrest of normal limb bud development in utero may be the cause. Genetic factors play a role, with family history being important.

The basic pathology is at the level of the subtalar joint with a cavus deformity (high arch) and metatarsus adductus (Fig. 17.8). The Achilles tendon is also tight, resulting in an equinus deformity.

Associated soft-tissue contractures occur on the medial side.

Clinical features

The condition is easily noted at birth as a fixed varus and equinus deformity of the hindfoot. The calf is underdeveloped when compared with the normal side.

The baby should be examined for associated syndromes or conditions (such as spina bifida or DDH).

Diagnosis and investigation

The diagnosis is a clinical one and X-ray images are usually taken after initial treatment or surgery.

Management

Conservative

Initial treatment is with serial manipulation and casting (Ponseti method), changed weekly for up to 3 months, achieving a 90% success rate.

Surgical

Surgery is reserved for those cases that fail to correct fully or for later recurrence.

Prognosis

Success rates with the Ponseti method are greater than 90% for avoiding comprehensive surgical release.

OSTEOGENESIS IMPERFECTA

Also known as brittle bone disease, osteogenesis imperfecta (OI) is a type I collagen disorder predisposing a patient to multiple fragility fractures.

Incidence

The condition is rare. In the United States, the incidence is approximately 1 in 20,000 live births.

Aetiology and pathology

There are four different types of OI. The primary abnormality is a defect in the synthesis of type I collagen, leading to either abnormal collagen or decreased quantities of collagen.

OI is usually inherited as an autosomal dominant condition (types 1 and 4), although sporadic and recessive cases can occur (types 2 and 3). 90% of cases have an identifiable genetic mutation.

Clinical features

The child may present with a low-energy fracture and the diagnosis is made subsequently, following examination and investigation.

Blue sclerae are pathognomonic and present in types 1 and 2 OI. Children are usually small with bony deformities (including

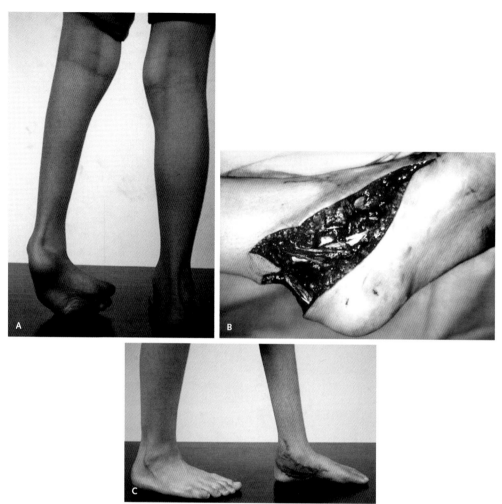

Fig. 17.8 (A) Untreated talipes equinovarus showing inversion contracture. (B) Intraoperative view showing release of soft tissues. (C) Postoperative image showing corrected deformity and soft tissue coverage. (With permission from Zuker RM, Bains RD. Gracilis flap. In Wei FC, Mardini S, eds. *Flaps and Reconstructive Surgery*. 2nd ed. Elsevier; 2017.)

scoliosis) and joint abnormalities. Associated features include deafness, joint laxity, altered dentition (brownish teeth), dysmorphic facies and valvular defects.

Diagnosis and investigation

X-ray images may show:

- multiple fractures (can lead to a 'saber shin' appearance of the tibia)
- deformity
- thin-looking cortices

Treatment

Conservative

Gentle handling of patients is needed to prevent fractures.

Bisphosphonates such as pamidronate can be given intravenously to try to improve bone strength.

Surgical

Intramedullary telescoping rods are the mainstay of treatment for the prevention of deformity and further fracture.

Established deformity is treated with osteotomy.

Prognosis

The outcome depends on the type of OI: some types, such as type 2, are lethal.

CEREBRAL PALSY

Definition

This is a nonprogressive upper motor neurone, neuromuscular disorder that results from injury to an immature brain.

Incidence

Incidence is 2 per 1000 births.

Aetiology and pathology

The cause is often unknown but can include prematurity, perinatal anoxia, perinatal infection, including meningitis and kernicterus.

Clinical features

There is a mixture of muscle weakness and spasticity. This can lead to characteristic joint deformities, contractures, fractures and hip subluxation. There may be athetosis and ataxia. This can be associated with varying degrees of cognitive impairment and emotional disturbance. Children may also develop seizures.

CLINICAL NOTES

Characteristic joint deformities associated with cerebral palsy

- Flexion at elbows and wrists with clasped fingers
- Adductor spasticity of the hips, resulting in a scissors stance
- Flexion at the hips and knees
- Equinus deformity of the feet

Diagnosis and investigation

Cerebral palsy is a clinical diagnosis based on a thorough birth and developmental history and is normally apparent within the first 2 years of life. MRI of the brain may show periventricular leukomalacia.

Management

Conservative

Depending on the severity of the disease, children will benefit from physiotherapy, occupational therapy, speech and language therapy and other forms of special needs care.

Surgical

In children who have not developed fixed contractures, intramuscular botulinum injections can temporarily reduce spasticity. For fixed deformity, soft-tissue release or tendon lengthening is required to improve function. Severe muscle imbalance can result in bone deformity, sometimes requiring corrective osteotomy.

NONACCIDENTAL INJURY

Nonaccidental injury (NAI) is becoming increasingly recognized and is often diagnosed late. A diagnosis is critical to prevent further harm, and in some cases, to prevent death.

Clinical features

The history is often vague, inappropriate or changes each time it is told. In young children (<2 years), it is rare for accidental fractures to occur, particularly in long bones. Delayed presentation is often a feature of NAI.

The child may have external features of abuse such as bruising (with bruises of varying age) in other areas of the body away from the fracture. The child may be withdrawn, particularly when the parents are present.

Diagnosis and investigation

In suspected cases, a skeletal survey or bone scan is performed to look for occult fractures. Certain fractures such as of the rib or tibial metaphysis are typical of NAI.

Conditions such as OI can be confused with NAI.

Management

The child should be admitted for protection if NAI is strongly suspected and the fracture should be treated in the usual way.

Paediatricians and social workers are involved from admission.

Prognosis

A child left in an abusive environment has a 5% risk of death.

PAEDIATRIC KNEE CONDITIONS

Osgood-Schlatter's disease

Definition

Osgood-Schlatter's disease is traction apophysitis of the tibial tuberosity.

Incidence

The condition is very common, usually in adolescent boys.

Aetiology and pathology

It occurs during a period of rapid growth and is related to the pulling force of the patellar ligament on the tibial tuberosity (Fig. 17.9).

It is more common in athletic individuals.

Clinical features

The patient complains of localized pain over the tubercle. The pain is usually made worse by activity and relieved by rest.

Clinically, a tender swollen tuberosity is found.

Diagnosis and investigation

Fragmentation and sclerosis of the tibial tuberosity are present. Sometimes a visible ossicle remains.

Management

Conservative

Treatment is rest if the knee is very inflamed, with simple analgesia and modification of activities. Parents are usually very worried and need reassurance that conservative management is usually successful in 90% of patients. The child may choose to put up with the pain and continue sporting activities and this has no detrimental effect and will not prolong the natural history of the disease process.

Surgical

Surgery is used only for a painful ossicle whereby it can be excised. This treatment is reserved for refractory cases in skeletally mature patients.

Prognosis

The natural history is complete resolution of symptoms after 2 years.

Osteochondritis dissecans

Definition

Osteochondritis dissecans is a small area of avascular bone on an articular surface, usually in the knee.

Incidence

The incidence is 4 per 1000. Presentation is between 10 and 15 years of age and is more common in boys.

Aetiology and pathology

The condition is most common in the knee (medial femoral condyle) but can affect other joints. It is thought to be due to repeated trauma in a susceptible patient.

Clinical features

The patient has intermittent ache, swelling and catching of the knee. The patient may complain of the knee giving way owing to acute sharp episodes of pain.

Diagnosis and investigation

X-ray images show a variably sized lesion on the medial femoral condyle, which is fragmented in the child, but in mature adults the lesion shows as a clear, demarcated sclerotic zone. The lesion can be attached or may be a loose body.

An MRI scan will help define the lesion. An isotope bone scan confirms the presence of activity and hence healing potential.

Management

Conservative

Activity modification with avoidance of sporting activity, restricted weightbearing and bracing, is adequate to allow small well-fixed lesions to heal. Younger age correlates with better prognosis.

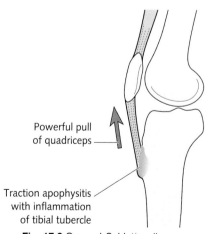

Powerful pull of quadriceps

Traction apophysitis with inflammation of tibial tubercle

Fig. 17.9 Osgood-Schlatter disease.

Surgical

Lesions that become detached or give significant persistent symptoms require surgical stabilization. If the fragment becomes a loose body, removal may be the only option.

Juvenile idiopathic arthritis

Definition

Juvenile idiopathic arthritis (JIA) is a chronic inflammatory condition in children primarily involving synovial joints. In JIA, symptoms persist for more than 6 weeks in patients younger than 16 years of age. It is a diagnosis of exclusion.

JIA has been classified into seven subtypes. This classification is based partly on the number of joints involved 3 months into the disease process. It is useful as a guide to prognosis.

CLINICAL NOTES

The subtypes of juvenile idiopathic arthritis
- Oligoarticular disease
- Extended oligoarticular disease
- Polyarticular disease: rheumatoid factor-negative
- Polyarticular disease: rheumatoid factor-positive
- Systemic-onset disease
- Enthesitis-related arthritis
- Psoriatic arthritis

Incidence and prevalence

Incidence is approximately 1 per 10,000 and prevalence is 10 per 10,000 children.

Clinical features

Joint disease

Children develop symptoms and signs of joint inflammation similar to those in adults, including joint pain, stiffness and swelling. Presentation depends on the joints affected and the age of the child. A 12-year-old with knee synovitis will complain of pain, whereas a 2-year-old may just be irritable and reluctant to mobilize. Paediatric Gait Arms Legs Spine (p-GALS) is a useful screening tool when examining children.

Joints from most frequently affected to least affected: knee > hand/wrist > ankle > hip > cervical spine.

Eye disease

Some forms of JIA can be associated with anterior uveitis. Acute anterior uveitis presents with pain and redness of the eye. Chronic anterior uveitis, however, is more insidious and can cause significant visual loss. All children with JIA need regular eye checks.

Constitutional symptoms

Fatigue, malaise and other systemic symptoms affect JIA patients, in particular those with systemic-onset disease. Growth retardation is an important consequence of prolonged inflammation in childhood.

Juvenile idiopathic arthritis subtypes

Oligoarticular disease

This is the most common subtype. Between one and four joints are affected, commonly in the lower limb. The prognosis is good and many children grow out of it. This group of patients has the greatest risk of developing chronic anterior uveitis.

Extended oligoarticular disease

Initially, fewer than four joints are involved, but these patients gradually develop polyarthritis after the first 3 months. The outcome is often poor.

Polyarticular disease

More than four joints are affected from an early stage. There are two types. Rheumatoid factor–negative arthritis targets small and large joints and tends to persist into adult life. Rheumatoid factor–positive arthritis is the equivalent of adult rheumatoid arthritis. It is seen mainly in teenage girls and frequently has a poor outcome.

Systemic-onset disease

This arthritis is characterized by prominent systemic symptoms. It was previously known as Stills disease. Patients present with a swinging fever, plus any of the following features:

- rash
- hepatomegaly
- splenomegaly
- anaemia
- lymphadenopathy
- serositis, especially pericarditis

The differential diagnosis includes infection and malignancy. Joint involvement may initially be mild or absent.

Enthesitis-related arthritis

Inflammation of entheses, e.g., Achilles tendonitis, is a prominent feature. Enthesitis-related arthritis encompasses juvenile ankylosing spondylitis. A positive family history of ankylosing spondylitis or related diseases is common and patients are often HLA B27-positive.

Psoriatic arthritis

This is usually oligoarticular and often involves weight-bearing joints. A personal or family history of psoriasis is common.

Investigations

The diagnosis of JIA is clinical. X-ray images are helpful in excluding other causes of joint pain, such as malignancy, but are usually normal in early JIA.

Blood tests are useful, but not diagnostic. Full blood count may reveal anaemia or thrombocytosis and the erythrocyte sedimentation rate and C-reactive protein are usually elevated. Serum rheumatoid factor should be measured. It is also important to know whether the patient has positive antinuclear antibodies, as they are associated with an increased risk of uveitis.

> **HINTS AND TIPS**
>
> All children with juvenile idiopathic arthritis should be seen by a rheumatologist.

Management

Physiotherapy

This is vital to maintain mobility and function. Hydrotherapy is commonly used and is popular with children. Splinting is sometimes required to prevent deformity.

Drug treatment

Initial treatment is with nonsteroidal antiinflammatory drugs and corticosteroid joint injections. Disease-modifying therapy with drugs such as methotrexate is used. Corticosteroids may be necessary in severe or systemic-onset disease. Biological agents, such as the antitumour necrosis factor drugs, are indicated for children with persistent major synovitis or unresolving systemic features.

Eye screening

Children should have their eyes examined regularly by an ophthalmologist.

> **HINTS AND TIPS**
>
> Eye screening is particularly important in young children with juvenile idiopathic arthritis, as they do not reliably report visual disturbance to their parents.

● Chapter Summary

- There are many normal variations of gait that do not need intervention. However, there are several conditions that require investigation and intervention.
- Developmental dysplasia of the hip should be picked up on examination after birth, but this is not always the case. An abduction brace such as a Pavlik harness can often treat it.
- Perthes disease is idiopathic avascular necrosis (AVN) of the femoral head and can cause significant osteoarthritis at a young age and can require pelvic osteotomy.
- Slipped capital femoral epiphysis should be picked up on X-ray examination and is most common between 11 and 14 years of age. The most common resting position of the leg is in fixed external rotation. It is also likely to happen on the other side. It often requires fixation in situ rather than reduction due to the AVN risk.
- Clubfoot or talipes equinovarus is often treatable in a cast and only rarely requires surgery.
- There are four different types of osteogenesis imperfecta and they can lead to multiple fractures due to weak bones. It should not be confused with nonaccidental injury.
- Knee pain is common in children and can be caused by hip problems. Osgood-Schlatter disease and osteochondritis dissecans can also cause knee pain.
- Cerebral palsy can have orthopaedic manifestations with a mixture of weakness and spasticity causing contractures.
- Juvenile idiopathic arthritis has several subtypes and is a chronic inflammatory condition involving synovial joints.

UKMLA Conditions
Ankylosing spondylitis
Cerebral palsy
Idiopathic arthritis
Nonaccidental injury

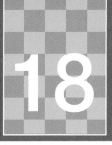
In this chapter we will discuss the principles of managing basic fractures, particularly of the wrist, hip and ankle. Advanced Trauma Life Support (ATLS) and the management of a multiply injured patient are both covered in Chapter 19.

INCIDENCE

Fractures are very common and most of us will have at least one during a lifetime. They occur in peaks during childhood and young adult life when risk-taking behaviour is more common, and again in old age, when osteoporosis has weakened bony structures meaning that simple accidents can cause significant fractures (see Chapter 11).

DEFINITIONS

The following are the terms used to describe fractures (Fig. 18.1):

- Fracture: loss of continuity of the cortex of a bone.
- Pathological fracture: a fracture through bone weakened by a preexisting pathological process.
- Simple: a bone fractured into two pieces.
- Comminuted: a bone in three or more pieces.
- Segmental: fractures at two levels of the same bone.
- Closed: a fracture with intact skin overlying it.
- Open: a fracture with a skin overlying it so that the fracture communicates with the outside world (formerly known as a compound fracture).
- Extraarticular: a fracture that leaves the adjacent joint entirely undamaged.
- Intraarticular: a fracture that involves a joint.
- Undisplaced: a fractured bone with its anatomy unchanged.
- Displaced: a fracture which has its component parts in a non-anatomical position. Displacement describes the position of the distal fragment in relation to the proximal fragment. A displaced fracture may have component parts that are translated, angulated, rotated or distracted for example.
- Fracture pattern: may be transverse, oblique or spiral.

The causes of pathological fractures are shown in the box.

UNDERLYING CAUSES OF PATHOLOGICAL FRACTURES

- Osteoporosis
- Tumour
  - Metastases (more common than primary bone tumours)
  - Primary bone tumour
    - Benign, e.g., osteoid osteoma, osteoblastoma, enchondroma
    - Malignant, e.g., osteosarcoma, Ewing sarcoma
  - Haematological malignancy
  - Lymphoma
  - Myeloma
- Infection
- Bisphosphonate use
- Metabolic bone disease
  - Osteomalacia/rickets
  - Hyperparathyroidism
  - Paget's disease
  - Osteogenesis imperfecta

In children, a fracture may occur through the growth plate (physis) and these injuries are classified as shown in Fig. 18.2.

When concentrating on the bone, it is easy to forget the soft tissues surrounding the bone. Soft-tissue integrity is vital, as it is the soft tissues that provide a healing environment to the injured bone. However, soft tissues are unable to heal without bony stability underneath. A fracture should be thought of as a soft-tissue injury with a broken bone inside; both must be carefully considered before healing can occur.

CLINICAL FEATURES

The patient almost always gives a clear history of an injury. Difficulties can arise if the patient cannot give a history, e.g., because of dementia in the elderly, intoxication or coma in major trauma (see Chapter 19). In cases where the history cannot be directly elicited, information must be obtained from a third person such as a carer, witness to the accident or ambulance personnel.

Patients will complain of pain, may be unable to weight bear and they may have noticed a deformity (e.g., 'my ankle pointed

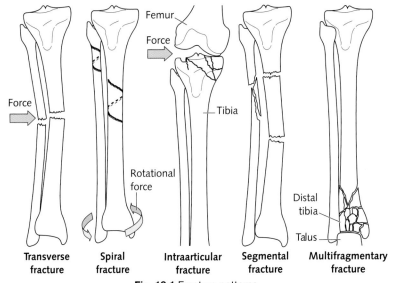

Fig. 18.1 Fracture patterns.

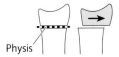

Type I
Fracture through physis only

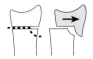

Type II (most common)
Fracture travels through physis but part of metaphysis is involved

Type III
Epiphyseal segment separated (intraarticular fracture)

Type IV
Fracture crosses physis and involves joint interface
Requires accurate reduction to prevent growth problems leading to deformity

Type V
Crush injury
Difficult to diagnose initially becomes obvious later when growth arrest occurs

Fig. 18.2 The Salter-Harris classification of fractures of the growth plate (physeal fractures).

the wrong way') which they may have had corrected at the scene of injury.

The patient should be examined as a whole for associated injuries as per ATLS guidelines, and then the injured limb should be examined. The affected limb will be swollen and bruised with significant localized tenderness on palpation.

It is very important to note and to document:

- Skin integrity (i.e., is the fracture open or closed, are there associated blisters or abrasion overlying the fracture, is there any significant soft tissue swelling (meaning closure after surgery may be challenging)
- Peripheral nerve function: any weakness or numbness distal to the injury
- Distal vascular status: assess peripheral pulses and capillary refill distal to the injury

Compare the abnormal limb with the normal limb.

DIAGNOSIS AND INVESTIGATION

Radiographs should be taken in at least two orthogonal planes (90 degrees to each other), usually anteroposterior (AP) and lateral, and include both ends of the injured bone. The anatomical area in question should be in the centre of the X-ray image (Fig. 18.3). Special views are required for certain fractures (e.g., scaphoid views).

CT scans are helpful to diagnose and categorize complex fractures and to plan surgery, as a 3D image can be constructed.

Magnetic resonance imaging (MRI) or isotope bone scans are occasionally used to diagnose a fracture where doubt exists or to assess associated soft-tissue injuries.

Describing X-ray images

This is something which requires a systematic approach and practice. When asked to comment on an X-ray image, always state:

- The name and age of patient, and date and time of X-ray examination (this proves that you are looking at the correct radiograph).
- Which anatomical region is shown, e.g., anterior-posterior (AP) X-ray examination of a pelvis lateral X-ray examination of a wrist.

Remember ABC:

- A is for *a*dequacy and *a*lignment (is the film rotated? And is it of acceptable quality, i.e., too light (overpenetrated) or too dark (underpenetrated)?).
- B is for *b*one:
  - State which bone is fractured, e.g., tibia.
  - State where in the bone the fracture is, i.e., metaphysis/diaphysis/epiphysis.
  - State whether the fracture is simple or comminuted.
  - Comment on the fracture pattern: transverse, oblique, spiral, segmental.
  - Describe the displacement of the fracture (Fig. 18.4).
  - Comment on whether the joint is involved or not: intraarticular/extraarticular.
  - Comment on whether the joint is congruent or dislocated/subluxated.
- C is for *c*overing soft tissues: look for air (may indicate an open fracture), foreign material, soft tissue swelling or joint fluid (haemarthrosis or lipohaemarthrosis (Fig 4.12)).

COMMUNICATION

When describing a fracture remember to add important clinical features of the patient which will aid surgical planning:

- The general medical condition of patient; are they currently well enough for an operation? What is their level of functioning usually? Do they walk with a walking aid or need carers to help with activities of daily living?
- Skin and soft tissue envelope – is it open or closed? (Fig. 18.5)
- Neurovascular status – with respect to the relevant named nerves distal to the fracture

---

MANAGEMENT

Initial management

A trauma patient must first be managed in an ATLS manner with an A–E approach. You must ensure there are no imminent life or limb-threatening injuries, and that the patient's general condition is optimized.

Then (with respect to relevant national guidelines such as the British Orthopaedic Association Standards for Trauma):

- For open fractures: take photographs with a workplace camera (important for surgical planning in conjunction with the plastic surgeons), remove any large debris, irrigate the wound with saline and cover the wound with sterile dressings before splinting the fracture. Ensure antibiotic cover and tetanus prophylaxis are administered (see Chapter 19).
- Immobilize the fracture: back-slab/splint/brace/sling where appropriate.
- Give adequate and appropriate analgesia – this will often mean opiates.
- Arrange imaging and further investigations.

Definitive management

The basic principles for the treatment of any fracture are:

- Reduction of any deformity (displacement, angulation, rotation), i.e., put the bones back into the correct place
- Stabilization (maintain reduction until healing occurs)
- Rehabilitation (rehabilitate the limb and the patient)

Reduction

Reduction can be performed in either a closed or open manner.

- Closed reduction is performed by manipulating the fracture into position without opening the soft tissue envelope. This can be done under sedation or a general anaesthetic.
- Open reduction is performed in the operating theatre and involves a surgical procedure to open the soft tissues down to the fracture site and to reduce the bones accurately under direct vision. It is usually accompanied by operative stabilization.

Intraarticular fractures are usually treated with open reduction so that the joint can be accurately and anatomically reduced, minimizing the risk of secondary osteoarthritis.

Stabilization

This can be achieved without an operation by external splinting, e.g., a plaster cast. Intraoperative fixation can be with percutaneous wires, open reduction and fixation with plates and screws, minimally invasive intramedullary nail for long-bone fractures or external frame fixation (Fig. 18.6).

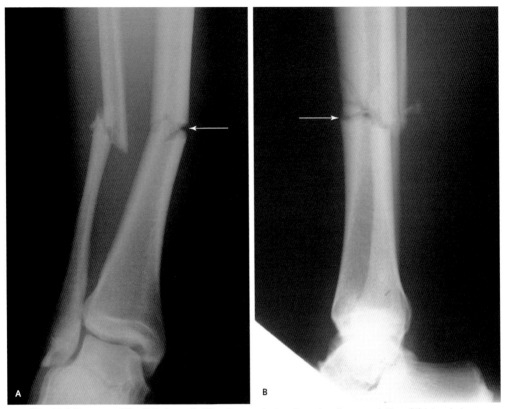

Fig. 18.3 Fracture of the tibia (*arrow*): (A) anteroposterior view showing angulation; (B) lateral view.

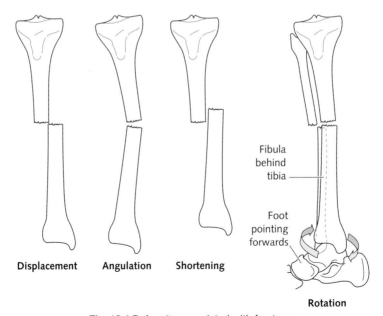

Displacement   Angulation   Shortening

Fibula
behind
tibia

Foot
pointing
forwards

Rotation

Fig. 18.4 Deformity associated with fractures.

Rehabilitation

Once the fracture is immobilized and stable, the limb can be mobilized and range-of-motion exercises can begin. One of the principles of operative stabilization is not only to allow early mobilization on the affected limb but also to reduce the more general risks of the patient being immobile (e.g., deep vein thrombosis (DVT), pulmonary embolism (PE), chest infection).

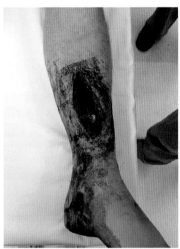

Fig. 18.5 An open tibial fracture. (With permission from Jones CB, Wenke JC. Open fractures. In Browner B, Jupiter JBM, Krettek C, Anderson P, eds. *Skeletal Trauma: Basic Science, Management, and Reconstruction.* 5th ed. Saunders, Elsevier; 2015.)

Rehabilitation of the limb may often take as much time as the fracture took to heal.

Following a hip fracture, for example, elderly patients require intensive input from physiotherapy, occupational therapy and sometimes social workers in order to become self-caring and safe prior to discharge.

COMPLICATIONS OF FRACTURES

Complications can be categorized as local or general, and immediate, early or late.

Immediate

Local

Initial fracture displacement can cause the skin to tear, resulting in an open fracture. Fracture fragments may press on or entrap nerves, producing a nerve palsy (common in the humerus, resulting in radial nerve palsy), or blood vessels, producing ischaemia (e.g., distal femur/proximal tibia; popliteal vessels).

Very occasionally, nerves and blood vessels are completely torn and urgent repair is needed.

General

Haemorrhage from fractures can be substantial, especially from the femur and pelvis, and in open fractures or multiply injured patients. Hypovolaemic shock may result (see Chapter 20).

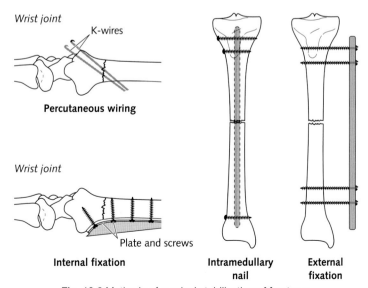

Fig. 18.6 Methods of surgical stabilization of fractures.

Early

Local

Compartment syndrome

Compartment syndrome is a true emergency in orthopaedics. It can occur anywhere that muscle is surrounded by a fascial compartment and results from excessive pressure developing within the fascial muscle compartment. The forearm and lower leg are the most common sites. While uncommon, if left untreated, the condition can be limb- or even life-threatening. Following an injury (within a few hours usually), swelling can cause the blood supply to the muscle to be impaired, causing muscle ischaemia. This occurs at the level of small vessels and peripheral pulses are usually still present. The patient will complain of extreme pain (much more than expected for the injury) and they will have a sharp increase in pain on passive stretching of the muscles in the compartment. Paraesthesia and pulselessness are late signs; in such cases irreparable damage has already occurred. The diagnosis is clinical (it is possible to confirm it with compartment pressure monitoring, but a normal reading does not rule it out). Any circumferential bandage or splint should be removed immediately, the limb raised to the level of the heart as the patient lies in bed and strong analgesia (IV morphine) given. If the pain does not settle within 30 minutes, surgical decompression (fasciotomy) is required at once.

> **RED FLAG**
>
> ## COMPARTMENT SYNDROME
>
> An emergency not to be missed:
> - Pain exceeding the expected level for the injury, particularly on passive stretch of muscles in the affected compartment. This is the first sign and the most important.
> - No pulses (late sign).
> - Paraesthesia (late sign).
> - Paralysis (late sign, poor prognosis of recovery).

Infection

This can occur early or late, following operative stabilization or open fracture. See Chapter 21.

Complex regional pain syndrome

See Chapter 4.

General

Thromboembolism

DVT can occur more commonly after any pelvic or lower-limb injury and resultant surgery. Prevention, in the form of mechanical agents (foot pumps, graduated compression stockings) or chemical agents (anticoagulants or antiplatelets), is routinely used perioperatively.

When examining a patient postoperatively, the affected limb will be swollen and may be painful because of the injury. It can be difficult to determine if there is an underlying DVT, and if in doubt, further imaging should be obtained in the form of an ultrasound. Patients are treated prophylactically with anticoagulation with lower-limb fractures unless contraindicated. Pulmonary embolism is a rare, but potentially fatal, complication of DVT.

> **CLINICAL NOTES**
>
> ### DEEP VEIN THROMBOSIS PROPHYLAXIS
>
> Used in all cases where prolonged immobility is likely and there are no contraindications. Local guidelines will vary.
> Mechanical: antiembolism stockings, pneumatic compression devices.
> Pharmacological: low-molecular-weight subcutaneous heparin injection, aspirin.

Fat embolism syndrome

This condition may occur after long-bone fractures (particularly of the femur) or intramedullary nailing of long bones. It occurs when fat from the medullary canal enters the circulation and embolizes to the lungs. Early stabilization of fractures reduces the risk and this may be with an external fixator as a temporary measure.

The patient presents with shortness of breath, petechial haemorrhages and sometimes confusion from low circulating oxygen levels, usually within 24 hours of injury or operation.

This condition is potentially very serious and, in some cases, fatal. Treatment is supportive with oxygen and fluids. The patient should be transferred to a high-dependency unit.

Late

Delayed union/nonunion

Some fractures are slow to unite or fail to do so despite adequate treatment. This can be due to injury factors or patient factors. Certain fractures (e.g., of the tibia) are more prone to this and it is more likely if the initial injury was high-energy or complicated by compartment syndrome. Further surgery and insertion of bone graft may be required to encourage the bone to heal. Some patients are more likely to suffer a delayed union or nonunion fracture. Included in this group are diabetics, smokers and immunosuppressed patients.

Malunion

The fracture heals but in an abnormal position. This can be due to inadequate reduction or stabilization of the fracture. The resulting deformity may reduce movement in an associated joint and predisposes to postoperative arthritis.

Osteoarthritis

Osteoarthritis, which is discussed in Chapter 11, is more common and may occur at a younger age, after intraarticular fractures.

Stiffness

Prolonged immobilization can lead to serious stiffness in the joints. This issue can also arise if there is a delay in starting physiotherapy and the recommended rehabilitation exercises. The joint may then be held in a resultant flexed position due to ligament and capsular contracture.

Growth disturbance

Fractures occurring through the growth plate in children can cause growth arrest. Growth arrest can be partial (i.e., one side of the limb grows, the other does not), leading to deformity, or complete, leading to shortness of the limb. Growth arrest can also be caused by placing wires/screws across growth plates and therefore transphyseal fixation devices should be kept to a bare minimum and removed once the fracture has healed. Treatment of such problems is complex. Young patients are usually followed up more closely than adults, when fractures and operations cross the growth plate, for this reason.

COMMON FRACTURES

Any bone can be fractured. Different fracture patterns and treatment options are extensive. It is beyond the realms of this book to cover all of them. We have selected the three most common fractures to discuss further: distal radius, hip and ankle fractures.

Distal radial fractures

These are common at all stages of life, from greenstick fractures in children to osteoporotic fractures in the elderly. They are usually the result of a fall on to an outstretched hand.

Clinical features

The patient will present with a grossly swollen and deformed wrist (the deformity will depend upon the type of fracture). Pain will be the main complaint and the patient will hold their wrist still so as not to exacerbate the pain. The patient may complain of altered sensation in the hand due to dysfunction of the median nerve if they develop an associated traumatic

carpal tunnel syndrome. The most common fracture is dorsally translated and dorsally and radially angulated. This is known as a Colles fracture. A distal radius fracture that is volarly translated and angulated is a Smith fracture (Fig. 18.7). Use of the eponymous names of fractures is becoming less common. Being able to describe the fracture on an X-ray is more important and reduces the risk of inter-reporter variability. Having an awareness of these eponymous terms will however be beneficial, as some people still use them.

HINTS AND TIPS
EPONYMOUS NAMES IN ORTHOPAEDICS
Care should be taken when using eponymous terms such as Colles or Smith to describe a fracture. Colles is a term that is often used incorrectly to describe any fracture at the distal radius with dorsal displacement, but its definition is a specific term describing a transverse, extraarticular fracture, 2.5 cm proximal to the radiocarpal joint with dorsal displacement and dorsal angulation.

Investigations

Wrist fractures are diagnosed by plain X-ray examinations. Heavily comminuted or intraarticular fractures may require a CT scan, for planning prior to theatre.

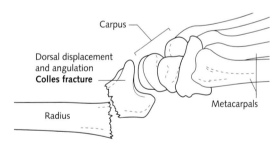
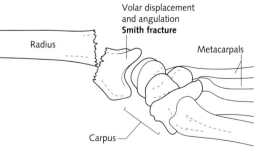

Fig. 18.7 Common distal radial fractures (*lateral view*).

Treatment

The fracture pattern and the age, comorbidity and function of the patient will influence treatment.

Undisplaced fractures of the wrist, minimally angulated fractures and angulated fractures in the elderly may require immobilization in a cast for 4 to 6 weeks or simply splintage if they are comfortable. Very comminuted and intraarticular fractures, and angulated fractures in higher demand, or more active, patients will require manipulation and K-wiring or open reduction and internal fixation.

Whichever treatment option is used, the wrist will often be stiff afterwards and require physiotherapy to restore a satisfactory range of movement.

Hip fractures

Hip fractures (femoral neck fractures) are very common. They particularly occur in elderly patients with osteoporosis. Femoral neck fractures can also occur as pathological fractures related to malignancy. They are rare in young patients, normally only occur after high-energy trauma, and are subject to different considerations. Hip fractures in the elderly have a huge impact on health resources, as well as having major implications for the patient with regard to mortality, disability and loss of independence. A hip fracture can be seen as a sign of frailty – approximately one-third of patients with a hip fracture will die within a year of injury.

Hip fractures can be broadly divided into (Fig. 18.8):

- intracapsular fractures
- extracapsular fractures (intertrochanteric, subtrochanteric)

The blood supply to the femoral head originates predominantly from the medial femoral circumflex artery which arises from the profunda femoris. The branches of the medial femoral circumflex artery travel from the capsular attachment along the intertrochanteric line to the femoral head and are closely attached to the posterior femoral neck. Consequently:

- In an intracapsular fracture (Fig. 18.9A), the fracture line is between the blood supply and the femoral head, potentially severing the blood supply to the head. This leads to a risk of avascular necrosis and nonunion.
- In an extracapsular fracture (Fig. 18.9B), the femoral head is in continuity with its blood supply and therefore there is usually little risk of avascular necrosis.

Aetiology

Most hip fractures are the result of a simple fall from standing height, in an elderly patient.

Clinical features

The patient will complain of severe pain around the affected hip or in the groin. This pain will be exacerbated by any attempt

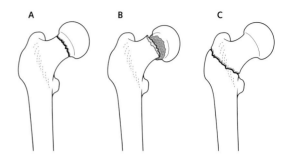

Fig. 18.8 Fractures of the femoral neck. (A) Undisplaced intracapsular fracture. (B) Displaced intracapsular fracture. (C) Extracapsular trochanteric fracture.

to move the leg. The patient will usually be unable to bear any weight on the affected side.

Classically, patients will have a shortened and externally rotated leg. They will be unable to raise the leg straight because of pain in the hip or groin. The patient might demonstrate tenderness on palpation over the greater trochanter or in the groin.

Diagnosis

Femoral neck fractures are usually diagnosed with plain film X-ray images (AP pelvis and lateral hip views). However, occult fractures might not be obvious on X-ray examination and further imaging such as a CT or MRI scan may be required.

Treatment

Nonoperative treatment with immobilization has high mortality and morbidity. In the vast majority of cases, femoral neck fractures are treated surgically. Postoperative patients are mobilized early to minimize these complications. Even when faced with a bed-bound nursing home resident, surgeons usually advocate operating to provide pain relief to allow the patient to transfer more comfortably.

Intracapsular fractures can be divided into undisplaced and displaced.

- Undisplaced fractures (Fig. 18.8A) have a low chance of disruption to the blood supply of the femoral head and can be treated with internal fixation (Fig 18.10). However, a third will develop avascular necrosis or a nonunion, and therefore patients must be followed up closely.
- Displaced fractures (Fig. 18.11) are normally treated with hemiarthroplasty; the femoral head is removed and the implanted artificial head will articulate with the normal acetabulum. A total hip replacement may be more appropriate in young or active patients where the femoral head and the acetabulum are replaced (Fig. 18.12).

Extracapsular fractures are trochanteric or subtrochanteric and are treated with internal fixation with either a dynamic hip screw (Fig. 18.10) or an intramedullary nail (Fig. 18.13).

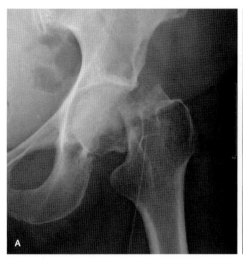
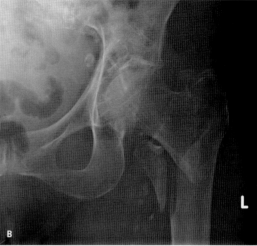

Fig. 18.9 (A) Intracapsular fracture with the fracture line potentially severing the blood supply to the head; (B) extracapsular fracture with blood supply intact.

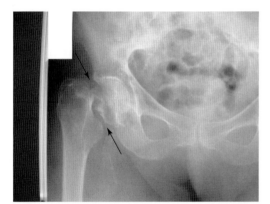

Fig. 18.10 Displaced intracapsular hip fracture *(arrows)*

CLINICAL NOTES

The subtrochanteric region is a common place for metastatic deposits. Be suspicious of an atypical fracture in this region in a young patient with a low-energy injury and consider getting preoperative imaging in the form of an MRI or bone scan ± a biopsy for tissue diagnosis.

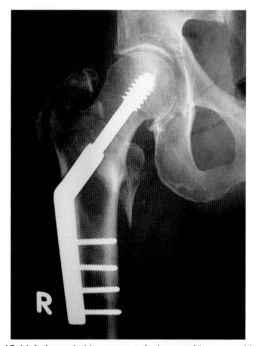

Fig. 18.11 A dynamic hip screw, a device used to secure hip fractures where the hip fracture is extracapsular as shown. The device is dynamic; the screw can collapse down as the fracture heals. (From Garden OJ, et al. Principles and Practice of Surgery. 8th ed. Elsevier; 2023.)

Ankle fractures

The tibia and fibula form a mortice in which the talar dome sits, supported by surrounding ligaments. Damage to the bones or ligaments can lead to instability in the ankle joint.

Clinical features

Following an injury, the patient will describe pain and swelling around the ankle (medially or laterally or both) and will be unable to bear weight. The ankle might be obviously deformed. There will be tenderness over fracture and any torn ligaments. The fibula can fracture anywhere along its length: palpate for tenderness along its entire length. A high fibular fracture results in an unstable ankle (a Maisonneuve fracture). It is important to check the neurological and vascular status of the foot.

Diagnosis

Diagnosis is made by X-ray. However, you should not wait for an X-ray examination before you reduce an obviously deformed ankle. If no fracture can be seen at the ankle in cases

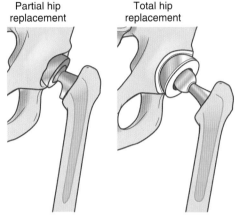

Fig. 18.12 Types of hip replacements. Partial hip replacement (hemiarthroplasty) and total hip replacement. (From Filson R, Harding MM. *Lewis's Medical-Surgical Nursing: Assessment and Management of Clinical Problems.* 12th ed. Elsevier; 2023.)

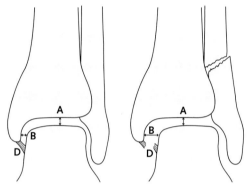

Fig. 18.14 Talar shift. If the medial clear space between the talus and tibia (B) is significantly greater than the joint space (A), talar shift is present. Talar shift is suggestive of disruption of the medial ligaments (D) and indicates the fracture is likely to be an unstable pattern requiring fixation. (A) Tibio-talar joint space; (B) medial clear space; (D) medial (deltoid) ligament.

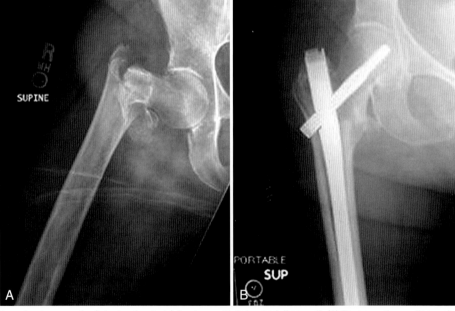

Fig. 18.13 Fixation of extracapsular (intertrochanteric) fracture with intramedullary nail. (A) Preoperative radiograph. (B) After fixation. (From Azar FM, Weinlein JC, Beaty JH. *Campbell's Operative Orthopaedics.* 14th ed. Elsevier; 2022.)

of significant ankle injury or if there is proximal fibular tenderness, a full-length tibia and fibula X-ray image is required.

Management

Fracture patterns thought to be stable can be managed conservatively with external splintage. Unstable ankle fractures – usually injuries that involve two of the three malleoli, in either a bony injury or ligamentous injury – require surgical stabilization. One indication of instability is of talar shift on X-ray (Fig 18.14).

● Chapter Summary

- Specific terminology is used when describing fractures and must be learnt to accurately describe a radiograph.
- Fractures can be pathological with an underlying cause, or due to trauma. Differentiating these is important for fixation technique and prognosis.
- Open fractures must be recognized and treated appropriately with antibiotics in the Emergency Department as per national and local guidelines.
- Recognize the specific problems of certain broken bones such as the hip. Understand that there are very few situations where a hip fracture will be left to heal without an operation due to the challenge of providing adequate pain relief and comfortable nursing care to a patient with a broken hip.
- Casting is often a good immobilization technique for fractures and can treat a vast majority of undisplaced fractures.
- Operative fixation is often indicated in unstable or very displaced fractures. Methods include open reduction and internal fixation, external fixation and intramedullary nailing.
- If a patient needs to undergo surgical fixation of a fracture, they are at risk of perioperative complications, the worst of which can be death, limb loss and compartment syndrome.
- Femoral neck fractures are divided into intracapsular and extracapsular fractures. These are managed differently, with different patients requiring different procedures.
- Wrist and ankle fractures can be treated operatively or nonoperatively, based on whether the fracture pattern is stable or unstable.

UKMLA Conditions
Compartment syndrome
Lower limb fractures
Lower limb soft tissue injury
Pathological fracture
Upper limb fracture
Upper limb soft tissue injury

UKMLA Presentations
Musculoskeletal deformities
Soft tissue injury
Trauma

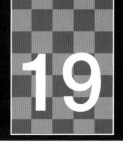
DEFINITION

'Trauma' can broadly refer to any injury a patient sustains. In the context of surgery, and orthopaedics in particular, a 'trauma patient' normally refers to a patient with a major isolated injury or a multiply injured patient. Over the last few decades, major changes have occurred in how trauma care is delivered, with the focus on a rapid delivery of standardized care in major trauma centres from dedicated trauma teams.

INCIDENCE

Trauma is the leading cause of death for those aged 1 to 44 years. Worldwide, 9 people die every minute and 5.8 million die every year, from trauma.

CLINICAL ASSESSMENT

Advanced Trauma Life Support

Advanced Trauma Life Support (ATLS) is a system that was developed in the United States for assessing and managing trauma patients in a logical and time-efficient fashion. It prioritizes examination and intervention by system so that most immediate threats to life are addressed first. The primary survey forms the foundation for the ATLS system and whilst its structure is rigid, it is designed to prevent inexperienced or overwhelmed minds from missing reversible, life-threatening pathology. The following box summarizes the primary survey process that should be remembered as 'ABCDE'.

PRIORITIES FOR ADVANCED TRAUMA LIFE SUPPORT

A: Airway maintenance with cervical spine control	**Assess airway for patency** **Cervical spine immobilization** (cervical collar with blocks + tape/ manual c-spine control)

- Talking in full sentences: patent airway
- Inspect for obstruction; food stuffs, teeth, vomit or chewing gum in the mouth, facial/neck trauma, stridor or abnormal breathing sounds
- Consider intubation in a patient with a reduced conscious state GCS <8)
- In patients with a higher but reduced GCS, a naso- or oropharyngeal airway adjunct may be employed
- Suction should be used but cautiously to avoid pushing any potential obstruction further
- Oedema: burns, heat/chemical/ smoke inhalation may cause upper airway obstruction
- High-flow oxygen must be given to all patients initially via a nonrebreather mask
- Protect the c-spine by minimizing excessive movement and immobilize with a cervical collar if indicated

B: Breathing and ventilation	**Assess breathing**

- Respiratory rate
- Oxygen saturation
- Inspect; visible wounds, symmetrical chest wall movements, respiratory effort, paradoxical breathing, neck vein distension (cardiac tamponade)
- Palpate; is the trachea central? Are both sides of the chest moving equally? Crepitus/tenderness: possible rib fracture
- Percussion: dull in haemothorax, hyperresonant in pneumothorax
- Auscultate for breath sounds bilaterally

C: Circulation with haemorrhage control	Assess circulation
	• Pulse: rate, character • Blood pressure • Capillary refill time: centrally at sternum or peripherally at nail bed • Note general condition of patient – are they pale and clammy? Any obvious bleeding sources? • Urine output: excellent guide to volume status • Make sure the patient has wide bore IV access, fluid resuscitation if needed and initial bloods are sent including a group and save for blood typing
D: Disability/ neurological status	Assess neurological status
	• GCS/AVPU • Blood sugar • Temperature; trauma patients get cold quickly so rewarming blankets are often needed • Pupil size and reactivity
E: Exposure and environmental control	Assess the rest of patient
	• Appropriate further examination may form part of primary survey or be delayed until secondary survey • The patient should be exposed from top to toe (whilst maintaining dignity and keeping the patient as warm as possible) and an examination from top to toe should be carried out

AVPU, *Alert, responds to verbal stimuli, responds to pain, unresponsive*; GCS, *Glasgow Coma Scale.*

The very first step is a brief initial 'end-of-bed' assessment and this can be carried out, in a compos mentis and co-operative patient, by asking them their name and what happened. Appropriate responses suggest a patent airway (A) with breathing adequate to generate speech (which requires a perfused brain) (B and C) and no major reduction in level of consciousness (D).

A – Airway with C-spine control

Lack of oxygenated blood delivered to the brain and other major organs causes rapid deterioration and death. A patent and protected airway (either by the patient themselves or by airway adjuncts) is a priority to avoid hypoxia. A definitive airway can be achieved either through intubation with a cuffed endotracheal tube or surgical techniques such as a cricothyrotomy or tracheostomy. A patient's airway can be compromised with:

• A decreased level of consciousness; Glasgow Coma Scale (GCS) <8 (secondary to, e.g., a head injury, hypoxia, hypovolaemia, drugs).
• Facial trauma.
• Neck trauma.
• Aspiration of vomit or broken teeth.
• Swelling of subcutaneous tissues associated with burns or smoke inhalation.

Cervical spine control

All high-energy trauma patients should be assumed to have unstable neck injuries until proven otherwise, especially in those with an altered level of consciousness or with injuries above the level of the clavicle. The cervical spine is not considered immobilized unless held manually or with an appropriately sized hard collar, sandbags and tape across the patient's forehead (triple immobilization). The patient should remain immobilized until the cervical spine can be cleared clinically and radiologically if required.

B – Breathing

Adequate ventilation is required to oxygenate blood and in turn, organs such as the brain. A quick way to determine adequate ventilation is to check mentation of the patient. Causes of ventilatory compromise include (Table 19.1):

• Central nervous system depression (head injury, alcohol, drugs, cervical spine injury).
• Tension pneumothorax (needs immediate decompression with a cannula in the second intercostal space midclavicular line, followed by formal chest drain).
• Open/simple pneumothorax requiring chest drain.
• Rib fractures/flail chest (a condition where fractures at both ends of a rib leave it floating and severely affect the ability of lung to create negative pressure and inhale).
• Massive haemothorax (blood in the thorax).

C – Circulation

Shock is defined as inadequate organ perfusion and therefore tissue oxygenation. The most common cause of this in the trauma patient is hypovolaemia secondary to haemorrhage.

It is important to recognize hypovolaemic shock so that treatment is not delayed. The patient should have their pulse

Table 19.1 Common causes of respiratory compromise in trauma

	Tension pneumothorax	Cardiac tamponade	Open pneumothorax	Haemothorax
Features	Tachycardia Tracheal Deviation Air hunger/respiratory distress Neck vein distension Hyper resonance Absent breath sounds Cyanosis: late sign Hypotension	Tachycardia Neck vein distension Hypotension Cyanosis	Tachycardia Air hunger/respiratory distress Hyper resonance: unilateral Absent breath sounds: unilateral Cyanosis Hypotension Search for open wound	Tachycardia Air hunger/respiratory distress Dullness to percussion Hypotension Cyanosis
Treatment	Large bore needle decompression to 2nd intercostal space midclavicular line	Needle pericardiocentesis: urgent discussion with cardiothoracic team	Occlusive dressing secured on three sides to create flutter type valve	Chest drain: 5th intercostal space just anterior to midaxillary line

Table 19.2 Physiologic response to haemorrhage

	1	2	3	4
Blood loss (mL)	<750	750–1500	1500–2000	>2000
Blood loss (%)	<15	15–30	30–40	>40
Pulse rate (beats/min)	<100	100–120	120–140	>140
Blood pressure	Normal	Decreased	Decreased	Decreased
Respiratory rate (breaths/min)	14–20	20–30	30–40	>35
Urine output (mL/h)	>30	20–30	5–15	Negligible
CNS symptoms	Normal	Anxious	Confused	Lethargic

(Adapted from Committee on Trauma. Advanced Trauma Life Support Manual. 10th edition. Chicago: American College of Surgeons; 2018.)

rate, blood pressure, capillary refill, urinary output and level of consciousness closely monitored. Clinical findings allow the remaining circulating blood volume to be estimated (normal is approximately 5L in adults). Blood pressure can be normal in a young person with up to 30% blood loss, but, as they decompensate, there is tachycardia, hypotension and confusion as shown in Table 19.2.

There are five areas to consider in identifying sources of potential blood loss to estimate the volume lost. These are known as 'blood on the floor and four more' – the chest, abdomen, pelvis, long bones (femurs) and on the floor (at the scene of the accident as well as in hospital).

Whilst hypovolaemic shock secondary to haemorrhage is most likely in a trauma patient, other causes can also occur. These include:

Cardiogenic shock

The heart is unable to maintain adequate cardiac output, usually because of infarction. Intravenous fluids may further overload the heart and positive inotropes such as noradrenaline (norepinephrine) may be required.

Neurogenic shock

This is due to peripheral vasodilatation secondary to injury to the central nervous system.

It is important not to overload such a patient with fluid in an attempt to raise the blood pressure (the blood pressure remains low because of loss of peripheral resistance). A systolic blood pressure of 100 mmHg is normally acceptable in these patients.

Septic shock

Peripheral vasodilatation occurs due to bacterial endotoxin release in severe infection. Patients require intravenous antibiotics, whilst simultaneously receiving haemodynamic support.

Anaphylactic shock

This occurs in patients already sensitized to an allergen. There is an aggressive immune response resulting in massive histamine release from basophils. The patient may rapidly deteriorate and develop generalized urticaria, with stridor (upper-airway narrowing), wheeze and shortness of breath. There is massive vasodilatation and tachycardia associated with hypotension. Treatment should be rapid, including emergency airway procedures, oxygen, nebulizers, intravenous fluids, intravenous hydrocortisone, antihistamines (chlorphenamine) and most importantly intramuscular or intravenous adrenaline (epinephrine).

In any type of shock, intravenous access should be gained as quickly as possible, and fluid resuscitation commenced. In the case of haemorrhage, this means a blood transfusion. Major haemorrhage protocols (which will recommend fresh frozen plasma and clotting factors to complement red blood cell transfusion) are present in all hospitals in the UK.

D – Disability/neurological status

Can be measured by GCS; scores range from 3 to 15. This should be monitored regularly to observe for deterioration in the patient's condition. A simpler method to determine level of consciousness is AVPU.

NEUROLOGICAL ASSESSMENT USING GCS	
Eyes	4 – Opens eyes spontaneously
	3 – Opens eyes in response to voice
	2 – Opens eyes in response to pain
	1 – Does not open eyes
Voice	5 – Normal speech, orientated to time, person and place
	4 – Confused speech
	3 – Inappropriate words
	2 – Incomprehensible sounds
	1 – No sounds
Movement	6 – Obeys commands
	5 – Localizes to pain
	4 – Withdrawal from painful stimuli
	3 – Abnormal flexion (decorticate posturing)
	2 – Abnormal extension (decerebrate posturing)
	1 – No movements

NEUROLOGICAL ASSESSMENT USING AVPU	
A	Alert
V	Responds to verbal stimuli
P	Responds to pain
U	Unresponsive

E – Exposure and secondary survey

Examine from head to toe for other injuries. This includes log-rolling the patient (with cervical spine control) to assess for trauma to the back and spine. A rectal examination should be carried out at this point to assess for sensation, anal tone and for blood on the examiner's glove (this can indicate internal bleeding or an open fracture where there is an associated pelvic fracture).

The secondary survey involves a full examination of all systems. It is important that the secondary survey does not begin until the primary survey is complete, initial management has begun and the patient is stable.

It is the aim of the secondary survey to find injuries not yet identified in the primary survey. The examination should be from top to bottom and should evaluate each body part, including revisiting all the areas previously covered in the primary survey. Injuries commonly missed are those in the extremities; these may well only become apparent a day or two after the initial injury once the patient is able to tell you specifically where they are sore.

COMMUNICATION

When taking a history from a multiply injured patient, the assessment should be rapid to avoid delays in diagnosing life-threatening conditions. Specifically ask about allergies, medications they are taking, their past medical history, the last time the patient ate or drank and the events surrounding the injury (sometimes called an AMPLE history). Seek a collateral history from others such as paramedics or people at the scene for clues about the mechanism (e.g., damage to the car) and to gain an idea of the patient's initial condition.

INVESTIGATIONS

A trauma series of X-ray images (taken in the resuscitation area) should include at least chest and pelvis films and, if indicated, cervical spine films. Major trauma patients will now often be directed rapidly to the CT scanner for imaging (from head to pelvis) as soon as it is safe for the patient to be moved out of the resuscitation bay. Blood tests include full blood count, urea and creatinine and clotting. Blood group should be typed and blood stored in case the patient needs blood transfusion.

TREATMENT

Treatment is guided initially by ATLS principles and early imaging which have both changed the way trauma is managed. Rapid access to blood transfusion products and quick transfer to dedicated operating theatres has reduced mortality. The concept of damage control surgery is now used in trauma and centres around the principle that trauma patients die from coagulopathy, hypothermia and metabolic acidosis (the 'lethal triad'), not from imperfect fixation of their fractures. Temporizing measures such as external fixators are used to stabilize fractures adequately, so the patient has time to improve physiologically before they undergo the definitive procedure.

OPEN FRACTURES

Definition

An open fracture is a fracture with an overlying soft tissue defect which allows the fracture to communicate with the outside world, and therefore potentially become contaminated with bacteria (see Fig. 18.5). Open fractures were formerly called compound fractures, but this term has dropped out of use.

Incidence

Incidence of open fracture is approximately 23 per 100,000 patients per year.

Aetiology and pathology

Most open fractures are the result of high-energy trauma and are associated with significant damage to soft tissues. They can also commonly occur when the fracture is grossly angulated or displaced and the sharp fracture end exits through the skin. The greatest risk to the bone is infection and the development of chronic osteomyelitis which can lead to amputation. There is also risk to the surrounding soft tissues which may be trapped behind bone ends and therefore ischaemic. Every effort should be made to protect the surrounding soft tissues whilst the patient is waiting for theatre.

Clinical features

Any wound around the fracture site should be assumed to communicate with the bone. Also look for evidence of compartment syndrome which is still possible in open fractures.

Management

The patient should be given broad-spectrum intravenous antibiotics as soon as possible, the wound should be photographed for the patient's medical notes and for surgical planning with plastic surgery, large debris removed and the wound should then be irrigated and dressed with saline-soaked swabs. Give tetanus prophylaxis if recommended by local guidance. The limb should then be splinted. The wound should be aggressively debrided in theatre as soon as possible (without putting the patient's health at risk) to minimize bacterial infection of the fracture. The fracture can then be stabilized with a suitable method of internal or external fixation either at the primary operation or as a delayed procedure.

> **CLINICAL NOTES**
>
> Open fractures should be treated as per British Orthopaedic Association Standards for Trauma (BOAST) guidelines:
> - Assess and document the neurovascular status carefully.
> - The limb should be realigned and splinted.
> - Wound should only be handled to remove gross contamination and to allow photography, then dressed with saline-soaked gauze and an occlusive film.
> - Intravenous antibiotics as soon as possible, ideally within 1 hour of injury.
> - Debridement should be performed along fasciotomy lines where possible, timing guided by the degree of and type of contamination.
> - Definitive soft tissue coverage should be achieved within 72 hours of injury.

SPINAL INJURIES

Definition

Spinal injuries include fractures and subluxations/dislocations of vertebrae. They also include damage to the spinal cord in the absence of a fracture.

Incidence

These are common injuries in high-energy trauma patients, especially in road traffic accidents or a fall from height. A spinal injury should always be suspected in the multiple injured patient. Overall, 10% to 20% of patients with a spinal fracture will have a second spinal fracture at another level. Patients with significant trauma to lower limbs are at risk of spinal fractures, for example, 10% of calcaneal fractures will have a concurrent vertebral fracture.

Aetiology and pathology

Spinal injuries often occur after road traffic accidents. Other examples of causative trauma include: neck injuries from diving into a shallow pool, thoracic injuries from hyperflexion and lumbar injuries after a fall from a height. Thoracolumbar injuries often occur as a result of wearing only a lap belt in a road traffic collision. In elderly patients with osteoporosis, low-energy trauma can result in simple wedge fractures.

The stability of the spine depends on the bony structures and the integrity of strong ligaments. The spine can be thought of as three columns (Fig. 19.1). Fractures involving one column only, such as anterior wedge fractures, are usually stable and can be treated conservatively. Fractures involving two or three columns, such as a high-energy burst fracture (Fig. 19.2), are often unstable. Injuries may involve the bony structures only, both ligaments and bones or purely ligaments. This means that even if the radiograph is normal, you cannot assume the spine is stable as a significant proportion of ligaments may be torn. However, this type of injury is extremely rare. If there is doubt, magnetic resonance imaging (MRI) will show the soft tissues and any potential damage.

CLINICAL NOTES

Potential spinal injuries must be managed with care and attention. To exclude injury, you need good X-ray images (and/or computed tomography) and a fully conscious patient. An MRI may be required to assess the soft tissues.

Clinical features

As part of the 'exposure' assessment in a trauma patient, a log roll and examination of the spine must be performed. A conscious patient will complain of pain at the level of injury (caution must be taken in patients with a decreased level of consciousness).

HINTS AND TIPS

Patients with facial or head injuries should be presumed to have a significant neck injury until proven otherwise.

Clinical examination of the spine may reveal tenderness, bruising, a boggy swelling or bony step. The patient should be log-rolled with cervical spine control to examine the thoracic and lumbar spine. Examine the limbs for abnormal neurology. A full neurological examination should include a rectal examination for anal tone and sensation (sacral nerves) and should be

Fig. 19.1 Anatomy of the spine divided into its three columns.

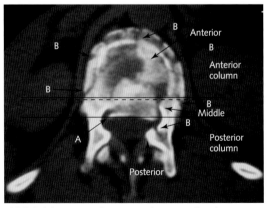

Fig. 19.2 Axial computed tomography scan showing an unstable two-column burst fracture (*arrows B*) with retropulsion of a bone fragment (*arrow A*) into the spinal canal.

documented on an ASIA (American Spinal cord Injury Assessment) chart to assess trends of neurological function. Knowledge of dermatomes and myotomes will guide you to the level of spinal cord injury if present.

Remember that spinal injury might cause bradycardia and hypotension (spinal shock). These patients should receive intravenous fluids cautiously.

Diagnosis and investigation

X-ray views of the cervical spine are needed: anteroposterior, lateral (to at least T1) and odontoid peg views.

X-ray views of the thoracic and lumbar spine are needed: anteroposterior and lateral views.

Remember, X-ray images can be normal, even with spinal cord trauma.

Further imaging may be required: computed tomography (CT) scan in the case of equivocal or inadequate X-ray images; MRI to look for ligament and spinal cord damage.

Treatment

Treatment depends on the stability of the fracture. The TLICS scoring system (Fig. 19.3) can guide in the decision between operative and nonoperative management.

Patients with stable fractures can be mobilized. Unstable fractures require immobilization (e.g., halo vest), bracing or possibly internal fixation. The patient's fitness for surgery must also be considered when deciding which patients should be recommended for operative/nonoperative management.

Prognosis

Patients with spinal cord damage and neurological symptoms have a poor functional prognosis and often require extensive rehabilitation on a spinal unit.

PELVIC FRACTURES

Pelvic fractures in the young, are high-energy injuries which can be associated with massive bleeding, urethral, bladder and abdominal injuries. In the elderly, pelvic fractures can occur from a simple fall, e.g., pubic rami fractures.

Incidence

Pelvic fractures in the young, are rare injuries and careful assessment of the polytraumatized patient is necessary to avoid

TLICS 3 Independent Predictors				
1	**Morphology** Immediate stability	• Compression • Burst • Translation/rotation • Distraction	1 2 3 4	**Radiographs** **CT**
2	**Integrity of PLC** Long-term stability	• Intact • Suspected • Injured	0 2 3	**MRI**
3	**Neurological Status**	• Intact • Nerve root • Complete cord • Incomplete cord • Cauda equina	0 2 2 3 3	**Physical examination**
Predicts need for surgery			03	Non-surgical
			4	Surgeon's choice
			>4	Surgical

Fig. 19.3 Thoracolumbar Injury Classification and Severity (TLICS) score. (From Gandham S, Annis P. *The principles of the advanced trauma life support (ATLS) framework in spinal trauma.* Orthopaedics and Trauma. 2020; 34(5): 305-314.)

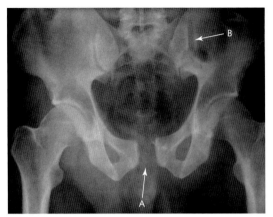

Fig. 19.4 X-ray image of an open-book pelvic fracture. There is widening at the symphysis pubis (*arrow A*) and the left sacroiliac joint (*arrow B*).

missing them. Hypovolaemia secondary to a pelvic fracture carries a high mortality.

Aetiology

The pelvis is a stable ring formed by the sacrum, ilium and pubis bones held together by strong ligaments. The basic mechanisms of injury are anteroposterior compression (blow from the front: Fig. 19.4), lateral compression (side impact), vertical shear forces (usually fall from height) or a combination of all three.

Clinical features

Clinical examination may reveal asymmetry to the pelvis or lower limbs and bruising and swelling around the pelvis itself. There may be blood at the urethral meatus (urethral tear) and bruising in the perineal or scrotal region. Rectal examination may reveal blood (bowel injury) or a boggy, high-riding prostate (urethral tear). Bone fragments may be palpable indicating

an open fracture. Do not assess pelvic stability by bimanual compression of the iliac wings, i.e., springing the pelvis, an outdated manoeuvre, as this may displace a significant clot and cause renewed bleeding.

Diagnosis and investigation

An anteroposterior X-ray image of the pelvis should be checked for fractures, symmetry and normal contours. This should be performed in binder initially and out of binder once the patient is stable. A CT scan will enable a more accurate identification of the fracture.

Emergency treatment

The patient should be managed according to ATLS protocol and resuscitated with intravenous fluids. Patients who either transiently respond or do not respond are likely to have ongoing bleeding. There might be haemorrhage from bones, the pelvic venous plexus and, less commonly, arteries.

Bleeding can be reduced by stabilizing the pelvis. This can be done immediately by applying a pelvic binder to close the pelvic ring and reduce its volume. If this fails, angiography and embolization of bleeding vessels or laparotomy with pelvic packing may be required. A pelvic external fixator can also be of use in certain specific situations. However, a well-placed binder is usually sufficient for immediate purposes.

Stable fractures require pain relief and mobilization. Unstable fracture patterns require surgical fixation.

Prognosis

Mortality can be high, especially when the patient has associated head, chest or abdominal injuries. Complications such as urethral tears, sciatic nerve damage or persistent sacroiliac pain can affect the quality of life and prognosis of the patient in the long term.

● Chapter Summary

- The most important step in managing any trauma patient is the ABCDE approach: this should be your first step.
- Open fractures should be managed with early antibiotics, reduction and splinting of the fracture. Photographs of wound should be acquired before dressings applied. External fixation may be required temporarily and plastic surgery might be required to close the wound.
- Spinal fractures should be assessed as either stable or unstable using the three-column theory and the TLICS scoring system. Any neurological deficit should be carefully documented and will influence operative decisions.

- Pelvic fractures can be life-threatening injuries and should be addressed as part of the primary survey. A pelvic binder can be a life-saving piece of kit in managing trauma patients.
- Managing major trauma requires a team approach and should be practiced on a regular basis. Courses such as the ATLS are mandatory for doctors treating trauma to keep practice up to date.

UKMLA Conditions
Compartment syndrome
Lower limb fractures
Lower limb soft tissue injury
Spinal cord compression
Spinal cord injury
Spinal fracture
Upper limb fractures
Upper limb soft tissue injury

UKMLA Presentations
Back pain
Neck pain/stiffness
Trauma

Infection of bones and joints | 20

INTRODUCTION

Infection of any kind needs to be recognized and treated promptly to avoid potentially fatal complications. In this chapter we will discuss osteomyelitis (infection in a bone), septic arthritis (infection in a joint) and tuberculosis.

OSTEOMYELITIS

Infection of bone can be caused by direct inoculation (exogenous spread) or blood-borne bacteria (haematogenous spread).

In childhood or adolescence, osteomyelitis is usually caused by the haematogenous spread of bacteria and is most likely to be found in the metaphysis or epiphysis of long bones. In adults, the source is more likely to be exogenous, most commonly due to infection developing after surgery or after a penetrating injury (particularly in the case of an open fracture).

Incidence

Osteomyelitis is becoming more uncommon in modern medicine. The exact incidence is unknown.

Aetiology and pathology

The most common infecting organism overall is *Staphylococcus aureus*; other pathogens are shown in Table 20.1. If unusual

Table 20.1 Common pathogens in osteomyelitis

Patient's age	Common organisms
Newborns (younger than 4 months)	*Staphylococcus aureus, Streptococcus* (group A and B), *Enterobacter*
Children (4 months to 4 years)	*Staphylococcus aureus, Streptococcus* (group A), *Enterobacter, Kingella kingae*
Children (4 years to adult)	*Staphylococcus aureus, Streptococcus* (group A), *Haemophilus influenzae, Enterobacter*
Adult	*Staphylococcus aureus, Streptococcus, Enterobacter*
Immunocompromised	*Staphylococcus aureus, Salmonella, Pseudomonas, Bartonella, Mycobacterium tuberculosis*, fungal infection

organisms are present, or a patient has recurrent unexplained infections, consider specific predisposing factors, as listed in the box; for example, patients with acquired immunodeficiency syndrome (AIDS) are more likely to develop fungal infections.

CLINICAL NOTES

Conditions associated with osteomyelitis

Congenital	Acquired
Sickle cell disease	Diabetes
Haemophilia	Renal failure
	Intravenous drug use
	Malnutrition
	Immunosuppression
	HIV/AIDS

AIDS, *Acquired immunodeficiency syndrome*; HIV, *human immunodeficiency virus*.

The three most common causes of osteomyelitis are:

- acute haematogenous osteomyelitis
- posttraumatic osteomyelitis
- postoperative osteomyelitis

Acute haematogenous osteomyelitis

This form of osteomyelitis is usually seen in children, in the metaphysis or epiphysis of long bones. Vertebral bones are the most commonly affected bones in adults. Blood supply to bone is initially via the endosteum and periosteum.

The pathogenesis of acute haematogenous osteomyelitis is as follows (Fig. 20.1):

1. Bacteria settles in the metaphysis of a long bone causing inflammation. Pus forms within the bone.
2. Pus escapes through the Haversian canals to form a subperiosteal abscess. Pus is now present on both sides of the bone, causing this part of the bone to die.
3. Pus may collect in the joint causing an associated septic arthritis
4. Dead bone, called sequestrum, harbours infection. Periosteal new bone, called involucrum, forms around the sequestrum as the body tries to fight the infection.

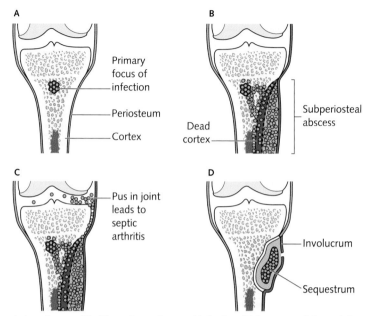

Fig. 20.1 Sequence of events in osteomyelitis. The primary focus of infection (A) has spread through bone, causing the death of cortical bone and formation of a subperiosteal abscess (B). Infection can spread into the joint (C), causing septic arthritis. Death of a segment of bone (sequestrum) occurs (D), and the area is surrounded by new subperiosteal bone (involucrum).

Acute osteomyelitis can easily become chronic if the sequestrum is neglected or not completely excised at surgery.

Posttraumatic osteomyelitis

An open fracture means the skin and soft tissues have been injured and there is a communicating tract down to bone. This allows bacteria direct access to the bony surfaces. Large dirty wounds associated with high-energy injuries are more likely to result in posttraumatic osteomyelitis. Urgent surgical debridement and lavage are required to remove contaminated material and necrotic tissues, to reduce the risk of subsequent osteomyelitis. Inadequate or delayed surgery will lead to osteomyelitis due to bacteria colonizing bone. In these circumstances, the fracture in question will often fail to heal and will become an infected nonunion; a difficult to treat sequelae.

Postoperative osteomyelitis

Many operations in orthopaedics involve using implants such as joint prostheses or plates and screws. These foreign bodies can harbour infection if bacteria are introduced at the time of surgery, or colonize the implant from systemic spread at a later date. Since there is obviously no blood supply to the implants, antibiotics have no way of being delivered to the implant, and eradication is almost impossible without surgery. For this reason, orthopaedic surgeons are fastidious about aseptic techniques in the operating theatre and routinely use antibiotics as prophylaxis. Despite this, infection still occurs and might spread around the implant, devitalizing bone.

Other conditions associated with osteomyelitis

The above three causes of osteomyelitis are the most common, but osteomyelitis also occurs in the other conditions listed in the earlier box.

Bone and joint infection are common among intravenous drug users. These patients are often malnourished and immunosuppressed (sometimes due to being human immunodeficiency virus (HIV)-positive). They may be repeatedly using dirty needles for injecting deep under the skin, often neglect small abscesses, and are therefore at risk of opportunistic infections developing into serious problems.

HINTS AND TIPS

Acute osteomyelitis and chronic osteomyelitis behave differently. Acute osteomyelitis occurs rapidly (e.g., in an open fracture) and can cause the patient to become unwell quickly. Chronic osteomyelitis can develop over weeks and months and the patient may appear 'well' with inflammatory markers that are only slightly raised. Both usually need to be treated with long courses of antibiotics.

Clinical features

Acute osteomyelitis causes pain, fever and loss of function (often a limp if the lower limb is involved).

It is more common in the tibia and femur. The limb will be tender to palpate, erythematous and possibly swollen.

At the extremes of age (neonate, infant or elderly), the symptoms and signs are often nonspecific (such as general malaise). These patients can be seriously ill and it can be extremely difficult to pinpoint the exact site of the problem.

Occasionally, a patient presents with multiple sites affected or there may be another focus of infection that has spread from or to bone, for example, infective endocarditis. This is called seeding of infection.

In postsurgical and posttraumatic osteomyelitis, the wound will be painful, red and inflamed. Normally following surgery, once postoperative pain has settled, patients are comfortable and can mobilize without pain. If pain persists or increases, infection is a possible cause. Wounds will continue to leak and eventually break down or there will be dehiscence. If left untreated, a sinus will result.

A limb with chronic osteomyelitis will be swollen and have thickened, woody skin. Here the focus of infection remains within the bone as sequestrum and the infection can remain quiescent for a period of time (maybe many years) and then flare up unexpectedly, often producing an abscess. A chronic discharging sinus can result.

Diagnosis and investigation

The diagnosis may be obvious on clinical examination, particularly if the history reveals a clear predisposing factor.

A raised white cell count (WCC), erythrocyte sedimentation rate (ESR) and C-reactive protein (CRP) are likely to be present on blood tests.

Initially X-ray images will be normal, but beyond 10 days, changes begin to appear. There will be lysis, periosteal elevation and eventually new bone formation. Later, sequestrum may be seen as a sclerotic area.

A Brodie's abscess may be seen in the metaphysis of long bones (Fig. 20.2).

Early osteomyelitis can be detected before it can be seen on X-ray images by using a bone scan or white cell-labelled scan (shows increased uptake) or MRI.

It is very important to take microbiology specimens such as blood cultures, or a direct biopsy or pus samples in theatre if the patient is well enough, prior to starting antibiotics.

Management

Medical

The patient needs adequate analgesia, splinting of the affected limb and appropriate antibiotics. Most hospitals or health boards will have an antibiotic policy; however, consultation

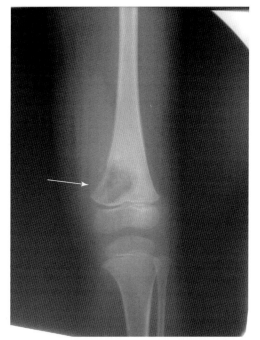

Fig. 20.2 Brodie abscess (*arrow*).

with the microbiologists in a multidisciplinary team meeting, is advisable as these can be complex infections to treat.

As most infections are with *S. aureus*, flucloxacillin is the most common first-line antibiotic, usually in combination with fusidic acid or rifampicin. The course is initially usually given intravenously for a number of weeks, with additional oral antibiotics if necessary. Once control of the infection has been established, and the patient stabilized, intravenous antibiotics may be switched to oral antibiotics if there is a suitable oral alternative.

Antibiotic-resistant strains such as methicillin-resistant *S. aureus* (MRSA) are becoming more prevalent and, if suspected, vancomycin or teicoplanin can be used instead after consultation with a microbiologist.

Antibiotics will suffice in cases where the patient does not have a driving collection or abscess and dead bone is not present.

Surgical

As well as medical treatment, the patient may require surgical debridement. If an accompanying abscess is present, this should be drained surgically. If a deep abscess such as a Brodie's abscess is present, this needs to undergo curettage back to healthy bone. Dead bone (sequestrum) needs to be removed, otherwise eradication is impossible.

In a chronic case, if the patient and surgeon decide to attempt to cure the infection, extensive surgery is required to remove all infected bone and implants if present. Techniques for doing this vary depending on the extent of involvement and the site. It is also possible simply to treat the flare-ups and suppress the infection with antibiotics when required, particularly in patients not fit for major surgery.

Complications

Complications occur if:

- Osteomyelitis persists.
- The physis is damaged in paediatric cases, leading to growth disturbance and deformity.
- The infection spreads to the joint, causing septic arthritis.

Prognosis

In cases of acute osteomyelitis, the outcome is usually good and the majority make a full recovery provided none of the above complications occur. In chronic cases following surgery or trauma, many surgical procedures are often required and amputation is not an uncommon outcome.

HINTS AND TIPS

Chronic osteomyelitis is very difficult to treat. It may remain dormant for many years and then flare up intermittently, causing pain and loss of function. These flare-ups are often managed with antibiotics. Some people cannot tolerate long-term loss of function of the limb, in which case amputation may be indicated.

COMMON PITFALLS

Patients with amputation can still go on to develop osteomyelitis in the remaining bone and soft tissue. Careful assessment with MRI is needed. Often psychological support with counselling is required.

CLINICAL NOTES

Amputation is a last resort in cases of severe infection and deformity. Upper limb amputation is generally better tolerated than lower limb. A below knee amputation is well tolerated by fitter patients, but an above knee amputation leaves no functioning joint and makes walking much more challenging. Every effort should be given to early intervention to prevent above knee amputation as much as possible.

SEPTIC ARTHRITIS

Septic arthritis is infection within a synovial joint.

Incidence

The condition is uncommon but is seen more often in children, young adults and the elderly. It is more common in the developing world and in patients with a predisposing reason to develop it. In children, it is less common than osteomyelitis.

Aetiology and pathology

Infection reaches a joint via the haematogenous route, direct spread from osteomyelitis in the metaphysis (common in children) or penetrating trauma/surgery. Associated conditions are similar to those for acute osteomyelitis (see box: Clinical Notes, Conditions associated with osteomyelitis), with the addition of rheumatoid arthritis and crystal arthropathy. In all groups, *S. aureus* is the most common causative pathogen; however, certain organisms are more common at different ages. *Haemophilus influenzae* used to be the most common infecting organism in infants prior to the introduction of the vaccination programme. In sexually active young adults, *Neisseria gonorrhoeae* is more common.

In haematogenous septic arthritis, the bacterium settles in the synovium, which may be already inflamed due to trauma or disease. Proliferation of bacteria causes an inflammatory response by the host with numerous leukocytes migrating into the joint. The variety of proteolytic enzymes and breakdown products produced damages the delicate articular cartilage very quickly (within hours) and, if left treated, permanent damage will ensue (Fig. 20.3).

Clinical features

The patient will have an acutely hot swollen joint with a fever and be systemically unwell (see Chapter 6). An infant or young child will be distressed, unwell and difficult to assess. There may be a history of recent systemic infection such as otitis media.

Septic arthritis is more common in the hip and knee but can present in any synovial joint.

Even slight movement causes intense pain and weight-bearing will not be tolerated. Patients typically resist any movement at the joint and hold it rigidly still. If the joint is superficial, an effusion is palpable.

In neonates and infants, the diagnosis may be less obvious, particularly if the joint is deeply situated, such as the hip. These patients may be seriously unwell, and systemically compromised.

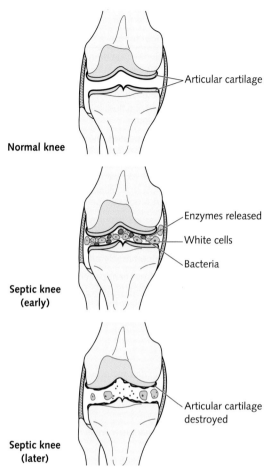

Normal knee

Articular cartilage

Enzymes released

White cells

Bacteria

**Septic knee
(early)**

Articular cartilage
destroyed

**Septic knee
(later)**

Fig. 20.3 Sequence of events in septic arthritis.

Diagnosis and investigation

- WCC, CRP and ESR will be elevated in typical cases.
- X-ray images will be normal initially and show joint destruction late.
- If available, ultrasound scanning is useful to see if there is a joint effusion when the hip is the suspicious joint.

- Any joint suspected of infection must be aspirated (prior to antibiotic administration) and the fluid sent for urgent Gram stain, culture and examination for crystals.

Management

Similar to osteomyelitis, relieve pain by giving analgesia and splinting the limb if necessary. Aspiration should be performed at the earliest opportunity, before the commencement of antibiotics. Give appropriate antibiotics as directed by the microbiology team, depending on the age of the patient and any predisposing illnesses. Treatment can be either medical with serial aspirations or surgical with arthroscopy or arthrotomy and washout, both in conjunction with antibiotics. If infection is serious, whether the patient is young or old, the chances of full recovery are slim once the articular cartilage is destroyed. Further procedures, often in the form of arthroplasty, may be needed in the future to return to normal function.

Complications

- Seeding of infection can occur to the spine or other organs.
- Recurrence of infection.
- Joint destruction with long-term arthritis or even ankylosis (bony fusion across the joint).
- Avascular necrosis (particularly in the hip).

Prognosis

If treated promptly, prognosis is good, but if joint destruction occurs, prognosis is very poor. Septic arthritis, if missed or left untreated, can even be fatal.

TUBERCULOSIS

Incidence

Tuberculosis (TB) is common in global terms and causes significant morbidity and mortality in Africa and Asia.

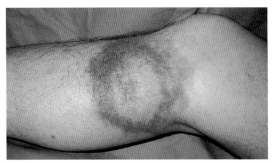

Fig. 20.4 Erythema migrans. (From Ball JW, et al. *Seidel's guide to physical examination*. 10th ed. St. Louis, Elsevier; 2023.)

TB has made a comeback in the UK, with over 10,000 cases per year, most of which are in the Asian community or immunocompromised patients, but it is increasingly seen in all communities.

Aetiology and pathology

TB is due to Mycobacterium tuberculosis or M. bovis infection.

Histologically, the classic appearance is of granulating caseating necrosis.

Musculoskeletal TB results when primary TB becomes widespread or when later reactivation or reinfection occurs (immunosuppressed patients).

Clinical features

Patients have general symptoms of ill health, such as malaise, weight loss, cough and loss of appetite. The most common musculoskeletal sites affected by TB are the spine, hip and knee.

Unlike other orthopaedic infections, TB presents with gradual symptoms of pain and may be initially diagnosed as osteoarthritis or inflammatory arthritis.

Diagnosis and investigation

The two most common tests for TB exposure are the Mantoux and Heaf tests, which are skin hypersensitivity tests.

For confirmation, large samples of bone or synovial fluid are required, which need to be cultured (Löwenstein-Jensen medium) for a prolonged period (6 weeks).

If mycobacterial infection is suspected, samples should be submitted to a Ziehl-Neelsen stain to look for acid/alcohol-fast bacilli. Remember to ask for this specifically when requesting a Gram stain.

X-ray images show variable amounts of joint destruction with periarticular osteopenia.

In the spine, vertebra plana may be found with almost complete collapse of the vertebral body (see Fig. 9.11).

Not only should TB pertaining to the area of interest be investigated but it is likely that this TB has seeded from elsewhere, so a full workup looking for a primary source of TB is imperative.

Table 20.2 Stages of Lyme disease

Stage	Clinical features
Early	Within the first month of exposure to Lyme disease, a distinctive target lesion known as erythema migrans will appear (see Fig. 20.4). The patient will also experience flu-like symptoms at this early stage.
Early disseminated	If left untreated, the disease will spread to other organs through the blood and lymphatics. Clinical features include AV node block, palpitations, cranial nerve palsies, radiculitis and viral meningitis. Heart block can be fatal.
Late	Late-stage features include arthritis, encephalitis and peripheral neuropathy. Arthritis presents as pain and swelling, most commonly affecting the knee joint.
Posttreatment	After treatment patients often experience chronic fatigue. This is a fibromyalgia-like condition.

Treatment

Drugs commonly used are rifampicin, isoniazid, pyrazinamide and ethambutol. Multidrug therapy is required.

A spinal abscess may need surgical drainage with stabilization of the spine.

Ankylosed joints from previously treated TB can be replaced (usually the hip).

LYME DISEASE

Lyme disease is a multistage, tick-borne disease that is most commonly caused by the spirochete bacterium, *Borrelia burgdorferi*. The clinical manifestations of Lyme disease are split into the following stages: early disease, early disseminated disease, late disease and a posttreatment stage.

Table 20.2 details the clinical manifestations found at each stage.

When taking a patient history, it is essential to think about the patient's expose risk to Lyme disease. Many patients will not remember having been bitten by a tick, therefore, it is important to consider if they have recently been in an area that carries an increased risk of Lyme disease. The initial screening test looks for the presence of antibodies to *B. burgdorferi*. This may not be present in early disease but will present in late disease. To conform diagnosis, western blot analysis will be carried out. Fig. 20.5 details the treatment plan for patients with Lyme disease.

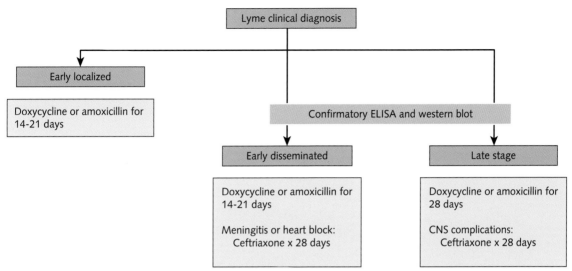

Fig. 20.5 Treatment given at the distinct stages of Lyme disease. (From Spec A, et al. *Comprehensive Review of Infectious Diseases*. Elsevier; 2020.)

● Chapter Summary

- Musculoskeletal infections can become serious diseases rapidly. They require prompt identification with a high clinical suspicion in the right patients, quick diagnosis on blood cultures and direct samples and timely treatment. Patients are usually managed by a multidisciplinary team with microbiology, infectious diseases and medical and/or surgical colleagues working together.
- The most common causative organism for septic arthritis in all ages is *Staphylococcus aureus.* An aspirate of the joint should be sent to culture to confirm the offending organism so antibiotic therapy can be tailored.
- Osteomyelitis can develop either posttraumatically, postsurgically or from haematogenous spread. Sequestrum and involucrum are terms relating to the effect of infection on bone and its response.
- The clinical features of septic arthritis in children and adults are redness, swelling, pain, difficulty moving the joint, difficulty bearing weight and systemic upset and in some cases sepsis.
- Septic arthritis should be investigated and treated aggressively. Arthroscopic washout of a large joint or open washout of smaller joints may be indicated to save cartilage.
- For the diagnosis of bone and joint sepsis, inflammatory markers, X-ray imaging and aspiration should be used as diagnostic methods.
- Tuberculosis differs from other infections in orthopaedics in that it can lie dormant for a number of years before reactivating and can cause significant collapse of the spine.
- Tuberculosis can be found in the skeleton. The patient should be managed in conjunction with infectious diseases physicians and a primary focus should be looked for.
- Lyme disease is a not uncommonly seen tick-borne disease. Diagnosis can be difficult as patients may not remember being bitten, but the characteristic target lesion is a defining clinical sign if present.

UKMLA Conditions
Lyme disease
Osteomyelitis
Reactive arthritis
Septic arthritis

UKMLA Presentations
Acute joint pain/swelling
Fever

Malignancy 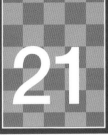 21

This chapter covers bone tumours (benign and malignant; primary and secondary). A tumour may be diagnosed after investigation of a patient's presenting problem, but may also be discovered incidentally as a lesion on X-ray examination, when the X-ray image was taken for another reason. Examples include a chest X-ray image taken for respiratory disease showing a lesion in the clavicle or a pelvic X-ray image taken for hip disease showing a showing a lesion in the proximal femur.

Benign lesions are quite common. Thankfully, primary bone malignancies are extremely rare. Secondary bone tumours are common in the elderly. It is important to remember that infection and metabolic bone disease can mimic bone malignancy.

BENIGN TUMOURS/DISORDERS

- Osteochondroma.
- Osteoid osteoma.
- Enchondroma.
- Bone cysts.
- Fibrous dysplasia.

MALIGNANT TUMOURS

- Primary:
  - osteosarcoma
  - Ewing sarcoma
  - chondrosarcoma
- Secondary (metastatic):
  - breast
  - lung
  - prostate
  - renal
  - thyroid
- Haemopoietic diseases:
  - myeloma
  - leukaemia
  - lymphoma

TUMOUR MIMICS

- Infection
  - osteomyelitis
- Metabolic bone disease
- Paget's disease

While the clinical features, treatment and prognosis will depend upon the specific pathology, the way a suspected bone tumour is initially approached is largely the same irrespective of which type it turns out to be. We will address the general approach to the history, examination and investigation of bone tumours and then discuss the individual pathologies separately.

HISTORY

The following points must be elicited in the history, looking for clues as to the diagnosis.

Age of patient

Certain lesions such as bone cysts are more common in children and other benign bone lesions such as enchondroma usually occur in young adults.

Overall, primary malignant tumours are rare and metastatic bone disease is a disease of the elderly.

Pain

Pain that is severe and does not respond to simple analgesia, is particularly worse at night, suggests a malignant process. Pain that steadily worsens and is not related to any trauma is suspicious.

Swelling

Benign lesions are more likely to present with swelling, particularly osteochondroma, a lesion commonly found around the knee.

Malignant tumours may have pain and swelling, but it is rare for a bone tumour to present with swelling only.

General health

General features of ill health such as tiredness, weight loss, poor appetite and fever suggest a systemic illness such as malignancy, a haemopoietic disorder or infection.

Primary bone malignancy is unlikely to present with widespread features of malignancy as patients will usually present with pain and swelling before these general features have developed.

It is important to ask about any other areas of pain in the musculoskeletal system, particularly if considering widespread metastatic disease.

Medical history

A history of known cancer is extremely important when dealing with such a patient. The lesion should be treated as a metastatic lesion until proven otherwise.

Breast malignancy can be dormant for many years prior to representing with metastases.

EXAMINATION

Site of symptoms

Different lesions are more common in certain locations, for example, enchondromas are more common in the hand.

Secondary bone metastases tend to be found in the central skeleton and proximal aspects of limbs (hips and shoulders).

Limb examination

On initial examination, the affected limb will usually appear normal.

Tenderness and swelling would be present in:

- impending or actual fracture associated with a bone metastasis
- osteomyelitis
- osteoid osteoma
- malignant primary bone tumour

Malignant secondaries or bone lesions from haemopoietic diseases rarely show any external features.

Examination of a lump is a particularly important skill in the context of suspected musculoskeletal malignancy and will be considered here in detail.

When examining a lump or swelling, the following should be considered and your findings should be described in a logical sequence such as this:

Site of lump

Size

Sinister pathology should be suspected in any lump larger than 5 cm.

Depth of lesion

Is the lesion within the skin, in the subcutaneous tissue, tethered or deep to the fascia? Painful deep lesions are suspicious and need investigation.

Skin

Is the skin inflamed or abnormal over the lesion?

Consistency

Is the lesion soft, firm or hard? A lipoma is often described as firm.

Diffuse or discrete

Some swellings are large without clear margins and appear to merge with the surrounding structures, whereas others have borders which are more easily palpable.

Surface

Is the surface of the lesion smooth or irregular?

Mobile or fixed

A discrete mass may be fixed to the underlying structures, e.g., a ganglion, or more mobile, such as lipoma.

Fluctuance

Fluctuant lesions contain fluid, such as a Baker's cyst.

Pulsatile

Pulsatile and expansile lesions are commonly found to be vascular aneurysms.

Transillumination

Fluid-filled lesions (e.g., ganglion) will transilluminate when tested with a pen torch if the fluid is clear.

CLINICAL NOTES

DIFFERENTIAL DIAGNOSIS FOR A PALPABLE LUMP WITH REGARD TO ANATOMICAL LOCATION

Skin or subcutaneous:
- Cyst
- Lipoma
- Rheumatoid nodule

- Bursitis
- Neurofibroma
- Ganglion
- Neuroma
  Joint:
- Joint effusion
- Ganglion
- Baker cyst
  Bone:
- Osteophytes
- Bone tumour
  Muscle/deep soft tissues:
- Sarcoma
- Lipoma

Patients commonly present with lumps, bumps and swellings. The majority of these are benign; when diagnosing these, the main consideration is to rule out malignant causes.

Generalized

In secondary malignancy with unknown primary, it is important to examine the common sites of primary malignancies that spread to bone:

- Breast (for lumps, nipple changes, skin changes, nipple discharge).
- Chest (for evidence of a lung lesion).
- Abdomen (for a renal mass, or evidence of haemopoietic disease such as liver and spleen enlargement); this should be completed with a PR exam (looking for prostate changes).
- Thyroid (locally for a lump and systemically for generalized features of thyroid disease).

INVESTIGATION

The X-ray examination

It is important to obtain two views taken at 90 degrees (orthogonal) to one another and to obtain full-length views of the entire bone (to ensure there are no further lesions along the same bone).

Most benign lesions need no further investigation and repeat X-ray examinations after 6 months are useful to ensure the bone lesion does not change in appearance and develop any sinister features.

Practice describing bone defects and lesions whenever possible. The following should be covered when describing a lesion.

1. Name and age of patient.
2. Site, i.e., which bone and where in the bone.
   - The lesion can be in the diaphysis (shaft), metaphysis (cancellous bone between the growth plate and shaft) or epiphysis (between the growth plate and the joint).
   - The lesion can primarily affect either the cortex or medulla of the bone.
3. Appearance
   - Lytic (e.g., breast metastasis; Fig. 21.1), sclerotic (e.g., prostate metastasis), mixed or calcified (enchondroma).
   - Ground glass (fibrous dysplasia; Fig. 21.2).
   - Abnormal bony architecture, e.g., postosteomyelitis.
4. Zone of transition
   - A well-defined border between the lesion and the normal bone suggests a benign slow-growing lesion (i.e., it is clearly demarcated).
   - A broad, irregular or indistinct zone of transition where the change from abnormal to normal is poorly defined suggests a malignant process (Fig. 21.3).
5. What is the bone doing in response?
   - A significant periosteal reaction, with a Codman triangle (elevation of periosteum; see Fig. 21.7B), onion skinning (Fig. 21.4A) or sunray spicules (Fig. 21.4B), is a feature of malignancy.
   - Note that infection can also cause a periosteal reaction.
6. What is the lesion doing to the bone?
   - Cortical destruction is typical of a malignant process.
   - Cortical thinning does occur in benign disease due to expansion.

Further investigation

Further investigation is necessary if there is any doubt about the diagnosis or to confirm or to exclude malignancy.

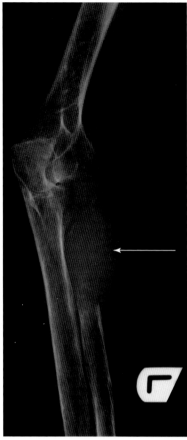

Fig. 21.1 This lytic lesion (proximal radius) is suggestive of malignancy (*arrow*).

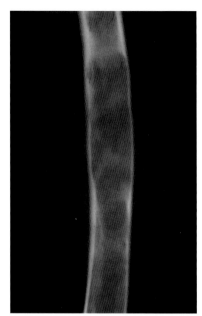

Fig. 21.2 Fibrous dysplasia. (Reproduced with permission from Hochberg, MC, Silman, AJ, Smolen, JS et al., eds. *Rheumatology*. 5th ed. London: Mosby; 2011.)

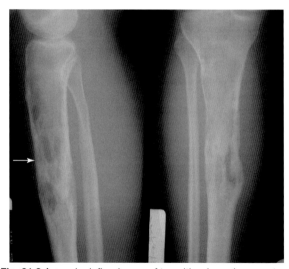

Fig. 21.3 A poorly defined zone of transition (*arrow*) suggests malignancy.

> ### COMMUNICATION 💬
>
> It is not uncommon for patients with a lesion on X-ray examination to find they have metastatic disease from an unknown primary. Make sure this news is broken in the right way, preferably once all the information is available, a plan has been made and with relatives and nursing staff present.

Blood tests

- A full blood count may show anaemia of chronic disease.
- Liver function tests could be deranged if liver metastases are present.
- The calcium profile is often elevated in generalized malignancy and alkaline phosphatase is elevated in Paget's disease.
- C-reactive protein (CRP) and erythrocyte sedimentation rate (ESR) are elevated in infection or malignancy.
- A very high ESR suggests myeloma. It is confirmed with serum electrophoresis and urinary Bence Jones proteins.
- Prostate-specific antigen (PSA) is elevated in prostate malignancy.

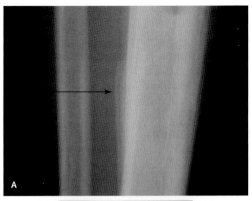

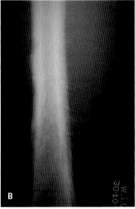

Fig. 21.4 Primary bone tumour showing: (A) onion skinning (*arrow*) and (B) sunray spicules.

- Carcinoembryonic antigen (CEA) is elevated in bowel carcinoma.

Isotope bone scan

This is a very useful tool to detect further lesions in malignancy or to establish whether a lesion is metabolically active (i.e., 'hot' on bone scan). Infection will show up 'hot', as will malignant lesions.

Of the benign lesions, only osteoid osteoma will show increased uptake.

Computed tomography

Computed tomography (CT) is used to confirm osteoid osteoma.

Magnetic resonance imaging

Magnetic resonance imaging (MRI) can detect early metastatic lesions before features are apparent on X-ray images.

It is also used to define the extent of malignant bone tumours and can help to distinguish between benign and malignant lesions.

Biopsy

It can be very difficult to be certain of the diagnosis in some cases. A biopsy will prove whether the tumour is benign or malignant and exclude infection as the cause.

PRIMARY BONE TUMOURS

Primary tumours of bone can be benign or malignant.

Benign bone tumours

Enchondroma

An enchondroma is a benign bone lesion of cartilaginous origin.

Incidence

Enchondromas are relatively common, occurring usually in adulthood.

Aetiology and pathology

Enchondromas develop from aberrant cartilage (chondroma) left within bone ('en'). They are usually found in the metaphysis of long bones (femur or humerus) but are also common in the hand (Fig. 21.5).

Clinical features

An enchondroma is usually asymptomatic and may be found incidentally. Large lesions causing cortical erosion can be painful and the patient may notice a swelling, particularly in the hand.

Diagnosis and investigation

Typical features on X-ray examination show a well-demarcated calcifying lesion in the metaphysis of the bone. Serial X-ray images may be obtained to make sure the lesion is not growing rapidly.

Treatment

Usually no treatment is required, but if the lesion is significantly painful or associated with fracture, excision or curettage may be performed.

Osteochondroma

Incidence

This is the most common benign bone lesion, presenting from childhood through to adult life.

Aetiology and pathology

The lesion develops from aberrant cartilage remaining on the surface of the cortex. It is usually found around the knee, most commonly on the distal femur (see Fig. 21.5).

The pathological appearance is of a bone lesion continuous with the cortex of the bone, capped with hyaline cartilage. It can be sessile or pedunculated (see Fig. 21.5).

Clinical features

The majority are asymptomatic, presenting incidentally or as a swelling. Rarely, pain or pressure effects on nerves or vessels occur.

Diagnosis and investigation

The typical appearance of a pedunculated lesion in continuity with the cortex clinches the diagnosis. If there is doubt, CT or MRI may be used.

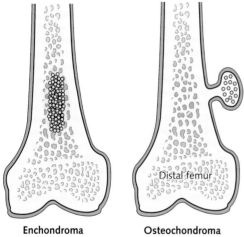

Enchondroma   Osteochondroma
Fig. 21.5 Benign cartilage tumours.

Treatment

Usually no treatment is needed; rarely, excision is carried out, if symptomatic.

Prognosis

It is extremely rare for either osteochondroma or enchondroma to undergo malignant change.

Osteoid osteoma

Osteoid osteoma is a painful, self-limiting benign bone lesion.

Incidence

The lesion is uncommon, usually presenting between 5 and 30 years of age.

Aetiology and pathology

It is caused by a nidus of osteoblasts located in the cortex of bone and is usually found in the tibia, spine or femur.

Clinical features

Patients have intense pain, particularly at night. Tenderness over the lesion is usual. In the spine, scoliosis may be present.

Diagnosis and investigation

X-ray images show a radiolucent nidus surrounded by a dense area of reactive bone (Fig 21.6A). CT scans confirm and accurately locate the lesion (Fig. 21.6B).

Treatment

Pain is typically relieved by nonsteroidal antiinflammatory drugs which can be employed while the tumour regresses

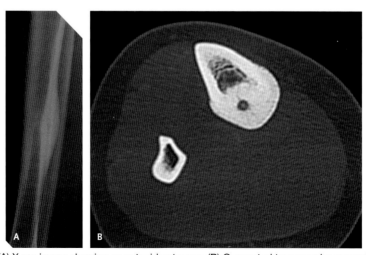

Fig. 21.6 (A) X-ray image showing an osteoid osteoma. (B) Computed tomography scan will confirm.

naturally. If required, CT-guided ablation is now preferred over surgical excision.

Prognosis

This tumour is eventually self-limiting.

Fibrous dysplasia

This is not strictly a bone tumour. It is a deficiency in bone development whereby abnormal scar tissue develops in place of normal bone.

Incidence

The true incidence is unknown as many patients are asymptomatic, but fibrous dysplasia is thought to be relatively common, usually presenting by the age of 30 years.

Aetiology and pathology

It is most commonly found in the skull, jaw, ribs and proximal femur and is caused by developmental abnormality of bone with numerous fibrous proliferations.

Clinical features

The condition is usually asymptomatic, discovered as an incidental finding, but can present with pain, swelling, deformity or fracture.

Diagnosis and investigation

A typical ground-glass appearance is diagnostic (Fig. 21.2).

Treatment

No treatment is usually required, but if the dysplasia is significant, curettage and bone grafting can be performed.

Malignant primary bone tumours

Primary malignant bone tumours are very rare. We will discuss some of those most likely to be encountered.

Osteosarcoma

Incidence

There are approximately 5 cases per million children under 15 years of age. Presentation is more commonly seen in adolescence and young adulthood or in the elderly where they develop in Pagetic bones.

Aetiology and pathology

Paget's disease or radiation can predispose a patient to osteosarcoma, but most cases occur sporadically. The tumour is highly malignant. Local spread occurs quickly, destroying the cortex, but the tumour can also metastasize.

The most common location is around the knee; other sites include the proximal humerus and femur.

Clinical features

The patient presents with pain and sometimes swelling. Clinically, there is usually warmth over the affected area and there may be a palpable mass. 10% to 20% of patients present with pulmonary metastases.

Diagnosis and investigation

X-ray images (Fig. 21.7) may show:

- An ill-defined lesion with an indistinct zone of transition (Fig. 21.7A)
- Sclerotic or lytic areas within the lesion
- Cortical destruction
- A Codman triangle (elevation of periosteum; Fig. 21.7B)

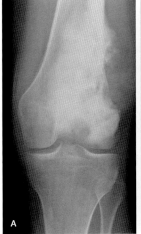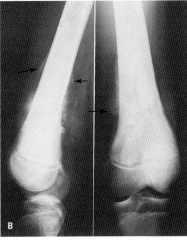

Fig. 21.7 X-ray images of osteosarcoma. (A) Ill-defined lesion. (B) Codman triangles (*arrows*).

- Sunray spicules (calcification within the tumour but outside the bone)

Biopsy might be necessary to confirm the diagnosis. Further investigations such as CT and MRI are required to stage the lesion.

Treatment

A combined multidisciplinary team approach is adopted.

Preoperative chemotherapy followed by limb salvage surgery is performed if possible. Amputation is occasionally required.

Prognosis

Five-year survival is 60%.

Chondrosarcoma

Incidence

Chondrosarcomas are more prevalent with age, with most tumours arising after the age of 40 years. The peak incidence is approximately eight cases per million at the age of 80 years. Men are more commonly affected than women.

Aetiology and pathology

A chondrosarcoma can be either a primary lesion or a secondary conversion of a benign cartilaginous tumour such as osteochondroma or enchondroma. Chondrosarcomas can be separated into low grade and high grade. Little difference can be seen histologically between a low-grade chondrosarcoma and a benign cartilaginous lesion. High-grade chondrosarcomas demonstrate a more abnormal cell structure and are consequently more aggressive. The most common areas of growth are in the pelvis, proximal femur, proximal humerus and proximal tibia.

Clinical features

Similar to osteosarcoma, the main clinical features are that of pain and localized swelling. On examination, there might be a bony mass palpable.

Diagnosis and investigation

X-ray images usually show a lytic lesion with cortical destruction and central calcification. Low-grade lesions may resemble benign cartilaginous lesion. CT or MRI may be required to investigate the lesion further.

Treatment

A multidisciplinary approach is once again adopted. Chemotherapy and radiotherapy are less effective. Wide excision of the lesion is sometimes possible, as chondrosarcomas are slow-growing and metastasize late in the disease; however, amputation may be the only viable option.

Prognosis

Prognosis is grade-dependent: 5-year survival for low-grade lesions is 90%, whereas for high-grade lesions it is 5%.

Ewing sarcoma

Incidence

Ewing sarcoma is less common than osteosarcoma with around 3 per million per year. It occurs most commonly between 5 and 25 years of age.

Aetiology and pathology

Histologically, this is a small-cell sarcoma. It occurs as frequently in flat bones as in long bones, being most common in the femur or tibia (long bone), pelvis or vertebra (flat bones).

These tumours are highly malignant and often large at presentation.

Clinical features

Patients present with pain and may be unwell with fever, malaise, anorexia and weight loss. Clinically, the area is warm and swelling may be present.

Diagnosis and investigation

Diagnosis is usually made from X-ray examination (Fig. 21.8). It usually appears as a lytic lesion with a laminated periosteal reaction (onion skinning). CT and MRI help to stage the lesion. Biopsy may be necessary.

Treatment

A combined multidisciplinary team approach is adopted.

Preoperative chemotherapy and radiotherapy followed by limb salvage surgery are performed if possible.

Prognosis

Five-year survival is 60%.

SECONDARY BONE TUMOURS

Incidence

Secondary bone tumours are the most common bone-destroying lesions in the older patient.

Aetiology and pathology

The tumours most likely to metastasize to bone are:

- breast
- lung
- prostate

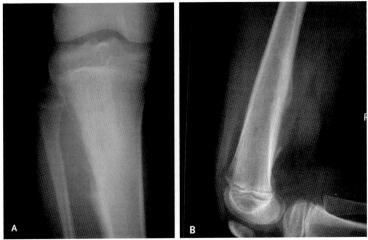

Fig. 21.8 X-ray images of Ewing sarcoma. (A) demonstrating lysis and periosteal reaction in a proximal tibial lesion. (B) demonstrating periosteal reaction in a distal femoral lesion.

- kidney
- thyroid

Metastatic lesions are most commonly found in the spine, pelvis, ribs and proximal long bones. The mechanism of metastasis is shown in Fig. 21.9. Bone is destroyed by metastatic disease causing lytic lesions, and weakened, predisposing to fracture. Most metastases appear osteolytic, but those from prostate cancer appear sclerotic.

Clinical features

Patients with a known primary

The patient has a clear history of previous malignancy, which in the case of breast carcinoma may have been many years previously. Unrelenting bone pain in the axial skeleton then makes the patient seek medical help. Night pain that does not respond to simple analgesia is often a feature. There may be constitutional symptoms such as weight loss and malaise.

Patients with no known primary

The patient presents with bone pain as described above but with no history of previous malignancy. In this case it is important to ask about symptoms suggestive of a primary malignancy (e.g., cough and haemoptysis (lung), urinary symptoms (prostate)). Patients often do not have any symptoms of the primary. Clinical examination should concentrate on likely sources of primary tumours. Therefore, the following should be examined:

- breast
- chest
- prostate (per rectum)

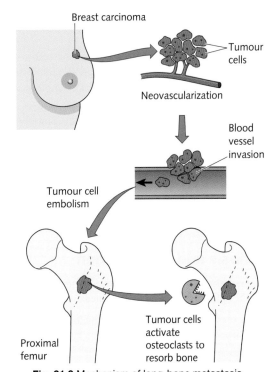

Fig. 21.9 Mechanism of long-bone metastasis.

- thyroid
- abdomen (kidney)

Fracture

The patient usually has a history of bone pain preceding the event (usually minor trauma) that caused the fracture.

Spinal cord compression

Patients with malignancy can appear to be 'off their legs' with weakness and/or altered sensation at a demonstrable spinal level (change in neurological signs corresponding to the specific vertebral level affected). There may be a history of preceding spinal bony pain and then weakness, numbness and loss of bladder and bowel control (cauda equina syndrome). An MRI scan is urgently needed to assess the spinal cord and radiotherapy may shrink the tumour, preserving spinal cord function.

Diagnosis and investigation

Any bone-destroying lesion could be due to infection or malignancy. The following should be investigated:

- Check the white cell count and inflammatory markers (CRP and ESR). These are elevated in infection but may also be elevated in malignancy (myeloma).
- Further blood tests may identify the primary such as CEA or PSA.
- Plain X-ray images may show an osteolytic, sclerotic or mixed lesion.
- If strong clinical suspicion exists then an MRI scan is more sensitive.
- Cortical thinning suggests impending fracture.
- A bone scan will be 'hot' and is useful to exclude further distant lesions.

- In an unknown primary, further investigation to find the primary is warranted (Fig. 21.10).

Treatment

Treatment depends on the primary and on the life expectancy of the patient. A multidisciplinary approach is required involving oncologists.

Conservative

- Adequate analgesia and splintage.
- Radiotherapy is used frequently for bony metastatic pain.
- Chemotherapy may have a role in certain tumours.
- Hormonal therapy is useful in some primaries such as breast cancer.
- Intravenous bisphosphonates are now being used to inhibit osteoclastic resorption of bone.

Surgical

- Intramedullary fixation of long bones is performed for fracture or impending fracture. This should be discussed carefully with the patient, but even in palliative care it can be a pain-relieving procedure to preserve mobility in a patient's final months of life.
- Joint arthroplasty is sometimes used around the hip and shoulder.
- Spinal decompression and stabilization can be used for acute cord compression.

HAEMOPOIETIC DISEASES

Lymphoma and myeloma can present with bone destruction.

Lymphoma

Incidence

Lymphoma is rare but can occur at any age.

Aetiology and pathology

Lymphoma is a malignant haematopoietic tumour usually occurring secondarily but rarely primarily in bone. Primary

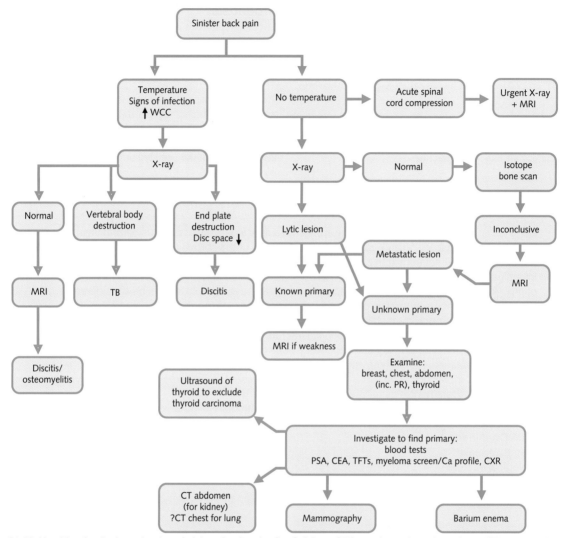

Fig. 21.10 Algorithm for the investigation of sinister back pain. *Ca*, Calcium; *CEA*, carcinoembryonic antigen; *CT*, computed tomography; *CXR*, chest X-ray examination; *MRI*, magnetic resonance imaging; *PR*, per rectum; *PSA*, prostate-specific antigen; *TB*, tuberculosis; *TFTs*, thyroid function tests; *WCC*, white cell count.

bone lymphoma has a better prognosis. It can occur in any bone, most commonly the pelvis, spine and ribs, but also around the knee.

Diagnosis and investigation
- X-ray images show a long lesion with mottled bony destruction.
- Isotope bone scanning excludes further lesions.
- Biopsy confirms the diagnosis.

Treatment
Chemotherapy and irradiation are commonly used together.

Myeloma

Incidence
This is a rare tumour, occurring between 50 and 80 years of age.

Aetiology and pathology
Lesions are due to a plasma cell malignancy and are usually found in the spine, ribs or clavicle.

Clinical features
Bony pain is common and there may be a pathological fracture. Systemic symptoms of fatigue and fever are very common.

Diagnosis and investigation

Patients will have a high ESR and may have hypercalcaemia. Serum electrophoresis for immunoglobulins and urinary analysis for Bence Jones proteins confirm the diagnosis.

X-ray images show classic punched-out lytic lesions. MRI and CT procedures are of less use than X-ray examinations.

Treatment

Chemotherapy is the mainstay with surgical stabilization or radiotherapy for impending fracture.

Prognosis

Overall prognosis is poor, with survival averaging 2 years.

LEUKAEMIA

The last malignancy to mention is leukaemia: a malignancy of white blood cells.

Leukaemia is the most common malignancy of childhood and about one-third of patients have bone pain. Leukaemia can also present with an acutely hot, swollen joint very similar to septic arthritis.

● Chapter Summary

- Bone lesions seen on X-ray images may appear as subtle lucencies or obvious deformities.
- Features of malignancy on an X-ray include; involvement of the cortex, periosteal reaction (Codman triangle) and indistinct transition zone.
- Investigation for a patient with an incidental bone lesion visible on X-ray examination will often take the form of an MRI scan. Primary malignancy causing bony metastases should always be considered.
- Primary bone tumours should be classified into benign and malignant.
- Tumours that commonly metastasize to bone are breast, lung, prostate, thyroid and renal.
- Bone metastasis may present as pathological fractures or simply as regional pain.
- Available treatments for primary and secondary bone tumours may involve primary excision, a wide local excision, amputation, radiotherapy and chemotherapy.
- Spinal cord compression is possible if metastases are present. If suspected, it should be investigated with MRI scanning. Treatment is usually with radiotherapy.
- Haemopoietic diseases such as myeloma can present with bone destruction.

UKMLA Conditions
Metastatic disease
Pathological fracture
Spinal cord compression

UKMLA Presentations
Back pain
Bone pain

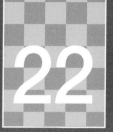
INTRODUCTION

This chapter will discuss injuries to the menisci of the knee, ligamentous injuries of the knee, patellar dislocation, shoulder dislocation and ankle sprain.

KNEE INJURIES

Meniscal injuries

The menisci are two semicircular fibrocartilage structures that lie between the femoral and tibial articular surfaces (Fig. 22.1). The medial meniscus is C-shaped and the lateral meniscus is more circular. They act as shock absorbers and are prone to injuries caused by the large forces crossing the knee.

Incidence

Meniscal injuries are common, usually occurring in young adult patients who participate in sports where a quick change in direction is required. They also occur in older patients as a degenerative process rather than a sporting injury.

There is a higher risk of a meniscal tear where the anterior cruciate ligament (ACL) has previously been torn.

Pathology and aetiology

The medial meniscus is more commonly injured because it is fixed, in comparison to the more mobile lateral meniscus.

Meniscal tears can be traumatic (as in sporting injuries) or degenerative:

- Traumatic tears. The meniscus is normal and injury usually occurs after landing or twisting with the knee flexed. This can be associated with a ligamentous injury, such as an ACL tear. A chronically unstable knee is prone to further tears.
- Degenerative tears. These occur in an older population through abnormal cartilage. They may occur with little or no injury.

Types of meniscal tears (Fig. 22.2)

1. Bucket handle. The tear extends over a distance, remaining attached at the anterior and posterior horns. A locked knee results when a large bucket-handle tear flips over and becomes trapped in the joint, resulting in loss of complete extension.
2. Radial.
3. Horizontal cleavage.
4. Flap/parrot beak.
5. Radial tear with an associated meniscal cyst.

It is clinically important to establish how peripheral the tear is. Very peripheral tears occur through tissue with a rich blood supply and are amenable to repair, as these tears can heal. Meniscal tears further away from the blood supply (i.e., more central) cannot heal.

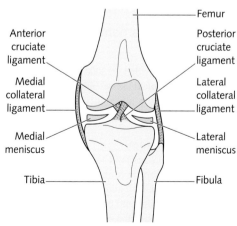

Fig. 22.1 Basic anatomy of the knee.

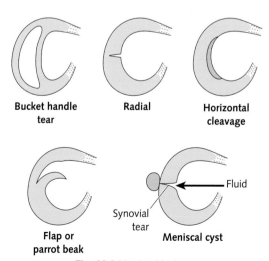

Fig. 22.2 Meniscal lesions.

Meniscal cysts result from synovial fluid being pumped into the meniscal tear. A valve effect means the fluid in the cyst cannot drain back into the knee (see Fig. 22.2).

Clinical features

Patients usually sustain this injury while playing sport, with the incident occurring during a tackle or when twisting or changing direction.

A patient may present immediately after injury with a painful locked knee or with a gradual chronic nagging pain with associated swelling over months or years following a minor injury. In the chronic setting, the symptoms are often intermittent.

Mechanical symptoms such as locking and giving way suggest meniscal pathology. A 'clicking' joint does not necessarily mean there is pathology and many normal knees 'click'.

A more major injury with acute swelling and instability suggests associated ligamentous injury.

Examination may reveal:

- Joint line tenderness: an important part of the examination and is usually positive in a patient with a torn meniscus.
- A locked knee (patient's knee is in flexion and cannot extend out straight).
- A palpable effusion.
- A large acute effusion can sometimes be caused by a very peripheral tear but should raise suspicion of another cause such as ligament injury or fracture.
- A meniscal cyst, which may be palpable over the lateral joint line.

A variety of special tests are described for meniscal tears (such as McMurray's test) and none are totally reliable. A good history is often the best tool in diagnosing meniscal pathology.

Diagnosis and investigation

In most cases, the diagnosis is made on the basis of history and examination.

X-ray images are normal and are performed to exclude fracture in the acute setting and osteoarthritis in the chronic setting.

MRI is used to confirm the presence of torn menisci, but as there is an associated false positive rate the most accurate way to confirm the diagnosis is with arthroscopy of the knee.

Management

Conservative

Initially rest, ice, compression, elevation (RICE) is used for an acutely swollen knee. Early physiotherapy is essential to encourage movement after the initial injury. Conservative management may be all that is required if the symptoms settle.

Surgical

If the patient has ongoing problems following conservative management or has a large tear or a tear amenable to repair, surgery is usually recommended. Surgery is now performed using arthroscopic techniques. For peripheral bucket-handle or vertical tears, meniscal repair has the advantage of retaining the meniscus.

For tears not amenable to repair, meniscal resection is commonly performed. Partial meniscectomy removes the damaged portion only, leaving a stable rim and reducing the risk of osteoarthritis in the future.

Prognosis

Patients usually recover well following treatment, however, removal of a significant portion of a meniscus can lead to osteoarthritic changes developing later down the line because of increased load on the articular surface of the knee.

Ligamentous injuries of the knee

Anterior cruciate ligament

Incidence

ACL tears are common with 1 in 3000 people, per year, being affected. Around half of all knee injuries are ACL injuries. Females are more likely to injure their ACL than males, in a 4.5:1 ratio.

Aetiology and pathology

The ACL is the primary restraint to anterior tibial translation and rotation. The mechanism of injury is usually a twisting or valgus strain of the knee, with adduction at the hip, commonly occurring in football, skiing and basketball (Fig. 22.3).

The knee is usually extended or slightly flexed with the foot fixed. Associated injuries to the medial collateral ligament (MCL)

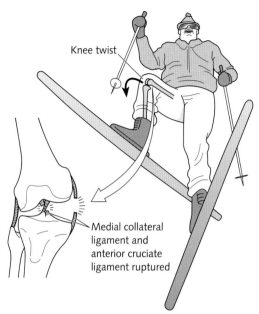

Fig. 22.3 Mechanism of injury in anterior cruciate ligament rupture.

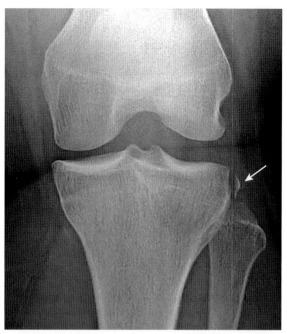

Fig. 22.4 Segond fracture. This is an avulsion fracture of the knee involving the lateral aspect of the tibial plateau (*arrow*). It is frequently (75% of cases) associated with disruption of the anterior cruciate ligament (ACL). (From Herring W. *Learning Radiology: Recognizing the Basics.* 5th ed. Elsevier; 2024.)

and either meniscus are common (the unhappy triad). The patient often hears a pop or feels 'something go' inside the knee.

ACL-deficient knees are susceptible to further meniscal tears and chondral injuries.

Clinical features

With an acute ACL rupture, the patient will be unable to play on and may have to be carried from the field.

Swelling typically occurs within the timeframe of minutes to hours, unlike meniscal tears, which swell over 24 hours. This is because the ACL is more vascular than the menisci and will therefore cause a haemarthrosis more quickly. Clinically, patients therefore have a tense effusion after the acute injury.

Once initial symptoms have settled, the patient may complain of giving way of the knee. Many patients present a long time after injury with symptoms of instability. This occurs when the patient tries to turn rapidly. Patients will frequently report being able to run in a straight line but not being able to twist and turn. This giving way or instability is pain free.

The anterior drawer test (see Chapter 2) and Lachman test are positive.

Diagnosis and investigation

The majority can be diagnosed clinically from history (mechanism of injury, with a 'pop' heard or felt and an immediate haemarthrosis) and examination. In some patients, it is difficult to achieve positive examination findings (especially acutely) and in those patients an MRI scan is used to confirm the diagnosis.

Arthroscopy is the most reliable diagnostic tool and findings do not always match the MRI. X-ray images will usually be normal but can show a Segond fracture which is pathognomonic for an ACL tear (Fig. 22.4).

Management

Conservative – Initial treatment is with RICE and physiotherapy. In the absence of instability, most patients can modify their activities and manage well following a rehabilitation programme concentrating on quadriceps and hamstrings strengthening.

Surgical – ACL reconstruction is indicated for functional instability of the knee. This can be performed either through open or arthroscopic surgery using a hamstring tendon or patellar tendon autograft or allograft. Meniscal tears can also be addressed at the time of surgery.

Posterior cruciate ligament

The posterior cruciate ligament (PCL) is the primary restraint to posterior movement of the tibia on the femur.

Incidence

As the PCL is stronger than the ACL, PCL injuries are rarer. Around 5% to 20% of knee injuries are PCL injuries.

Aetiology and pathology

PCL injuries require a significant force to occur either in sporting activities or from road traffic accidents (dashboard injury; Fig. 22.5). It is an injury often sustained by goalkeepers in football; the mechanism of injury being such that the knee is held in a flexed and static position as an oncoming attacking player forces the tibia backwards. The PCL can also rupture when the knee is forcibly hyperextended. Most PCL tears occur in combination with other ligamentous injuries and, rarely, injuries to the popliteal artery. It is important to check the distal vasculature in suspected cases of high-energy trauma and PCL rupture, as the knee may have been dislocated at the time of injury (see box: Clinical notes, Knee dislocation).

CLINICAL NOTES

KNEE DISLOCATION

(Note, not a patellar dislocation which is commonly referred to by laypeople as a 'knee dislocation'.)

This is a rare injury but carries significant morbidity. It is usually the result of high-energy trauma and can result in devastating neurological and vascular injury with a 50% vascular injury rate in anterior and posterior dislocations. The knee will need to be reduced urgently and bony and ligamentous injuries reconstructed after an interval. It is rare to recover preinjury function after a dislocated knee.

Clinical features

The patient will have a substantial injury to the knee and will usually be unable to bear weight. Swelling is usually less obvious than with an ACL injury. Patients complain less of instability than with ACL injuries. Clinically, patients will have a posterior sag sign and positive posterior drawer test. Careful assessment is needed to identify associated injuries such as lateral collateral ligament (LCL) injuries.

Diagnosis and investigation

All patients with suspected PCL injury should undergo an MRI scan.

Treatment

Conservative – Almost all isolated PCL injuries can be treated with rehabilitation alone.

Surgical – Patients with combined injuries or symptomatic instability require reconstruction.

Collateral ligament injuries

Incidence

MCL injuries are common injuries in isolation or combined with ACL injury, while LCL injuries are rare injuries. MCL injuries are more common in men than women.

Aetiology and pathology

In the case of MCL injuries, there is a valgus strain pattern of injury. The injury to the ligament can be complete or partial and is frequently associated with ACL injury. Isolated LCL injuries occur when a varus strain is placed on the knee (i.e., hit from the medial side; Fig. 22.6).

Clinical features

Collateral ligament injuries are usually sporting injuries; the patient may feel 'something go' but an effusion is not a feature of an isolated collateral ligament injury (they are extraarticular

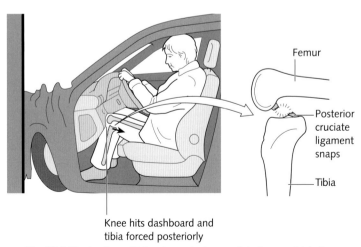

Knee hits dashboard and
tibia forced posteriorly

Fig. 22.5 Mechanism of injury in posterior cruciate ligament injuries.

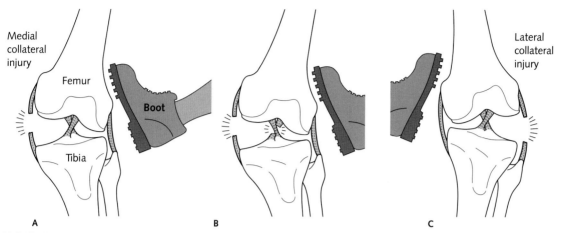

Fig. 22.6 Mechanism of injury in collateral ligament tears. (A) Valgus strain; (B) anterior cruciate ligament and medial collateral ligament rupture; (C) varus strain.

structures). The patient will complain of pain and possibly instability.

When the MCL is injured, there will be tenderness over the broad attachment of the MCL and opening of the joint on valgus stress. In the normal knee, the LCL is easily palpable as a cord-like structure. When the LCL is ruptured, the area is tender and indistinct. Opening of the joint on the lateral side will be present on varus stress.

Investigations
Radiographs should be taken as with any acute knee injury to look for an associated fracture from the trauma, however, an MRI is the imaging of choice to assess for a ligament injury and will be able to detect any other ligamentous injury.

Management
Many isolated injuries heal well with conservative treatment. Treatment is with physiotherapy and bracing for 6 weeks. Minor tears heal well without bracing.

Surgical repair or reconstruction is sometimes required for chronic unstable injuries.

Prognosis
The knee usually returns to normal after a period of rehabilitation.

Patellar dislocation

Introduction
The patella is prevented from dislocation by anatomical features such as a large lateral femoral condyle and the insertion of the vastus medialis oblique muscle and medial patellar femoral ligament (Fig. 22.7).

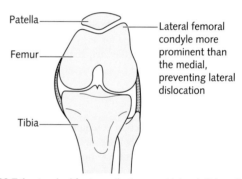

Fig. 22.7 Anatomical features that prevent lateral dislocation of the patella.

Incidence
Traumatic patellar dislocation is common and usually occurs in young adults due to the nature of their activities.

Aetiology and pathology
Patellar dislocation can be traumatic, chronic or habitual.

Traumatic dislocations occur during sports, usually with the knee slightly flexed with side impact. The dislocation occurs laterally and damage may occur to the joint surface as an osteochondral fracture. Structures along the medial border of the patella are torn.

Chronic subluxations or dislocations are traumatic but may require less force and are associated with anatomical malalignment.

Those suffering habitual dislocation are often young women with ligamentous laxity and a hypoplastic trochlea. This group suffers recurrent dislocations after minor injuries, or even during normal flexion, and is difficult to treat.

Clinical features

A first-time dislocation is extremely painful and the patient arrives in the emergency department with a history of 'a dislocated knee'. The patella might have spontaneously reduced if the knee was extended to allow transport. If not, it will be laterally situated.

There is often tenderness over the medial side of the knee and an effusion.

Later, when the acute injury has settled, the patient may have patellar apprehension evident on examination.

Patients who suffer habitual dislocation may show a J-sign on examination and additional evidence of generalized laxity in other joints such as fingers, thumbs, elbows and knees (hypermobility syndrome).

Patients who have chronic dislocations may have wasted or deficient vastus medialis.

Diagnosis and investigation

X-ray examinations should be made after reduction, including a tunnel and skyline view looking for any osteochondral defects. CT and MRI scanning can further help to plan surgery.

Management

Conservative

In acute cases, urgent reduction is required if this hasn't happened already. This is usually done in the emergency department. A short period on crutches may be helpful but long periods of immobilization are not helpful. Physiotherapy is the mainstay of treatment once pain and swelling allow, improving range of movement and quadriceps strength specifically to try to stabilize the patella. In first-time dislocations, conservative management may be all that is required.

Surgical

Large osteochondral fractures should be repaired or removed arthroscopically.

Recurrent dislocations may require surgical realignment. Repair or reconstruction of the medial patellofemoral ligament is carried out where physiotherapy has failed and persistent dislocation is causing symptoms.

SHOULDER DISLOCATION

Incidence

The shoulder is the most commonly dislocated large joint in the body.

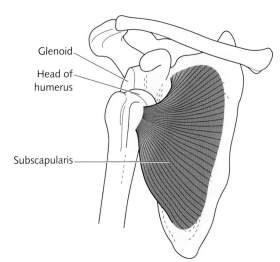

Fig. 22.8 Anterior dislocation of the humerus.

Labels: Glenoid, Head of humerus, Subscapularis

Aetiology and pathology

The shoulder is at risk of traumatic dislocation because the joint has very little inherent bony stability, with reliance instead on its capsule, labrum and rotator cuff muscles. Anatomically, the joint has sacrificed stability, in a small shallow glenoid, for an increased range of movement.

Dislocation can be anterior or posterior. Anterior dislocation (Fig. 22.8) accounts for 95% and usually occurs when the arm is forced back in a ball-throwing position of external rotation and abduction. In anterior dislocation, the labrum can be damaged anteroinferiorly, leaving a Bankart lesion predisposing to further dislocations. Recurrent dislocations cause a Hill-Sachs lesion due to impaction of the glenoid on the posterior part of the humeral head.

In older patients, a rotator cuff injury is more commonly seen than a Bankart lesion.

Posterior dislocations are far less common, occurring in fewer than 5% of cases. Posterior dislocations occur with high-energy trauma, epileptic seizures and electrocution.

Clinical features

The patient is often a sports player – typically rugby – and has an acute injury to the shoulder, as described above. The injury is intensely painful and the shoulder is held supported by the other arm (Fig. 22.9).

Examination findings include:

- Loss of normal shoulder contour
- A palpable glenoid
- Complete loss of movement

Check and document that the nerves of the upper limb (especially the axillary nerve) are functioning before and after any intervention.

Diagnosis and investigation

Anterior dislocation is usually obvious and confirmed with X-ray examinations (always performed to exclude a fracture).

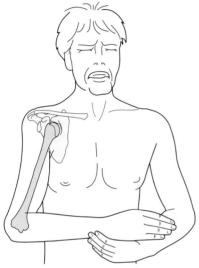

Fig. 22.9 Abnormal shoulder contour in anterior dislocation of the humerus.

Posterior dislocation is often missed as the initial anteroposterior X-ray image looks normal to the untrained eye. This should be suspected in any patient who has fixed internal rotation of the shoulder. The light bulb sign (Fig. 22.10A) should raise suspicion, but the diagnosis is made on axillary view (Fig. 22.10B) or CT scan.

CLINICAL NOTES

Injuries associated with a shoulder dislocation
Bankart lesion – a disruption of the anterior labrum
Bony Bankart lesion – fracture of the anterior glenoid
Hill-Sachs defect – impaction of the humeral head from the glenoid rim during dislocation
Axillary nerve injury
Rotator cuff tear

Treatment

Conservative

The dislocation needs to be promptly reduced in the emergency department under sedation.

Posterior dislocation often requires a general anaesthetic and may need open reduction.

Once the dislocation is reduced, the joint is rested in a collar and cuff and once the pain has settled, supervised early rehabilitation with a physiotherapist can commence.

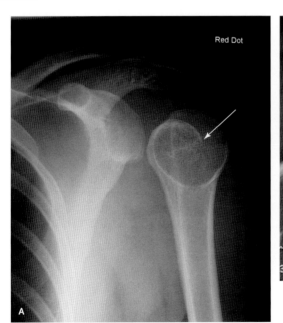

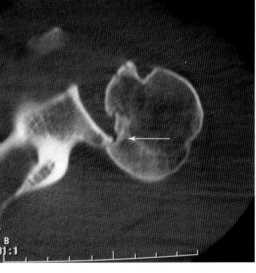

Fig. 22.10 Posterior dislocation of the shoulder. (A) Anteroposterior X-ray showing the light bulb sign (*arrow*); (B) computed tomography scan showing axial view. There is posterior subluxation of the head with impaction of the head from the glenoid rim (*arrow*).

Surgical

Surgery is reserved for recurrent dislocations to repair bone or labral defects.

Prognosis

Men have a higher rate of recurrence than females. The younger the patient at the time of first dislocation, the higher the recurrence rate (as high as 80% in teenage men).

In the more elderly population, shoulder stiffness is more of a problem than recurrence.

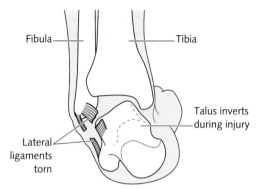

Fibula / Tibia

Talus inverts during injury

Lateral ligaments torn

Fig. 22.11 Ankle ligament rupture.

ANKLE SPRAIN

Incidence

Ankle sprains are very common injuries, lateral more so than medial.

Aetiology and pathology

These injuries are commonly found in sportspeople, but anyone can suffer a sprained ankle. The mechanism of injury is inversion or eversion with damage to the lateral ligament and medial ligament complexes, respectively.

In a lateral ligament sprain, the talus tilts in varus in the ankle mortice and the anterior talofibular and/or calcaneofibular ligaments are torn (Fig. 22.11). In a medial ligament sprain, the talus tilts in valgus in the ankle mortice and the deltoid ligament complex is torn.

Clinical features

The patient experiences pain and may feel 'something go'; swelling occurs rapidly.

Clinically, the patient has a variable amount of swelling and tenderness over either the lateral or medial ligament complex.

Chronic ankle instability leads to the joint giving way repeatedly.

Patients may have instability of the ankle joint with a positive anterior drawer test and opening of the lateral side.

Diagnosis and investigation

X-ray examinations are performed only if there is bony tenderness or inability to bear weight (Ottawa ankle rules).

CLINICAL NOTES

The Ottawa ankle rules suggest that an X-ray is required if:

- There is any pain over either malleoli or any one of the following:
  - Bony tenderness along the distal 6cm of the posterior edge of the tibia or the tip of the medial malleolus, OR
  - Bony tenderness along the distal 6 cm of the posterior edge of the fibula or tip of the lateral malleolus, OR
  - An inability to bear weight both immediately and in the emergency department for four steps.

Management

Conservative

All sprains are initially treated conservatively with analgesia, RICE and physiotherapy.

Surgical

Arthroscopy of the ankle is sometimes performed for associated large osteochondral injuries.

Ligament reconstruction is rarely required for a chronically unstable ankle.

● Chapter Summary

- A locked knee is often caused by a meniscal tear but can also be caused by loose bodies in the joint.
- Meniscal tears are often treated conservatively, but if chronically symptomatic, they can be either repaired or excised by arthroscopic techniques.
- The classic history for an ACL tear is one of twisting trauma to the knee or valgus strain, with adduction at the hip. A popping sensation is often felt with a rapid onset of effusion.
- Collateral ligaments supply lateral stability to the knee and can be injured with any significant valgus or varus stress.
- The patella does not normally dislocate because strong ligaments hold it in line; however, in those with lax ligaments, such as in connective tissue disorders, patellar dislocations are much more common.
- The shoulder is a ball and socket joint where the majority of stability comes from muscular and ligamentous attachments. It is more prone to dislocation than other joints due to its large range of motion and shallow depth.
- Shoulder dislocations are most frequently anterior–inferior and should be managed with reduction under sedation as soon as safely possible.
- Surgical treatment in the form of reconstruction for ACL rupture is indicated in high functioning individuals with good rehabilitation potential. It is possible to lead a normal life without an ACL.
- Ankle sprains are frequent and rarely require surgical intervention. However, X-ray examination should be performed in selected cases to confirm there is no bony injury.

UKMLA Conditions
Lower limb soft tissue injury
Upper limb soft tissue injury

UKMLA Presentations
Acute joint pain/swelling
Chronic joint pain/stiffness
Limp
Soft tissue injury

Soft tissue disorders

INTRODUCTION

Soft tissue disorders are common and are responsible for many days of absence from work. They contribute significantly to the workload in primary care, emergency departments, rheumatology clinics and orthopaedic clinics. This chapter will discuss their presentation, diagnosis and management.

COMMON TENDON PATHOLOGIES

The three main pathologies that affect tendons are:

- tendinopathy
- tenosynovitis
- tendon rupture

Tendinopathy

Definition

Pain arises from strain or injury to tendons and their insertions to bone. The term enthesopathy is used to describe cases with a significant periosteal component, such as lateral or medial epicondylitis.

Aetiology and pathogenesis

Some tendinopathies occur from overuse in, for example, labourers, musicians, athletes and some occur idiopathically. The pathophysiology of tendinopathy is multifactorial but not completely understood. Inflammation is thought to play a role.

Clinical features

The most frequent sites of tendinopathy are:

- shoulder
- elbow
- ankle (Achilles tendon)
- wrist
- hip
- knee

Patients complain of pain that is worsened by active movement. Examination findings include:

- Tenderness of the tendon and its insertion.
- An increase in pain when active movement is performed against resistance.
- Soft tissue swelling (not always present).

Examples

Shoulder

Biceps tendonitis and calcifying tendonitis (usually involving the supraspinatus tendon) both give rise to shoulder pain.

Tennis elbow

Commonly occurs with repetitive movements that mimic a backhand in tennis (pronation or supination in full extension). The common extensor origin, at the lateral epicondyle, is tender and pain is exacerbated by resisted wrist extension (Fig. 23.1A).

Golfer's elbow

Much less common than tennis elbow. Occurs with overuse of flexion and pronation. The common flexor origin, at the medial epicondyle, is tender and pain is exacerbated by resisted wrist flexion (Fig. 23.1B).

Investigation

Tendinopathy can be diagnosed clinically and investigations are often unremarkable. Radiographs may show abnormalities, such as calcification in chronic rotator cuff disease. Ultrasound scan and magnetic resonance imaging may also detect changes in the tendon and surrounding tissue.

Management

The interventions shown below may lead to improvement of symptoms. The strategies at the top of the list should be employed early in the disease process, whilst those at the bottom should be reserved for resistant cases:

- rest or avoidance of precipitating cause
- nonsteroidal antiinflammatory drug (NSAID) therapy
- physiotherapy
- local corticosteroid injection
- surgery

Tenosynovitis

Definition

Tenosynovitis is inflammation of the synovial lining of a tendon sheath. It can be infective (as in flexor sheath infection) or noninfective. Here we will discuss noninfective tenosynovitis.

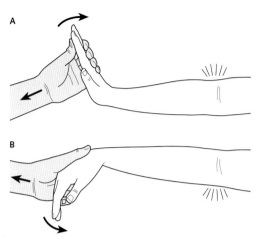

Fig. 23.1 The pain of tennis elbow is exacerbated by resisted wrist extension (A). The pain of golfer's elbow is exacerbated by resisted wrist flexion (B).

Aetiology

The two main causes are:

- inflammatory arthritis
- trauma

Trauma is usually a result of repetitive or unusual movement.

Clinical features

Patients present with pain in the region of the affected tendon. Common sites of tenosynovitis are the abductor pollicis longus and extensor pollicis brevis tendons (de Quervain tenosynovitis) and finger flexors. On examination, the tendon is swollen and tender and crepitus may be felt on palpation.

A trigger finger or thumb results from tenosynovitis of the flexor tendons. A nodule can develop on the tendon in response to constriction of the tendon sheath. The nodule catches as it enters or leaves the flexor tendon pulleys and a snapping or flicking movement of the digit occurs on flexion or extension. In severe cases, the digit may be held in flexion, requiring the patient to release the triggered digit with the other hand.

Management

Treatment includes rest, splinting and local corticosteroid injection. Surgical decompression of the tendon sheath may be required in chronic cases.

Tendon rupture

Aetiology

Tendon rupture may result from chronic inflammation and degeneration or trauma. For example, rupture of the extensor tendons of the fingers is often seen in rheumatoid arthritis.

Clinical features

The resulting clinical features are loss of movement at the joint to which the tendon provides power, deformity and sometimes swelling. Patients who suffer a rupture of their Achilles tendon will describe feeling a blow to the back of their leg and resultant inability to plantar flex at the ankle. After rupture of the long head of the biceps tendon, a bulge formed by the biceps muscle belly is seen in the upper arm – the so-called popeye sign (Fig. 23.2).

Extensor tendon rupture at the distal phalanx can occur after a direct blow to the fingertip, causing aggressive flexion of the distal interphalangeal joint. It results in an inability to extend the flexed distal interphalangeal joint (mallet finger; Fig. 23.3).

CLINICAL NOTES

When reviewing a patient with a suspected Achilles tendon rupture, Simmonds test is often used. With the patient supine and their foot hanging off the end of the bed, the calf is squeezed. If plantarflexion at the ankle does not occur, Simmonds test is positive and this indicates the tendon is ruptured (Fig. 23.4).

Management

Sometimes no intervention is required, such as a long head of biceps tendon rupture, because function is preserved with other muscles; in this case, short head of biceps, brachialis and supinator. Sometimes splintage is all that is required: a mallet splint in the case of a mallet finger or an equinus boot for an Achilles tendon rupture. However, surgery is often required to restore function. This may require direct repair of the tendon or a tendon transfer.

BURSITIS

Bursae are small sacs made of fibrous tissue that are lined with synovial membrane and secrete synovial fluid. They reduce friction where ligaments and tendons pass over bone. Inflammation of a bursa (bursitis) can be idiopathic, part of a systemic inflammatory disease or due to injury or infection. Common types of bursitis include olecranon bursitis, prepatellar bursitis and trochanteric bursitis. Some are notifiable industrial disorders.

Olecranon bursitis

This can be precipitated by excessive friction at the elbow, for example, by resting the elbow on a desk.

Idiopathic and traumatic cases are usually only painful when pressure is applied to the bursa; movement of the elbow is not usually impaired. On examination, the bursa is distended and tender.

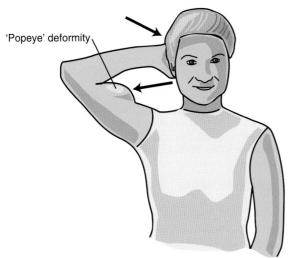

Fig. 23.2 Popeye deformity after rupture of the long head of biceps. (From Waldman SD. *Physical diagnosis of pain: an atlas of signs and symptoms*. 2nd ed. Philadelphia, Saunders; 2010.)

'Popeye' deformity

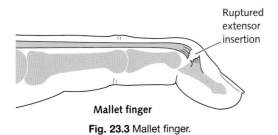

Ruptured extensor insertion

Mallet finger

Fig. 23.3 Mallet finger.

Bursal fluid should be aspirated only in cases of sepsis, to guide antibiotic treatment in a sick patient. The bursa should not be routinely aspirated as the patient can develop a chronic sinus. Local corticosteroid injection can help in resistant non-septic cases, but in most cases antiinflammatory medication and rest are preferable. Infection should be treated with appropriate antibiotics.

COMMUNICATION

Soft tissue lesions are commonly precipitated by injuries caused by overuse. It is therefore important to ask patients about their work and leisure activities.

CLINICAL NOTES

While aspiration of a prepatellar or olecranon bursitis may be useful in the treatment of recalcitrant infection, this should be as a last resort. The bursa itself will continue to make bursal fluid whilst any created tract is trying to heal, and this may lead to sinus formation. The patient must consent to this procedure and be made aware of the risk.

Prepatellar or infrapatellar bursitis

This type of bursitis is common in people such as cleaners, carpet fitters, plumbers or electricians, who spend a lot of time kneeling. A hot, red swelling develops anterior to the patella (prepatellar bursitis) or patella tendon (infrapatellar

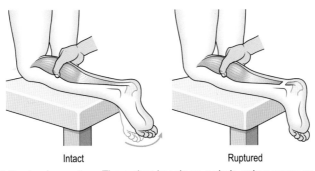

Intact   Ruptured

Fig. 23.4 Simmonds test for Achilles tendon rupture. The patient kneels on a chair, or lays prone on the examination couch, allowing the foot of the affected side to hang freely. If a rupture is present, the foot will not plantarflex when the calf muscle is squeezed. (From Jenkins P, Shields DW, White TO. *McRae's Elective Orthopaedics*. 7th ed. Elsevier; 2023.)

bursitis). Active knee extension is usually painful but possible (unlike in septic arthritis). Treatment involves rest, NSAIDs and analgesia. Recurrent episodes may require surgical excision of the bursa. Antibiotic therapy should be given in infective cases.

Infected bursitis that fails to settle with antibiotics requires formal incision and drainage.

Trochanteric bursitis

The trochanteric bursa is located lateral to the greater trochanter of the femurs and allows motion of the fascia lata over the trochanter. When this bursa becomes inflamed, the patient will develop pain over the affected trochanter, exacerbated by movement. Patients will often complain of hip pain; however, careful questioning and examination will identify pain localized to the trochanter as opposed to the groin or buttock pain of hip joint pathology. Treatment consists of physiotherapy in the first instance, with steroid injections used in more severe cases. Persistent and debilitating trochanteric bursitis may require surgery to excise the bursa.

DUPUYTREN CONTRACTURE

Definition

Dupuytren contracture is a common condition, characterized by fibromatosis (benign overgrowth of fibroblasts and myofibroblasts) of the palmar fascia, resulting in flexion contractures of the metacarpophalangeal and interphalangeal joints of one or more fingers.

Fibromatosis might affect other areas of the body: the plantar fascia (Ledderhose disease), the penis (Peyronie disease) or knuckle pads (Garrod disease). It is important to ask whether the patient has any symptoms or deformity elsewhere.

Incidence

Dupuytren disease is common and occurs in around 30 per 100,000 people a year. Before the age of 55 years, the incidence of Dupuytren contracture is much higher in men than in women. After this age, the incidence is equal.

Aetiology

Several factors predispose to Dupuytren contracture. These are shown in the adjacent box. Historically, Dupuytren contracture was felt to be a disease of northern Europeans and whilst there is a preponderance, it is also common in those of Mediterranean or Japanese descent.

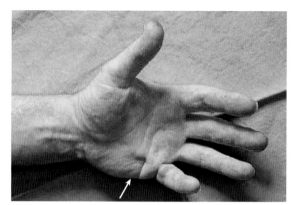

Fig. 23.5 Dupuytren contracture of the palmar fascia (*arrow*). (From Hochberg MC, Silman AJ, Smolen JS, et al., eds. *Rheumatology*. 3rd ed. St Louis: Mosby; 2003.)

CLINICAL NOTES

Factors associated with Dupuytren contracture
Family history of Dupuytren contracture (autosomal dominant inheritance)
Hepatic cirrhosis
Diabetes mellitus
Anticonvulsant therapy

Clinical features

The ulnar side of the hand is most commonly affected. Patients complain of an inability to extend one or more fingers, usually the ring and little fingers. It is rarely (perhaps never) painful. The fibromatosis may remain stable or progress. Progressive cases can result in marked deformity and loss of function, with the fingers held in a fixed position curled into the palm.

In early cases, nodules may be felt in the palm or on the palmar surface of the finger. In more advanced cases, flexion at the metacarpophalangeal joints is seen (Fig. 23.5) and the palm of the hand cannot be placed flat on a table (positive tabletop test). In severe cases, the proximal and distal interphalangeal joints are involved.

Management

Management ranges from conservative to operative. Nonoperative options include physiotherapy, injection of collagenase and needle aponeurotomy. Palmar fasciectomy is the most commonly performed surgical procedure. Complete correction of the deformity is more difficult the more advanced the disease. There is a risk of recurrence postoperatively.

Chapter Summary

- Tennis elbow affects the lateral epicondyle at the elbow.
- Golfer's elbow affects the medial epicondyle at the elbow.
- Tendon rupture can be either traumatic or degenerative due to repetitive insults (e.g., injury, inflammation). In some cases, such as in the Achilles tendon, it can be severely disabling.
- Bursitis is an inflammation of a bursa around a joint. It often settles down with antiinflammatory medication but it can occasionally become infected, requiring antibiotics or chronic, requiring excision.
- Dupuytren contracture involves a fibrous change in the palmar fascia causing thickening and fixed flexion of a digit. Multiple joints can be involved.

UKMLA Condition
Bursitis

UKMLA Presentations
Acute joint pain/swelling
Musculoskeletal deformities
Soft tissue injury

Most doctors during their career will treat orthopaedic patients undergoing surgery or who have had an orthopaedic procedure. It should be remembered that the surgical procedure is only a very small part of the overall surgical process. This chapter aims to take you through the patient's journey, starting with the preoperative period, through the basics of some orthopaedic surgeries, to postoperative management.

PREOPERATIVE ASSESSMENT

Patients undergoing elective surgery are seen a few weeks before surgery in the preoperative assessment clinic. It is important that concurrent medical problems are stabilized and new conditions identified, investigated and treated appropriately. Trauma patients are seen prior to surgery in a similar way to optimize their care prior to surgery, but usually the day before or on the day of surgery.

General approach to the preoperative patient

The following should be recorded:

- Baseline observations (e.g., blood pressure, pulse, temperature, respiratory rate): this will give clinicians the patient's normal values, but may also pick up, for example, an undiagnosed arrhythmia or undiagnosed hypertension.
- History, including past medical/surgical history and drug history: for example, the patient might be on warfarin for a metallic heart valve, and will need might need admission for perioperative bridging anticoagulation.
- Detailed systemic enquiry: to identify any other underlying medical problems which could be optimized prior to surgery.
- Examination: a detailed cardiorespiratory examination is important in regard to the anaesthetic, further examination should be carried out as per patient requirements.
- Blood tests (perhaps unnecessary in young, fit patients for simple surgery): full blood count (FBC), urea and electrolytes (U&E), liver function tests and clotting screen.
- Blood grouping should be carried out for all major joint surgeries and the patient's blood cross-matched preemptively if significant blood loss is expected.

- Urinalysis for urinary tract infection (UTI) if suspected. If a patient has a UTI, it should be treated prior to any orthopaedic operation that plans to leave metalwork in situ.
- Electrocardiogram (ECG) and chest X-ray examination (if indicated).
- Further investigations should thereafter be ordered if required, e.g., echocardiogram for a new heart murmur.

COMMUNICATION

Consent should be obtained from all patients who are able to consent. In trauma cases patients may not be able to consent and an incapacity form is usually used in the patient's best interests. In the case of elective surgery, consent is a process occurring over the weeks and months prior to the procedure, with a member of the team capable of carrying out the operation. The signing of the consent form should be the culmination of a detailed consent process starting on the first clinic visit.

Focussed approach to the preoperative patient

In the preoperative clinic the patient should be asked about their current symptoms as it may have been some time since they were first seen in clinic. The operative target (knee, hip, etc.) should be examined.

Note the skin condition of where the incision will be (there might be a current rash or skin breakdown over the operation site), the neurovascular status of the limb, range of movement and look for any distal infection. For example, a knee replacement procedure should not be carried out in a patient with an infected ingrown toenail.

IMMEDIATE PREOPERATIVE CARE

On the day of surgery, the patient will be seen again by their surgeon and anaesthetist. The procedure and anaesthetic will be explained again and the consent form checked with the patient.

Additional monitoring such as an arterial line and central venous line can be inserted in the anaesthetic room for patients expected to have a complicated anaesthetic or surgery.

A urinary catheter is an important consideration to keep the sterile field clean in incontinent patients, and to assess fluid balance in patients who may lose significant amounts of blood.

SURGERY

There are many types of surgery performed in orthopaedics, from large joint replacements to small soft tissue repairs, on all parts of the musculoskeletal system. It is far beyond the scope of this book to discuss them all, but instead, detailed here is an overview of several things a surgeon can do electively in orthopaedics.

Joint debridement

A diseased joint can be debrided surgically to improve range of movement or to reduce symptoms such as pain and swelling. Osteophytes are often removed in osteoarthritis (e.g., a cheilectomy of the first metatarsophalangeal (MTP) joint (Fig. 24.1)) but debriding a joint does not cure or stop the progression of the disease process.

Arthroscopy

Keyhole surgery techniques have become routine in recent years.

In the past, arthroscopy was seen as a diagnostic procedure, but now a number of operations are possible by purely arthroscopic means. Examples are rotator cuff repair in the shoulder and meniscal repair or anterior cruciate ligament reconstruction in the knee.

It is now commonplace for arthroscopy to be used on many joints, including the knee, shoulder, ankle, hip and wrist.

Joint excision (excision arthroplasty)

This operation has been mostly superseded by joint replacement. It is still occasionally performed for severe arthritis of the first MTP joint (Keller procedure) (Fig. 24.2) and also in the hip (Girdlestone procedure) to treat infection or as a salvage procedure for a failed hip prosthesis.

The operation leaves the joint unstable and it may still be painful.

Joint arthrodesis

Arthrodesis or fusion is performed to encourage the bones heal across a joint. Movement is obviously lost, but if the fusion is sound, the joint will be strong and pain free.

First metatarsophalangeal joint arthritis

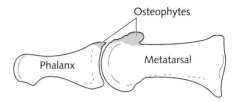

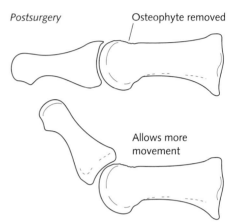

Fig. 24.1 First MTP joint cheilectomy.

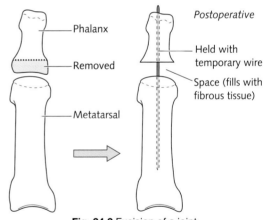

Fig. 24.2 Excision of a joint.

Bones are most commonly fused around the foot and ankle or hand and wrist, usually in patients with rheumatoid arthritis. Examples include ankle fusion, subtalar fusion and wrist fusion.

Fusion can be achieved by different means, such as:

- internal fixation such as screws, staples, and plates (Fig. 24.3A)
- intramedullary nail (Fig. 24.3B)
- external fixation (Fig. 24.7)

A bone graft may be used to encourage union.

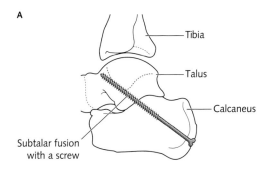

Subtalar fusion
with a screw

Tibia

Talus

Calcaneus

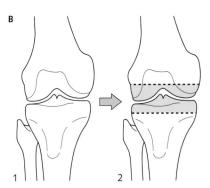

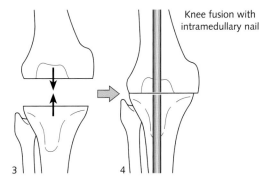

Knee fusion with
intramedullary nail

Fig. 24.3 Joint fusion. (A) Internal fixation. (B) Intramedullary nail.

Joint arthroplasty

Almost any joint can now be replaced. Pain is the primary reason to replace a joint.

The advantage of replacement over fusion is that movement is maintained and therefore function can return to near normal in some cases.

Implants are usually made from metal; however, the actual bearing surfaces can be made from a combination of a metal, high-density polyethylene or ceramic. The joint surfaces are highly polished for low friction.

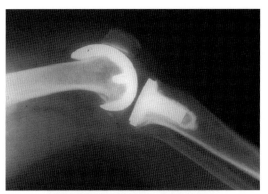

Fig. 24.4 Total knee replacement.

The joint components are either cemented in place or uncemented.

Joint replacements are available for almost any joint, although the most commonly performed are:

- knee (Fig. 24.4)
- hip (Fig. 24.5)
- shoulder

The majority of replacements should last more than 15 years, but this is partly dependent on the patient. A young patient is more likely to wear out a prosthesis due to having a higher functional demand.

The most common reasons for failure of an implant are loosening, infection and fracture (Fig. 24.6).

HINTS AND TIPS

INFECTED ARTHROPLASTY

Replaced joints are often red in the early postoperative phase and care should be taken before giving antibiotics if infection is suspected. Samples should be taken (preferably in theatre) unless the patient is septic, prior to giving antibiotics, because antibiotics will make any samples less likely to grow on culture. Ultimately, chronic infection in a joint replacement is unlikely to be cleared by antibiotics alone and often requires a two-stage revision.

Osteotomy/deformity correction

An osteotomy is an operation to cut a bone and realign a joint or deformity.

The most common place for this to occur is the first ray of the foot, in the case of hallux valgus. Osteotomies are also

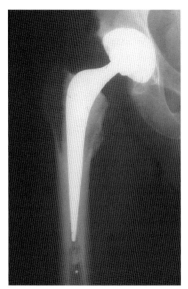

Fig. 24.5 Total hip replacement.

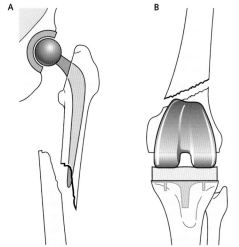

Fig. 24.6 Periprosthetic fracture of the femur: (A) at the hip; (B) at the knee.

performed at the knee to offload arthritic compartments in younger patients, reducing pain and postponing the need for arthroplasty.

Deformity can occur for other reasons such as malunion of fractures and congenital deformity (e.g., clubfoot) and correction of such deformity is an important part of orthopaedic surgery.

It is also possible to lengthen bones gradually with external fixation, usually in the form of circular frames with a variety of hinges and movable rods (Fig. 24.7).

Synovectomy

In the case of inflammatory arthritides, a synovectomy may be performed. The aim of this operation is to remove the synovial lining of the diseased joint or the tenosynovium around tendons. The procedure needs to be performed early and has three possible beneficial effects:

- reduction of swelling
- slowing of disease progression
- prevention of tendon rupture

Unfortunately, it is impossible to remove the whole synovium with synovectomy and symptoms often return. This procedure is commonly performed around the wrist.

POSTOPERATIVE CARE

General

Patients are taken to recovery until fully awake, then they are transferred to the ward. High-risk patients might need to be transferred to a High-Dependency Unit or Intensive Care Unit.

Regular recordings are made of blood pressure, pulse and oxygen saturation.

Adequate pain relief is very important.

After major surgery requiring an inpatient stay, patients will need:

- A full blood count and urea and electrolytes checked the day after surgery.
- X-ray examination of the operated joint.

Deep vein thrombosis (DVT) prophylaxis is continued until patients are fully mobile. Once patients are well, every effort is made to mobilize them and encourage early safe discharge. A multidisciplinary approach is needed to achieve this with input from physiotherapy, occupational therapy, social workers, nursing staff and sometimes physicians.

Home modifications might be required for patients after joint arthroplasty, but they generally return to having very good function.

Local

Elevation of the operated limb, for example, in a Bradford sling (for an arm), or on a stack of pillows or on a Braun frame (Fig. 24.8) for a leg, is very important to reduce swelling.

Distal neurovascular observations are performed to check the perfusion and function of the limb distal to the operation.

Physiotherapy is encouraged as soon as possible to mobilize the limb.

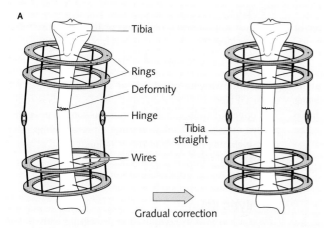

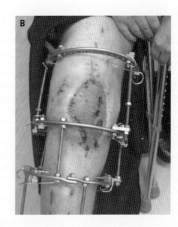

Fig. 24.7 Deformity correction with frames. (A) The use of an external fixator frame to achieve gradual correction of a deformity over several weeks. Note that the frame is also bent but straightens out as the bone is corrected. (B) Ilizarov frame on a fractured tibia. (With permission from Sala F, Catagni M, Pili D, Capitani P. Elbow arthrodesis for post-traumatic sequelae: surgical tactics using the Ilizarov frame. *J Shoulder Elbow Surg* 2015;24(11):1757–1763.)

COMPLICATIONS

Any surgical procedure has risks and complications and knowledge of these helps minimize and prevent them.

Patients need to be made aware of these important complications before informed consent is obtained.

Complications are divided into:

- local (specific to that operation)
- general (common to any operation)

We further subdivide complications here on the basis of the time that has elapsed after surgery into:

- immediate (within 24 hours)
- early (days/weeks)
- late (months/years)

General respiratory

Chest infections

Complications affecting the respiratory system are very common postoperatively.

A chest infection typically presents early in the first few days after an operation, with fever and shortness of breath. Elderly patients may also be confused.

There may be signs of consolidation on examination and a low PO_2.

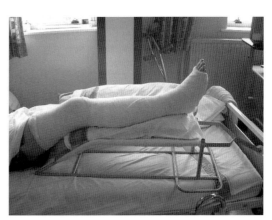

Fig. 24.8 Braun frame used to elevate a lower limb.

Treatment is with physiotherapy, nebulizers and most importantly, antibiotics.

Venous thromboembolism

Immobile orthopaedic patients with traumatized limbs are very susceptible to DVT. Risk is reduced by mechanical aids (foot pumps, graduated compression stockings) and chemical agents (heparin, enoxaparin, aspirin, warfarin) and early mobilization.

If the clot propagates and then breaks off, it travels to the lungs (a pulmonary embolus), which can be fatal. The patient becomes acutely short of breath and has pleuritic chest pain with signs of tachycardia, tachypnoea and a low PO_2. An ECG might show a sinus tachycardia, arrhythmias or the classic, but rare, S1Q3T3.

Treatment should be started immediately in the form of low-molecular-weight subcutaneous heparin if strongly suspected and the patient has suffered the sequelae of a PE or if the diagnosis is proven with a computed tomographic pulmonary angiogram (CTPA). If the diagnosis is ambiguous and the patient has no ill-effects of the suspected PE, the risks of causing bleeding at the operative site must be taken into account and in some cases, delaying treatment of the suspected PE should be delayed until the diagnosis is confirmed.

Cardiac

Myocardial infarction

Myocardial infarction (MI) is a relatively common postoperative complication, particularly in the elderly or those with preexisting heart disease. Patients do not always have typical central crushing chest pain radiating to the left arm associated with sweating and nausea and the cardiac event might be silent or occur during anaesthesia. This should be suspected in any patient with unexplained hypotension.

Diagnosis is made based on the patient's clinical presentation, ECGs and elevated troponin cardiac enzymes.

Initial treatment includes oxygen and aspirin. Further agents can be used based on advice from the physicians (there is difficulty in giving thrombolytic drugs to postoperative patients owing to the risk of bleeding at the operative site).

Left ventricular failure

This can result from a cardiac event or from aggressive fluid management over the perioperative period. It is important not to give too much fluid, particularly to elderly patients with little physiological reserve.

These patients present with shortness of breath and signs include a raised jugular venous pressure and bibasilar crackles. Simple measures such as sitting the patient up and giving oxygen can dramatically improve the patient's condition. Further treatment includes diuretics, morphine/diamorphine and nitrates.

Blood loss and blood transfusion

Most patients do not require a blood transfusion postoperatively, even after a total hip or knee replacement. Blood transfusions are associated with serious transfusion-related reactions, transmission of infections (hepatitis, human immunodeficiency virus (HIV), variant Creutzfeldt-Jakob disease), and immunosuppression and are expensive. Blood should therefore be prescribed sparingly. Most patients can tolerate a haemoglobin level of around 80 g/L, although higher values are often aimed for in those with known cardiac ischaemia.

Gastrointestinal

Bleeding

The most important complication of the gastrointestinal (GI) system is bleeding. The most common reason for this on orthopaedic wards is nonsteroidal antiinflammatory drug (NSAID) therapy.

Patients with haematemesis or melaena have a suspected upper GI bleed until proven otherwise. Diagnosis is confirmed with upper GI endoscopies performed as soon as possible. Supportive measures including starting a proton pump inhibitor, cross-matching blood, fluid resuscitation, careful observations and oxygen if required.

Referral to a gastroenterologist or surgeon is needed.

Paralytic ileus

This is a less serious complication presenting with abdominal distension and nausea. Operations or trauma to the spine predispose to ileus, which usually spontaneously corrects after a few days on intravenous fluids and a nasogastric tube.

Renal

Renal failure

Preexisting renal impairment is common in orthopaedic patients and the additional burden of a fracture or surgery with the associated blood loss, can tip the balance, causing renal failure.

Factors influencing the development of renal failure include drugs (diuretics, NSAIDs, antibiotics) and hypovolaemia. It is very important to keep patients well hydrated with enough fluid to prevent prerenal failure.

Careful monitoring of fluid input with hourly urine output and daily U&E measurements is important when assessing such a patient.

HINTS AND TIPS

FLUID BALANCE

Low urinary output postoperatively is almost always due to hypovolaemia and patients require fluids either orally or intravenously. It is very important to assess fluid balance carefully, so that diuretics are not given to such patients just to increase the output. This may instead precipitate renal failure.

Urinary tract infection (UTI)

Postoperative UTIs are very common. Diagnosis is made on urinalysis and a midstream urine sample sent to microbiology for analysis. Generic antibiotics are started after samples have been taken and refined once sensitivity results are known.

Local

Table 24.1 lists local complications, their timing, causes, signs and symptoms and management.

INFECTION

Infection is the major concern in elective orthopaedic surgery. Deep infection in joint replacement surgery is disastrous when it occurs as simple measures such as antibiotics and abscess drainage will not eradicate the infection. The patient may be worse off than before surgery and might require lengthy hospital stays with extensive further surgery and significant risks.

Table 24.1 Local complications of orthopaedic surgery

Postoperative timing	Complica- tion	Cause	Signs/symptoms	Management
Immediate up to first 24 hours	Tight cast	Swelling Dressing/cast too tight	Pain, tingling in toes/fingers Poor distal perfusion Numbness Ischaemia of limb	Elevation Split cast
	Compartment syndrome	Swelling in a closed fascial compartment (usually post fracture or post surgery)	Pain: pain on passive stretch Tense compartments Altered sensation	Fasciotomy
	Primary haemorrhage	Technical problem at surgical site, e.g., bleeding vessel Other risk factors include: major surgery, e.g., total hip replacement; drugs, e.g., warfarin; obesity	Haemodynamic instability Anxiety Slow capillary refill Tachycardia Hypotension Low urine output Confusion	Replace losses: fluids ± blood Reverse cause, e.g., warfarin Pressure dressing If heavy bleeding, re-examine wound
	Nerve injury	Usually retractor, e.g., sciatic nerve in hip replacement	Pain, weakness, paraesthesia	Wait and see - usually recovers
Early up to first 4 weeks	Secondary haemorrhage	Occurs at 5–10 days, usually secondary to infection	Bleeding with signs of infection	Treat infection Wound debridement and washout
	Infection (see Chapter 20)	Infection at time of surgery Can occur later with haematogenous seeding	Early: red, hot, swollen, discharging, temperature Late: persistent pain, loosening of prosthesis	Early: debridement and washout Late: removal of implant and debridement, reimplantation at second stage once infection treated
	Wound dehiscence (breakdown)	Within first week: usually due to poor surgical technique Later: invariably infection and poor healing	Wound gapes open Other features in keeping with infection may be present	Early: clean wounds are taken back to theatre for primary closure Later: treat infection as above
Late (in theory these can occur at any time)	Dislocation of total hip replacement	Patient: inappropriate patient activity Poor stem or cup position Excessive wear Infection	Severe pain, shortening External rotation (anterior) Internal rotation (posterior)	Reduce hip Abduction brace for 6 weeks if early Revision surgery if there is a problem with position of implant
	Periprosthetic fracture	Intraoperative: if a prosthesis is too big for the bone when inserted Late: loosening of the prosthesis, infection or trauma	Increased pain, deformity, unable to bear weight	Intraoperative: fixation of fracture Late: revision of prosthesis

Continued

Table 24.1 Local complications of orthopaedic surgery—cont'd

Postoperative timing	Complication	Cause	Signs/symptoms	Management
	Heterotopic ossification	Abnormal bone formation in soft tissues: more common in head-injured patients and with hip surgery or trauma	Stiffness	Surgical excision and immediate nonsteroidal antiinflammatory drugs or radiotherapy postoperatively
	Aseptic loosening	Loosening of prosthesis occurs because particle wear of the implant triggers macrophages. These cause osteolysis around the prosthesis	Pain, instability	Revision of the prosthesis

The risk of infection is minimized by the following preoperative, perioperative and postoperative factors.

Preoperative factors

- Cleaning the skin first with a nonsterile wash
- Avoidance of concurrent infection (e.g., UTI)
- Preoperative antibiotics on induction of anaesthesia
- A healthy, well-nourished patient

Perioperative factors

- Clean laminar airflow theatre (air is specially filtered)
- Adequate skin preparation and impervious exclusion drapes
- Sterile instruments and prostheses
- Careful surgical technique (including haemostasis)
- The use of antibiotic-loaded cement in joint arthroplasty

Postoperative factors

- Occlusive wound dressing, minimal dressing changes
- Prophylactic antibiotics for possible bacteraemia (e.g., during catheterization)
- Postoperative antibiotics

● Chapter Summary

- A preoperative assessment is vital prior to performing surgery because this is the stage at which potential perioperative problems can be identified and managed. A poor preassessment often causes delays or cancellations to an operating list.
- Arthroplasty for osteoarthritis and rheumatoid arthritis has been around for many years and is considered to be highly successful. If a hip replacement patient is fortunate enough to avoid complications, they are usually very happy with their outcome.
- Basic postoperative care involves regular observation and careful fluid management. Some patients may require a higher level of care. Postoperative blood tests are frequently done and most orthopaedic operations will require a postoperative X-ray examination.
- Complications of surgery are listed in detail in Table 24.1. These are very commonly found in exam questions and extra attention should be paid to learning them.
- Complications of orthopaedic surgery are reduced where possible. DVT prophylaxis is now standard, patients are mobilized quickly after surgery, anaesthetic nerve blocks are given preoperatively to reduce pain postoperatively and to speed up recovery, transfusions are given to keep blood counts above 80 g/L and many other changes are made to mitigate surgical risks.
- Infection is a devastating complication in arthroplasty and when chronic, necessitates the removal of all components and a staged revision.

SELF-ASSESSMENT

Rheumatology

Key findings	Diagnoses
Arthritis, dry eyes and mouth	Sjögren syndrome
Rheumatoid arthritis, painless red eyes	Episcleritis
Rheumatoid arthritis, painful red eye	Scleritis
Rheumatoid arthritis, splenomegaly	Felty syndrome
Rheumatoid arthritis, previous coal worker, now cough, SOB	Caplan syndrome
Difficulty swallowing, cold pale fingers	Limited cutaneous sclerosis (CREST syndrome)
Child, generalized pink rash, swollen knees	Still disease
Acute knee pain, X-ray – bright line above meniscus	Pseudogout
Rhomboid crystals, positive birefringent	Pseudogout
Sudden swollen and painful big toe joint	Gout/podagra
Needle-shaped, negative birefringent crystals	Gout
Rash, arthritis, pitting and lifting nails	Psoriatic arthritis
Knee pain, conjunctivitis, dysuria	Reiter syndrome
Bone symptoms, hearing loss	Paget disease of the bone
'Bamboo spine' on X-ray	Ankylosing spondylitis
'Butterfly' facial rash, arthritis in a young female	Systemic lupus erythematosus (SLE)
Antinuclear antibodies (ANAs)	SLE
Antineutrophil cytoplasmic antibodies (ANCAs)	Microscopic polyangiitis, eosinophilic granulomatosis with polyangiitis and granulomatosis with polyangiitis (c-ANCA)
Anticentromere antibodies	Limited cutaneous sclerosis (CREST syndrome)
Anti-Scl-70	Diffuse scleroderma
HLA-B27	Psoriatic arthritis, ankylosing spondylitis, IBD-associated arthritis, reactive arthritis

Orthopaedics

Key findings	Diagnoses
Obese boy, hip pain	Slipped upper femoral epiphysis (SUFE)
Boy, hip pain, gradual onset, X-ray shows collapsed femoral head	Perthes disease
Girl, postexercise knee pain	Osgood-Schlatter disease
Girl, knee pain climbing stairs	Chondromalacia

Continued

Key findings	Diagnoses
Prepubescent child, acute hip pain, nil else	Irritable hip (transient synovitis)
Young child, knee pain, periosteal elevation on X-ray	Osteosarcoma
'Onion skin' periosteal reaction	Ewing sarcoma
Unable to straighten finger tip	Extensor tendon injury (mallet finger)
Unable to flex finger at DIP	Flexor digitorium profundus damage
Unable to flex finger at PIP	Flexor digitorium superficialis damage
Claw hand	Ulnar damage
Fractured humerus and unable to extend wrist	Radial nerve damage
Anterior shoulder dislocation, now numb over upper lateral arm	Axillary nerve damage
Post accident, arm limp, extended, medially rotated, pronated	Brachial plexus damage (Erb palsy)
Bulge in upper arm in flexion at elbow	Rupture long head of bicep (Popeye sign)
Trauma to knee, now unable to flex toes, loss ankle jerk, loss sensation sole of foot	Tibial nerve damage
Shooting pain in toes in walking, tender at metatarsal heads	Morton neuroma
Arm adducted, internally rotated	Posterior shoulder dislocation
Arm abducted, externally rotated	Anterior shoulder dislocation
Painful joints in an elderly individual, worse with activity	Osteoarthritis

UKMLA Single Best Answer (SBA) questions

Chapter 1 Taking a history

1. A 55-year-old woman develops tingling and numbness in the radial 3.5 fingers of her right hand. Which is the most relevant part of her medical history to be considered in the diagnosis?
   A A family history of hypertension.
   B A drug history including nonsteroidal use.
   C A medical history of underactive thyroid.
   D A social history of working as an accountant.
   E A systemic enquiry revealing marked fatigue.

2. A 55-year-old woman presents with a fragility fracture. She undergoes a dual-energy X-ray absorptiometry (DEXA) scan revealing osteoporosis. Which of the following is the most important in terms of her medical history?
   A A family history of traumatic hip fracture.
   B Prednisolone 10 mg daily for several years for poorly controlled asthma.
   C Menopause aged 53 years.
   D Living in South America for several years.
   E A personal history of type 2 diabetes mellitus.

3. A 64-year-old man presents with severe pain in his fingertips and skin colour changes. What in his history would help differentiate between primary and secondary Raynaud disease?
   A A recent history of difficulty in swallowing.
   B A social history of alcohol misuse.
   C A family history of osteoarthritis.
   D A drug history of nifedipine use.
   E A medical history of chronic obstructive pulmonary disease (COPD).

4. A 44-year-old normally fit and well woman presents with bilateral swollen ankles and knee joints, which occurred a few weeks after a chest infection. The joints are warm and stiff for 2 hours upon waking. She has not been experiencing fever. She feels tired but is otherwise well. Her family history includes a brother with ankylosing spondylitis. What is the likely diagnosis based on the history?
   A Gout.
   B Rheumatoid arthritis.
   C Ankylosing spondylitis.
   D Reactive arthritis.
   E Septic arthritis.

5. A 43-year-old man presents to general practice with a 3-week history of pain and stiffness in his right knee. This is accompanied by obvious swelling of the distal fingers and a pitting pattern seen in the nails. Which feature of his medical history is the most important in helping to obtain a single diagnosis?
   A He smoked cigarettes as a teenager.
   B He has a BMI of 30 kg/m^2.
   C He has a past medical history of psoriasis that affects his scalp.
   D His father previously had acute arthritis affecting his knee after an episode of food poisoning.
   E He maintains a vegetarian diet.

6. A 21-year-old, female, university student presents to the GP with a 4-day history of a stiff left knee, fatigue, conjunctivitis and pustule formation on the palms of her hands. What is the most important question to ask to help obtain a diagnosis?
   A How is the pain affecting her activities of daily living?
   B Is she a smoker?
   C Is her diet high in protein?
   D Has she experienced any trauma to her knee in the past week?
   E Is she practicing safe sex if sexually active?

Chapter 2 Examining joints

1. A patient with an acquired foot drop will most likely present with which type of gait?
   A Trendelenburg.
   B Antalgic.
   C Circumduction.
   D Waddling.
   E High-stepping.

2. A young man experiences a wrist fracture while skiing. Afterwards, he is unable to lift his thumb off a table when the hand is placed flat. The tendon of which muscle has likely been damaged?
   A Adductor pollicis.
   B Extensor pollicis longus (EPL).
   C Abductor pollicis brevis.
   D Opponens pollicis.
   E Extensor digitorum.

3. A patient with a severe burning sensation in her hands presents with bilateral thenar and hypothenar wasting. The pain occurs over her thumb, index finger and middle finger. She has a history of hypothyroidism. What is the most likely cause of her symptoms and signs?

   A Carpal tunnel syndrome.
   B Hypothyroid-related peripheral neuropathy.
   C Peripheral vascular disease.
   D C8 radiculopathy.
   E Golfer's elbow.

4. A 55-year-old man presents to the emergency department. It becomes apparent that he has had a stroke. The next day you are asked to carry out a peripheral nerve examination on the patient. Which of the following findings will be present?

   A The Babinski reflex.
   B Medical research council (MRC) grade 3 power in the legs.
   C Obvious muscle wasting in the legs.
   D Visible muscle fasciculations in the legs.
   E Cogwheel rigidity.

5. A 25-year-old female arrives at the emergency department after she was injured playing football. Her right knee is red and swollen and you decide to carry out a knee examination. Part of the examination involves you flexing both knees to 90 degrees and comparing the contours of the knees. There is a visible sag of the right knee. Which soft tissue structure in the knee has most likely been damaged?

   A The medial meniscus.
   B The tendon of the popliteus muscle.
   C The lateral collateral ligament.
   D The posterior cruciate ligament.
   E The patellar tendon.

6. Which nerve is stretched when carrying out a straight leg raise to test for radiculopathy?

   A The sural nerve.
   B The femoral nerve.
   C The sciatic nerve.
   D The tibial nerve.
   E The saphenous nerve.

7. A 30-year-old professional rugby player presents to general practice with apparent muscle wastage of the deltoid muscle. He shows difficulty abducting and externally rotating his arm and there is a loss of sensation in a badge-like distribution over the inferior deltoid. He had recently suffered an anterior shoulder dislocation while playing rugby. Which nerve was damaged during his injury?

   A The median nerve.
   B The radial nerve.
   C The musculocutaneous nerve.
   D The supraclavicular nerve.
   E The axillary nerve.

8. A 47-year-old female presents to general practice with pain and swelling in her left shoulder. A rotator cuff injury is suspected and a series of tests are carried out. The patient shows inability to internally rotate her arm against resistance. Which muscle has most likely been injured?

   A Brachioradialis.
   B Subscapularis.
   C Teres minor.
   D Levator scapulae.
   E Supraspinatus.

Chapter 3 Investigations

1. A 33-year-old woman presents to her physician complaining of fatigue, myalgia and weight loss. She finds it more painful to bear weight compared with 6 months ago. She is losing her hair and there is a nonitchy rash over her nose and cheeks.

   Which test is most likely to confirm the diagnosis?

   A Anti–double-stranded DNA antibodies.
   B Erythrocyte sedimentation rate (ESR).
   C Skin biopsy of the rash.
   D Thyroid function tests.
   E MRI of her hips

2. A 68-year-old woman presents to her GP with fatigue. She has a history of rheumatoid arthritis and has recently had several flares requiring her medication to be increased. The GP performs some blood tests:

Liver function	
Alkaline phosphatase	78 (range 44–147)
Aspartate aminotransferase (AST)	138 (range 10–40)
Alanine aminotransferase (ALT)	179 (range 10–56)
γ-glutamyl transpeptidase (GGT)	36 (range 3–48)
Billirubin	17 (range 0–22)

What is the likely cause of the above results?

   A Primary biliary cirrhosis.
   B Methotrexate hepatotoxicity.
   C Acute viral hepatitis due to immunocompromised state.
   D Gallstones.
   E Alcohol.

3. A 28-year-old woman presents with Raynaud phenomenon, which ulcerated last winter, progressive tightness in her hands and small red dots on her chest that branch out like spiders.

   Which antibody is she likely to have?

   A Jo-1.

   B Anti-dsDNA.

   C Anti-SCL-70.

   D p-ANCA.

   E Histone.

4. A 45-year-old man is getting out of a car when he twists his leg and feels a pop in his knee. He is immediately unable to bear his weight and the joint proceeds to swell.

   Which investigation will be most helpful in arriving at a diagnosis?

   A Joint aspiration.

   B X-ray knee.

   C Ultrasound scan (USS).

   D MRI.

   E Erythrocyte sedimentation rate (ESR).

5. A 49-year-old woman presents to general practice with pain and stiffness in the small joints of her hands. She also has firm nodules on her elbows. Rheumatoid arthritis (RA) is suspected. Which of the following factors is the most specific to rheumatoid arthritis?

   A Jo-1 autoantibody.

   B Cyclic citrullinated peptide antibody.

   C Antibodies to myeloperoxidase (MPO).

   D C- Reactive protein.

   E Rheumatoid factor.

6. A 38-year-old woman visits the rheumatology clinic for her routine appointment. Urinalysis is carried out and the results show heavy haematuria and proteinuria. Her blood pressure is also measured at 170/90 mmHg. Which rheumatological condition is she most likely to have?

   A Systemic lupus erythematous.

   B Rheumatoid arthritis.

   C Gout.

   D Sjögren syndrome.

   E Reactive arthritis.

7. A 60-year-old man arrives at the hospital complaining of acute pain and swelling in his right knee. The joint is aspirated and the synovial fluid is examined under polarized light. The findings indicate a diagnosis of gout. What was found in the synovial fluid sample?

   A Irregular cysteine crystals.

   B Rhomboid-shaped calcium pyrophosphate crystals.

   C Needle-shaped monosodium urate crystals.

   D Irregular calcium oxalate crystals.

   E Needle-shaped calcium carbonate crystals.

8. A 19-year-old female presents to general practice complaining of increasing tiredness and dizziness. She looks pale. Before the onset of her symptoms she was fit and well. Her haemoglobin is low and a blood film is carried out which shows red blood cells that are abnormally small. What is the most likely cause of her abnormal blood results?

   A Low levels of folate.

   B Bleeding of the gastrointestinal tract.

   C Heavy menstrual periods.

   D Thalassemia.

   E Long-term use of NSAIDs.

9. Which inflammatory component will be found at low levels in active systemic lupus erythematous?

   A Cytokines.

   B Anti–double-stranded DNA antibody.

   C Lupus anticoagulant.

   D C-reactive protein.

   E Complement.

Chapter 4 Regional musculoskeletal pain

1. A 68-year-old woman presents with a history of acute-on-chronic lower back pain and fatigue. Which of the following additional findings when associated with the back pain would warrant urgent investigations?

   A A history of urinary incontinence.

   B A raised erythrocyte sedimentation rate (ESR).

   C A family history of psoriasis.

   D Abnormal thyroid function tests (TFTs).

   E A positive antinuclear antibody (ANA; 1:40).

2. A young woman presents to A&E after playing hockey. She twisted and felt a pop in her knee and now the joint is swollen, tense and tender. An X-ray examination of her knee is performed and a fluid level is seen within the joint. What does the history and radiograph imply?

   A A rheumatoid knee.

   B Ruptured anterior cruciate ligament (ACL).

   C Septic arthritis.

   D Patellar dislocation.

   E Pseudogout.

3. A 61-year-old retired bricklayer presents with chronic back pain. His pain is exacerbated by walking, particularly downhill, and radiates into his buttocks, thighs and calves bilaterally. Examination shows a stooped gait with

reduced motion in the lumbar spine. His symptoms are worsened by extension of the spine. What is the diagnosis?

A Prolapsed intervertebral disc.
B Mechanical back pain.
C Spinal stenosis.
D Spondylolisthesis.
E Spinal malignancy.

4. A 77-year-old man has bilateral shoulder pain, which is aching in nature, stiffness and difficulty in dressing. He is also fatigued, more so over the past 3 months. Which test is the most useful in establishing the diagnosis?

A Nerve conducting studies.
B Bilateral shoulder X-ray image.
C Urinary Bence Jones protein.
D Erythrocyte sedimentation rate (ESR).
E MRI of the neck.

5. Following a stroke, a patient develops severe hand pain, with skin changes, hypersensitivity and arm swelling. What is the diagnosis?

A Arterial insufficiency.
B Upper limb deep vein thrombosis (DVT).
C Factitious pain.
D Phantom-limb pain.
E Complex regional pain syndrome.

6. A 72-year-old man presents to his GP with the complaint of unilateral hip pain. When asked, he tells the GP that this pain has been going on for many years. It is worse on movement and towards the end of the day. He is frequently awoken from sleep with his hip pain. He knows that his mother had something similar around his age in her hip too. What investigation will give you the diagnosis of this man's pain?

A No investigation needed.
B Hip CT.
C Hip MRI.
D Pelvic and hip plain radiographs.
E Inflammatory markers including white cell count and CRP.

7. A 53-year-old ex-rugby player is seen in the orthopaedic clinic complaining of unilateral knee pain. The pain is worst on walking and he sometimes has the sensation of his knee locking. This pain has been going on for many months. His knee is not warm to touch or swollen, and he is most tender along the medial joint line. He is otherwise well with no systemic symptoms. What is the likely pathology causing his pain?

A Septic arthritis.
B A meniscal tear.
C Osteoarthritis.
D Gout.
E An ACL rupture.

8. A 22-year-old long-distance runner presents to the foot and ankle clinic having been referred in by her GP. She complains of hindfoot pain bilaterally which is centred over the weightbearing part of her heels. This radiates distally along the sole of her feet. She has tried resting her feet and running less but the pain persists. On examination the pain is reproducible by palpating over her heels. What is the likely pathology causing her pain

A Diabetic neuropathy.
B Achilles tendinopathy.
C Plantar fasciitis.
D Morton neuroma.
E Inflammatory arthritis.

Chapter 5 Widespread musculoskeletal pain

1. A 68-year-old woman presents with bilateral hip and shoulder pain. She has an elevated erythrocyte sedimentation rate (ESR; 68). She is prescribed steroids and a provisional diagnosis of polymyalgia rheumatic (PMR) is reached.

Two months later she is seen in clinic and despite the steroids she is still symptomatic, has developed synovitis and has lost 2 stone in weight.

What is the next investigation to consider?

A CT thorax, abdomen and pelvis.
B Vitamin D.
C Muscle biopsy.
D Check rheumatoid factor.
E Skeletal survey.

2. A 38-year-old woman presents with pain throughout the shoulders, arms and hip girdle. She has intermittent loose stools/constipation, low mood and severe fatigue.
Investigations show the following:

Erythrocyte sedimentation rate	9 mm/h (normal 0–29 mm/h)
Calcium	2.27 mmol/L (normal 2.20–2.70 mmol/L)
Vitamin D	78 nmol/L (normal 70–100 nmol/L)

Which of the following drugs would you consider using in treating her condition?

A Naproxen.
B Adalimumab.
C Pregabalin.
D Methotrexate.
E Oxycodone

3. A 42-year-old woman is unable to walk. She is tender over her greater trochanters, lower back and quadriceps. She is tearful and discloses a history of insomnia and intermittent paraesthesia. She has pain in 14/18 trigger points.

   Her initial blood tests are normal. Her chest X-ray and EKG is similarly unremarkable.

   What is the next best step?

   A MRI of the spine.
   B Autoimmune profile.
   C Electromyography.
   D Reassurance.
   E Intravenous immunoglobulins.

4. Which of the following are not typical features of fibromyalgia?

   A Altered sleeping pattern.
   B Pain in multiple tender points.
   C Altered bowel habit.
   D Headache.
   E Foot drop.

5. A 75-year-old male with known prostate cancer presents to the GP with worsening back pain. He is referred to the radiology department at the hospital where an X-ray reveals that the cancer has metastasized to the vertebrae. Which of the following features will most likely be seen in his blood results?

   A Low alkaline phosphatase.
   B Detectable anti-CCP antibodies.
   C High serum calcium.
   D High serum parathyroid hormone.
   E Detectable p-ANCA.

6. A 42-year-old female presents to general practice complaining of widespread pain that is not improving with analgesia. She complains of lethargy, poor sleep and she is finding it difficult to concentrate at work. She is asked when the pain started, but, she breaks down into tears, explaining that the pain has been getting worse since her husband left her 6 months ago.

   What is the most likely diagnosis?

   A Fibromyalgia.
   B Osteoarthritis.
   C Systemic lupus erythematous (SLE).

D Rheumatoid arthritis.
E Polymyalgia rheumatica.

7. What is the most likely cause of paraneoplastic rheumatic syndrome out of the following options?

   A Ganglioneuroma.
   B Melanoma.
   C Rheumatoid arthritis.
   D Acute myeloid leukaemia.
   E Polymyalgia rheumatica.

8. Which of the following aspects of a rheumatological examination will show positive findings in a case of fibromyalgia?

   A Palpation of the spinous processes.
   B Schober test.
   C Tinel test.
   D Palpation of trigger points.
   E Straight leg raise.

Chapter 6 An acute, hot, swollen joint

1. A 62-year-old diabetic woman presents with an acutely hot swollen right knee. She has recently been treated for a foot ulcer. She is febrile. Her bloods show a white cell count of 15.5 and a C-reactive protein of 113. What will her joint aspirate most likely show?

   A Gram-positive cocci.
   B Gram-negative bacilli.
   C Needle-shaped negatively birefringent crystals.
   D Rod-shaped positively birefringent crystals.
   E Blood.

2. A 25-year-old man presents with an acute monoarthritis of the left knee. He has a history of an itchy, flaky rash affecting the knees and his lower back. He has had painful distal finger joints in the past. How would you start to treat his condition?

   A Antibiotics.
   B Disease-modifying antirheumatic drugs (DMARDs).
   C Paracetamol.
   D High-dose steroids.
   E Topical emollients.

3. A 48-year-old man presents with acute arthritis of the right ankle. The joint is red and inflamed and he has difficulty bearing weight on it. Erythrocyte sedimentation rate 9 mm/h (normal 0–29 mm/h), calcium 2.27 mmol/L (normal 2.20–2.70 mmol/L), vitamin D 78 nmol/L (normal 70–100 nmol/L). Which of the following features would favour gout rather than septic arthritis?

   A A low-grade fever.
   B A high C-reactive protein (CRP).

C A previous history of right ankle swelling and pain.

D A history of immunosuppression.

E A family history of rheumatoid arthritis.

4. A 60-year-old female with a background of hypertension, peripheral vascular disease and type 2 diabetes, has been diagnosed with her first episode of gout by means of joint aspirate. She is quite concerned and asks you about which lifestyle modifications will help reduce her risk of a flare-up. Which of the following would you recommend to reduce her likelihood of a flare-up?

A Reducing alcohol intake of all types of alcohol.

B Cutting out drinking spirits.

C Stopping her diuretics.

D Adhere to a calorie restriction diet to lose weight fast.

E Increase seafood intake.

5. A 32-year-old female presents to the emergency department with an acutely hot, swollen and erythematous knee. She was gardening 36 hours ago and cut her knee with some shearing scissors while kneeling. Presently, she cannot move her knee. On arrival at hospital her observations are as follows: respiratory rate 24 breaths per minute, heart rate 110 beats per minute, blood pressure 95/55 mmHg and temperature 38.1°C. What is the most important step in her immediate management?

A Blood cultures.

B IV fluids.

C Paracetamol.

D IV antibiotics.

E Oxygen.

6. A 65-year-old female presents to her GP having been recently diagnosed with acute pseudogout on admission to hospital. She was discharged a few days ago, but was found to be hypercalcaemic in hospital. She was asked to follow up with her GP for further investigation of a possible underlying disorder. Which of the following are associated with pseudogout?

A Lung cancer.

B Paget disease.

C Hyperthyroidism.

D Multiple myeloma.

E Hyperparathyroidism.

Chapter 7 A child with a limp

1. Which of the following is not a risk factor in the development of Perthes disease?

A Delayed bone age.

B Hypothyroidism.

C Low socioeconomic group.

D Low birthweight.

E Family history.

2. A 13-year-old overweight boy presents with severe right hip pain, with a background of 2 weeks of groin pain. There is no history of trauma and he is otherwise well. He is unable to bear his own weight, holds his hip in external rotation and flexion and has a decreased range of motion in all axes because of pain. Inflammatory markers are normal. What is the likely diagnosis?

A Perthes disease.

B Septic arthritis.

C Neck of femur fracture.

D Osteoarthritis.

E Slipped capital femoral epiphysis.

3. A 3-year-old girl is brought to A&E by her mother with a 24-hour history of a left leg limp. Her mother states there is no history of trauma. The child localizes the pain to her groin. The patient has an unremarkable medical history, although her mother notes she had a common cold last week. On examination, the child is apyrexial and is systemically well. She is refusing to bear her weight fully and has a decreased range of motion in all axes secondary to pain. X-ray examination shows no abnormality and her blood tests are normal. What is the likely diagnosis?

A Transient synovitis.

B Septic arthritis.

C Slipped capital femoral epiphysis.

D Perthes disease.

E Malignancy.

4. A 7-year-old boy is brought to A&E by his father having been in pain for 6 hours and with reduced range of motion in his hip. He was recently admitted with pneumonia. He appears very unwell and is febrile. His pulse is elevated and he is clammy to the touch. What is the most appropriate next step?

A Aspiration of the painful joint.

B Await blood tests and await culture results to direct treatment.

C Ultrasound scan hip.

D Immediate resuscitation and IV antibiotics.

E X-ray examination of both hips.

5. An 11-month-old child is brought to the emergency department with a 24-hour history of pain in her left leg while having her nappies changed. She cannot tolerate any movement of the leg. Her mother states that she was left in her partner's care for the first time yesterday and hasn't been right since. The baby is not drowsy,

does not have a temperature and the rest of her observations are normal except for a high heart rate. What is your concern?

A   Septic arthritis.
B   Transient synovitis.
C   Nonaccidental injury.
D   Developmental dysplasia of the hip.
E   Osetomyelitis.

6.   A 13-month-old baby presents with a limp as the child begins to walk. The left leg looks shorter than the right. The child has a waddling gait but is not in obvious discomfort. What is the most likely diagnosis?

A   Slipped capital femoral epiphysis.
B   Developmental dysplasia of the hip.
C   Congenital talipes equinovarus.
D   Osteomyelitis.
E   Pes planus.

7.   A 12-year-old boy has been unwell for a few months with pain and swelling in his right knee. He has also been more tired than usual and not himself. On further questioning, it becomes clear that other joints are involved. The right knee is swollen with a small effusion. At presentation, he is noted to have decreased visual acuity in his right eye.

A   Transient synovitis.
B   Psoriatic arthritis.
C   Rheumatoid arthritis.
D   Systemic lupus erythematosus.
E   Juvenile idiopathic arthritis.

8.   A 14-year-old boy is a keen footballer and presents with bilateral knee pain that is worse on movement and very tender if touched. On examination, he is well and has tenderness over the tibial tubercle just beneath the patellar ligament.

A   Osgood-Schlatter disease.
B   Chondromalacia patella.
C   Patellar tendinitis.
D   Patellar tendon rupture.
E   Perthes disease.

9.   A 7-year-old boy presents with a 1-year history of right knee pain, gradually increasing. He has a pronounced limp and has been off school for 1 month. On examination the right knee is normal but the hip is irritable and abduction is markedly decreased. X-ray images show sclerosis of the femoral head.

A   Septic arthritis.
B   Transient synovitis.

C   Osteomyelitis.
D   Perthes disease.
E   Slipped capital femoral epiphysis.

10.   An 8-week-old baby girl is very ill on the paediatric intensive care unit. She has features of sepsis, including a raised temperature and WCC and blood cultures have grown Staphylococcus aureus. There is no obvious focus of infection. An ultrasound scan of both hips is normal.

A   Septic arthritis.
B   Osteomyelitis.
C   Transient synovitis.
D   Juvenile idiopathic arthritis.
E   Rheumatoid arthritis.

Chapter 8 Back pain

1.   In the case of a prolapsed vertebral disc, pain is caused when the nerve root is compressed by:

A   Annulus fibrosis.
B   Posterior longitudinal ligament.
C   Ligamentum flavum.
D   Nucleus pulposus.
E   Interspinous ligament.

2.   Which of the following is a sign of impending cauda equina syndrome?

A   Severe unilateral sciatic-type pain.
B   Bilateral sciatic-type pain.
C   Prolonged duration of symptoms.
D   Leg pain and altered sensation.
E   Muscle weakness.

3.   Which is the most important investigation in diagnosing impending cauda equina syndrome?

A   Blood test including urea and electrolytes, C-reactive protein and white cell count.
B   MRI scan.
C   CT scan.
D   X-ray examination.
E   White cell count scan.

4.   A 72-year-old male presents with back pain and mild weakness in both legs. An X-ray examination is performed and shows a sclerotic lesion in the L5 vertebrae. What is the most likely underlying diagnosis causing this man's problem?

A   Multiple myeloma.
B   Malignant sarcoma.
C   Metastatic prostate cancer.
D   Metastatic lung cancer.
E   Paget disease.

5. A 56-year-old diabetic patient with chronic renal failure is admitted for dialysis. He also complains of new back pain. The patient becomes unwell with a raised temperature, a white cell count of 22.5 × 109/L, C-reactive protein 125 mg/L and erythrocyte sedimentation rate 79 mm/h. The renal physicians treat him for line sepsis but he fails to respond. One week later, an X-ray examination of the lumbar spine shows loss of disc space between L3 and L4 with bony destruction of the end plates. What is the most likely diagnosis?

   A Acute on chronic renal failure.
   B Pyelonephritis.
   C Spinal tumour.
   D Osteomyelitis.
   E Discitis.

6. A 30-year-old man complains of low back pain after digging at work. The pain does not radiate and is worse on movement. He feels well and examination shows muscle spasm, reduced movements and some tenderness across the lower lumbar spine. How do you manage him?

   A Advise antiinflammatories, stretching and to continue gentle activity in the first instance.
   B Advise bed rest for 1 to 2 weeks.
   C Order an X-ray of his lumbar spine and take bloods for inflammatory markers.
   D MRI lumbar and sacral spine.
   E Organize a steroid injection at the most painful spinal level.

7. A 15-year-old boy presents with increasing low back pain for 1 year. He is a county-level fast bowler and is training to play at a higher level. The pain does not radiate and is worse after prolonged activity. Examination shows a well boy with well-maintained spinal movements and normal neurology. Pain is significant on extension. Oblique X-ray images of the lumbar spine show a typical Scottie dog appearance with a pars defect at L5–S1. What is the diagnosis?

   A Scoliosis.
   B Ankylosis spondylitis.
   C Prolapsed intervertebral disc.
   D Spinal stenosis.
   E Spondylolisthesis.

8. A 62-year-old male, who works as a brick-layer develops bilateral leg pain when walking long distances, especially when walking uphill. He has a background of intermittent back pain, type 2 diabetes, ischaemic heart disease and hypertension, when he sits and rests, the pain settles. On direct questioning he says leaning over does not make the pain in his legs better when it comes on. How would you like to investigate him further?

   A MRI lumbar spine.
   B X-ray lumbar spine.
   C Exercise tolerance test.
   D Ankle-brachial pressure index.
   E CT angiogram of lower limbs.

Chapter 9 Altered sensation and weakness

1. A distal radius fracture with significant dorsal angulation is most likely to cause altered sensation in the distribution of which nerve:

   A Ulnar nerve.
   B Superficial radial nerve.
   C Medial cutaneous nerve of the forearm.
   D Median nerve.
   E Axillary nerve.

2. A 56-year-old woman with rheumatoid arthritis presents to her GP with a 6-month history of altered sensation and pain in both her hands, the right worse than the left. She describes pins and needle in her index, middle and ring fingers and pain at night, which frequently wakens her from sleep. She also describes decreased grip strength. On examination, there is wasting of the thenar eminences and percussion at the wrist crease exacerbates her symptoms. What is the diagnosis?

   A Cervical radiculopathy.
   B Cubital tunnel syndrome.
   C Peripheral neuropathy.
   D Carpal tunnel syndrome.
   E Transient ischaemic attacks.

3. A patient presents with numbness in the hand, worse at night, in the radial three digits. It passes off rapidly, but she has begun to notice loss of fine movements in the hand. Which of these tests will be most helpful in confirming the diagnosis?

   A Blood tests including urea and electrolytes, C-reactive protein and full blood count.
   B MRI cervical spine.
   C Nerve conduction studies.
   D X-ray examination of the wrist.
   E CT of the brain.

4. A 67-year-old lady with a previous history of myocardial infarction presents with numbness and tingling in her left arm for only 6 hours duration. She is mildly confused and has 60% power in the left arm with numbness throughout. What is the likely diagnosis?

   A Transient ischaemic attack (TIA).
   B Carpal tunnel syndrome.
   C Brachial plexus injury.

D   Prolapsed cervical disc.

E   Ulnar nerve entrapment.

5. A 40-year-old man is tackled heavily during a rugby game and lands awkwardly on his left shoulder. His shoulder has lost its normal contour and he finds all movements painful. He notices some tingling over the outer aspect of his upper arm. Which nerve are you concerned about?

A   Radial nerve.

B   Median nerve.

C   Ulnar nerve.

D   Musculocutaneous nerve.

E   Axillary nerve.

6. A 65-year-old heavy smoker complains of weakness in his left hand. He has had a persistent cough for the last 3 months and has lost 13 kg in weight. On examination he has wasting of the small muscles of the hand. The doctor also notes that he has a constricted pupil on the left side with drooping of the eyelid and dry skin over the left side of his forehead. What diagnosis are you concerned about?

A   Pancoast tumour.

B   Carpal tunnel syndrome.

C   Oropharyngeal cancer.

D   Stroke.

E   Bell palsy.

7. A 26-year-old man crashes his motorbike at 40 mph. He sustains a spiral fracture to the mid-shaft of his right humerus. He has altered sensation over the first dorsal web space of his right hand and has weakness of extension of his wrist, fingers and thumb. Which nerve has he injured?

A   Radial nerve.

B   Median nerve.

C   Ulnar nerve.

D   Musculocutaneous nerve.

E   Axillary nerve.

8. A 40-year-old woman develops a sudden onset of severe neck pain after turning suddenly. This is associated with pain in her middle finger and weakness straightening her arm. She has no significant past medical history. What imaging modality will most readily confirm your suspected diagnosis?

A   X-ray.

B   CT.

C   MRI.

D   Ultrasound.

E   Bone scan.

Chapter 10 Osteoarthritis

1. Which of the following is not a typical finding from an X-ray examination in osteoarthritis?

A   Lytic bone lesions.

B   Joint space narrowing.

C   Sclerosis.

D   Cyst formation.

E   Osteophytes.

2. A 77-year-old man sees his GP for left knee pain, gradually worsening over a month. He is now struggling to bear weight on it and the joint appears slightly swollen. The pain is achy and is affecting his ability to walk. He has now started to experience pain at night.

What would an X-ray examination reveal?

A   Erosions.

B   Osteophytes.

C   Hairline fracture.

D   Osteopenia.

E   Soft tissue swelling.

3. An 80-year-old woman complains of worsening pain in her hands for 6 months. She finds it difficult to button up her clothes and her hands ache after gardening and doing household chores.

What might you expect to find on clinical examination?

A   Ulnar deviation.

B   Boutonniere deformity.

C   Heberden nodes.

D   Dupuytren contracture.

E   Metacarpophalangeal (MCP) swelling.

4. A 65-year-old former factory worker presents to his physician with pain in his hips. He has trouble sitting and standing. The pain increases after walking and radiates to his knees. Resting makes it better.

What is the next most appropriate step in his management?

A   Glucosamine.

B   Joint replacement.

C   Trial of steroids.

D   Physiotherapy.

E   Joint injection.

5. Which of the following options is a risk factor for the development of osteoarthritis?

A   Being a professional cyclist.

B   Being vegetarian.

C   Being male.

D Having previous partial meniscectomy surgery.

E A diagnosis of osteoporosis.

6. A 50-year-old man presents to the GP with a 5-week history of knee pain that is not present in the morning, however, it worsens after walking for extended periods of time. From the patient's history, it is clear that he has osteoarthritis (OA). What must be done to confirm a diagnosis of OA?

A An X-ray.

B No further testing is required to diagnose the patient with OA.

C An MRI scan.

D Joint aspiration.

E A DEXA bone scan.

7. A 71-year-old female has been diagnosed with osteoarthritis for the past 5 years. The pain in her left hip has been gradually getting worse. She is currently on nonopioid analgesia and is waiting for hip arthroplasty. The general practitioner reviews the patient's medication and decides to prescribe a weak opioid. Which of the following drugs would be appropriate?

A Tramadol.

B Ibuprofen.

C Paracetamol.

D Oxycodone.

E Hydromorphine.

8. A 65-year-old patient with a 7-year history of osteoarthritis presents to the emergency department with pain in their left knee that has worsened over the past few hours. The knee looks obviously red and is warm to touch. The patient complains of feeling dizzy. They are sweating and they look pale. What investigation should you carry out first from the following list?

A X-ray scan of the knee.

B Do a full knee examination.

C MRI scan of the knee.

D Aspiration of the knee joint.

E Check the patient's urea and electrolytes.

Chapter 11 Rheumatoid arthritis

1. A 65-year-old woman with stable rheumatoid arthritis (RA) notices loss of sensation in the lateral 3.5 fingers, palmar aspect.

Which is the most appropriate therapy for this more recent condition?

A Splinting.

B Oral steroids.

C Methotrexate.

D Physiotherapy.

E Vitamin B_{12}.

2. A 48-year-old woman presents with 8-week onset of bilateral stiffness and intermittent swelling of the metacarpophalangeal joints. She is otherwise fit and well. On further questioning, she admits to similar episodes over the previous 2 years.

She is anti-CCP and rheumatoid factor positive, with high erythrocyte sedimentation rate and C-reactive protein. X-ray images show erosive arthropathy.

What is the next most appropriate management step?

A Physiotherapy.

B MRI of the hands.

C Start disease-modifying antirheumatic drugs (DMARDs).

D Hydrotherapy.

E Start nonsteroidal antiinflammatory drugs (NSAIDs).

3. An 86-year-old woman goes to her GP with pain in her fingers and toes for 6 months. It is intermittent and her fingers feel stiff and tender. Stiffness is greatest when she wakes and eases as the day goes by. She has also noticed firm subcutaneous lumps forming on the extensor side of her elbow. Her medical history states she has had bleeding from a duodenal ulcer.

Which of the following would be best avoided in this woman?

A Hydroxychloroquine.

B Methotrexate.

C Paracetamol.

D Naproxen.

E Sulfasalazine.

4. A variation in which gene appears to be the most closely associated with the development of rheumatoid arthritis?

A HLA-DQ2.5.

B HLA-B27.

C PALB2.

D MLH1.

E HLA-DR4.

5. A 60-year-old female with a 15-year history of rheumatoid arthritis arrives at the hospital to undergo an elective hysterectomy. What important step should be taken before the patient is given a general anaesthetic?

A Cessation of methotrexate usage 1 week before surgery.

B A full musculoskeletal examination.

C X-ray imaging of the cervical spine.

D Double dosing of oral steroids 3 hours before surgery.

E Assessment of rheumatoid factor and anti-CCP levels.

6. A 63-year-old female attends her routine rheumatology appointment at the outpatient clinic. She complains of feeling lethargic and breathless recently. She has taken methotrexate to control her rheumatoid arthritis for the past 10 years, and sometimes she takes NSAIDs when her symptoms worsen. Routine tests are carried out which show that she has a macrocytic anaemia. What is the most likely cause of these abnormal blood results?

A A 10-year history of methotrexate usage.

B Use of NSAIDs.

C Heavy menstrual bleeding.

D Hashimoto thyroiditis.

E Presence of a chronic disease.

7. What immune component does the biological therapy rituximab target?

A IL-23.

B IL-6.

C Janus kinase enzymes.

D TNF-α.

E B cells.

8. A 55-year-old female presents to the rheumatology clinic complaining of continued joint pain and stiffness despite therapy with methotrexate and sulfasalazine. The rheumatology consultant decides to review the patient's medication and prescribes rituximab. What should the rheumatology consultant do before prescribing rituximab?

A Stop prescription of methotrexate and sulfasalazine.

B Communicate the increased risk of lung adenocarcinoma when using rituximab.

C Check for retinal damage due to previous use of methotrexate.

D Check HIV, tuberculosis, varicella and hepatitis status.

E Assess for signs of systemic lupus erythematous.

Chapter 12 Spondyloarthropathies

1. A 22-year-old man develops an acute swelling of his left knee and ankle with painful heels. There was no trauma.

A week previously he had conjunctivitis and a fever.

Blood and urine samples are taken for culture.

Which of the following is NOT the likely pathogen?

A *Haemophilus influenzae.*

B *Chlamydia trachomatis.*

C *Salmonella typhi.*

D *Neisseria gonorrhoeae.*

E *Escherichia coli.*

2. A 53-year-old woman complains of bloody diarrhoea and abdominal pain. She experiences low-grade fever, nausea and weight loss. A colonoscopy is conducted, which shows ulcerative lesions in her rectum.

During this period her shoulders become progressively stiffer and she develops pain and swelling in her right knee. The intensity of the pain has worsened with her bowel symptoms.

What is the most appropriate immediate management for this woman?

A Nonsteroidal antiinflammatory drugs (NSAIDs).

B Corticosteroids.

C Panproctocolectomy.

D Biologic therapy.

E Sulfasalazine

3. A 45-year-old man presents to his GP with joint pain and stiffness in both wrists, knuckles and distal interphalangeal joints. There is a slight degree of swelling in the right and left middle fingers, giving them a sausage-like appearance. The GP notices dry skin around his hairline and back of his ears.

Which of the following nail changes is he most likely to have?

A Keratoderma blennorrhagica.

B Koilonychia.

C Onycholysis.

D Leuconychia.

E Paronychia.

4. Which of the following is not associated with ankylosing spondylitis?

A Amyloidosis.

B Apical lung fibrosis.

C Aortic incompetence.

D Anticardiolipin antibody.

E Acute anterior uveitis.

5. Which of the following types of spondyloarthropathy is most closely associated with HLA-B27 positivity?

A Psoriatic arthritis.

B Enteropathic arthritis.

C Reactive arthritis.

D Undifferentiated spondyloarthritis.

E Ankylosing spondylitis.

6. The NICE guidelines (2019) define some key features of ankylosing spondylitis that clinicians should look out for to aid diagnosis. Which of the following is not a key feature of ankylosing spondylitis?

A Back pain that has been present for more than 3 months.

B Symptoms that wake the patient during the night.

C The patient is 30 years old or older.

D Back pain that is worse in the morning and improves with movement.

E Symptoms that respond to NSAIDs within 48 hours of use.

7. A 45-year-old man with previously diagnosed ankylosing spondylitis arrives at the rheumatology clinic for his routine appointment. The rheumatology consultant wants to assess the patient's spinal mobility. Which scoring system would be most appropriate?

A BASMI.

B CHA$_2$DS$_2$-VASc.

C PEST.

D BASFI.

E DAS 28.

8. A 50-year-old female presents to the GP with a 4-month history of pain and stiffness in the joints of her fingers accompanied by a rapid loss of function. Upon examination, the joints of the fingers appear deformed and there are obvious nail changes. Her past medical history includes hypertension, type 2 diabetes and psoriasis. What name is given to this likely disease process?

A Reactive arthritis.

B Symmetrical polyarthritis.

C Asymmetrical oligoarthritis.

D Arthritis mutilans.

E Enteropathic arthritis.

9. The inflammatory process seen in psoriatic arthritis is associated with activation of IL23. Which drug could be prescribed to target this particular immune component?

A Infliximab.

B Ustekinumab.

C Tocilizumab.

D Rituximab.

E Methotrexate.

Chapter 13 Connective tissue diseases

1. A 58-year-old man presents to the respiratory clinic with breathlessness. He is found to have a raised pulmonary artery pressure. High-resolution CT of the chest shows pulmonary fibrosis.

He also complains of painful discolouration of his fingers when outdoors, has evidence of skin thickening in the fingers and hands with hard deposits under the skin, and small red spider-like lesions on the chest and face.

What is the most likely explanation for the findings?

A Systemic lupus erythematosus (SLE).

B Systemic sclerosis.

C Linear scleroderma.

D Paraneoplastic syndrome.

E Multiple sclerosis.

2. A 48-year-old woman complains of dry eyes, dry mouth and lethargy. There is evidence of oral candidiasis and dental caries. She also complains of pains in multiple joints. Her GP questions what her diagnosis may be. Which is the most likely test to confirm the diagnosis?

A HIV test.

B Schober test.

C Schirmer test.

D Transoesophageal echocardiogram.

E Trendelenburg test.

3. A 67-year-old man presents to the GP complaining of difficulty in rising from a chair. He has also noticed the development of erythematous plaques over his knuckles and a lilac discolouration of his eyelids. The GP decides to order some tests to confirm the diagnosis.

Which test has the highest diagnostic yield?

A Erythrocyte sedimentation rate (ESR).

B Antinuclear antibodies.

C Chest X-ray.

D X-ray of the affected joints.

E Serum creatine kinase levels.

4. A 35-year-old woman is admitted as an emergency to A&E with breathlessness, haemoptysis, chest pain and signs of shock. She receives thrombolysis and is seen to improve. Contrast CT of the pulmonary arteries confirms bilateral pulmonary emboli.

She gives a history of stillbirth in the past and a retinal vein occlusion.

What is the most appropriate next investigation for this woman?

A Antiphospholipid antibody.

B Anti–double-stranded DNA antibody.

C Antineutrophil cytoplasmic antibody (ANCA).

D Prothrombin time.

E Syphilis serology.

5. A 40-year-old female with systemic lupus erythematous (SLE) has severe systemic disease, affecting multiple organs. Which of the following would not be found upon further investigation?

A Raised aspartate aminotransferase (AST) and alanine aminotransferase (ALT).

B ST-segment elevation on electrocardiogram.

C Normocytic anaemia.

D Heavy proteinuria.

E Eosinophilia.

6. Systemic sclerosis or scleroderma can be classified as either diffuse or limited disease. What are the key features of limited systemic sclerosis?

   A Calcinosis, Raynaud phenomenon, oesophageal disease, sclerodactyly, telangiectasia.

   B Corneal irritation, haemoptysis, enthesitis, serositis, transverse myelitis.

   C Cirrhosis, regurgitation, enthesitis, systemic inflammation, thenar eminence wasting.

   D Dactylitis, enthesitis, Raynaud phenomenon, uveitis, conjunctivitis.

   E Bursitis, restless leg syndrome, enthesitis, serositis, telangiectasia.

7. A 56-year-old male is being treated in the intensive care unit for renal failure, associated with severe hypertension. He presented to the emergency department 2 days previously with a severe headache and blurred vision. He has been known to have a rheumatological condition for the past 3 years. Which rheumatological condition is this most likely to be?

   A Sjögren syndrome.

   B Rheumatoid arthritis.

   C Systemic sclerosis.

   D Giant cell arteritis.

   E Systemic lupus erythematous.

8. A 27-year-old male presents to the GP with a continuous cough, vague chest pain, joint pain affecting multiple joints and erythematous patches on the knees. His symptoms have been getting worse over the past few months. He is sent to the hospital where a lung biopsy reveals granuloma formation in the lungs. What condition does this patient have?

   A Systemic sclerosis.

   B Systemic lupus erythematosus.

   C Chronic obstructive pulmonary disorder.

   D Polymyositis.

   E Sarcoidosis.

Chapter 14 The vasculitides

1. A 63-year-old man presents with a headache for 3 days. It is severe and unilateral, only affecting the left side of his head. It radiates to his scalp.

   He has no visual disturbance or pain in his jaw on eating, but feels sore when he brushes his hair.

   The pain is constant, with only temporary relief from analgesia.

   What investigation is most useful in confirming the diagnosis?

   A Temporal artery biopsy.

   B Erythrocyte sedimentation rate (ESR).

   C Antineutrophil cytoplasmic antibody (ANCA) screening.

   D Ultrasound scan.

   E MRI of the aortic arch.

2. A 60-year-old woman comes to the GP with stiffness, fatigue and muscle pains affecting her shoulder and hips. The onset was over several days. On examination, she is slow to rise from a chair, has difficulty in raising her arms and cannot undo her bra strap. She also complains of a right-sided headache, which isn't made better by simple analgesia and which is progressively worsening.

   What should you do immediately?

   A Check erythrocyte sedimentation rate (ESR).

   B Refer for temporal artery biopsy.

   C Refer for muscle biopsy.

   D Administer prednisolone.

   E Administer a nonsteroidal antiinflammatory drug.

3. A 40-year-old male presents to the GP with an unusual collection of symptoms. He has been experiencing recurrent nosebleeds and crusting around his nose. He has pain and stiffness in multiple joints and upon examination, has a widespread vasculitic rash. The patient is referred to the rheumatology department where they carry out a series of blood tests. Anti–proteinase-3 (PR3) antibodies are detected. What disease does this patient most likely have?

   A Granulomatosis with polyangiitis (formerly Wegener granulomatosis).

   B Giant cell arteritis.

   C Polyarteritis nodosa.

   D Eosinophilic granulomatosis with polyangiitis (formerly Churg-Strauss syndrome).

   E Behçet disease.

4. A 60-year-old female arrives at the emergency department acutely confused and vomiting frequently. Upon examination she is clearly dehydrated and hypotensive. The only notable feature in her past medical history is that she has been treated with prednisolone for the past 18 months after receiving a diagnosis of polymyalgia rheumatic, but has now stopped therapy. What is the most important initial step in the treatment of this patient?

   A Give adrenaline.

   B Give IV hydrocortisone and saline.

   C Give IV saline and insulin.

   D Give IV fludrocortisone.

   E Request a CT head.

5. A 3-year-old boy presents to the emergency department with a high fever and a vasculitis rash. Upon examination his cervical lymph nodes are palpable and his tongue has the same appearance as the skin of a strawberry. What is the main treatment given in this condition?

A Oral prednisolone.

B Azothioprine.

C Supportive treatment with analgesia, rest and rehydration.

D Tocilizumab (IL-6 blocker).

E Intravenous immunoglobulins and low-dose aspirin.

6. A 16-year-old boy presents to the GP with a palpable purpuric rash over his legs and buttocks, new abdominal cramping and arthritis in his left hip joint. A urine dipstick test is carried out which shows signs of proteinuria and haematuria. After consultation with the rheumatology team the patient is prescribed paracetamol and it is advised that he goes home, gets rest and drinks plenty of water. What would most likely precipitate this presentation?

A Norovirus infection.

B Gonococcal urethritis.

C Streptococcus throat infection.

D Oral candida.

E Impetigo skin infection.

7. A 54-year-old male presents to the GP with a 2-month history of weight loss, night sweats and diarrhoea. He explains that he has had a runny nose and a wheeze recently. He compares it to hay fever. The rheumatology department assessed his bloods and found MPO ANCA to be present. Which other component will be markedly raised in this patient's blood?

A Eosinophils.

B Anti-CCP antibody.

C Complement (C3).

D Basophils.

E PR3 ANCA.

Chapter 15 Metabolic bone disease

1. An 85-year-old presents to his GP with lower back pain for 2 days. Over the previous 3 years he has noticed his shirts seem to be getting longer but not looser. He had a rib fracture a year ago after slipping off a chair.

Blood tests are performed, which show the following:

Calcium: 2.38 mmol/L (normal 2.12–2.65 mmol/L)

Phosphate: 1.1 mmol/L (normal 0.8–1.4 mmol/L)

Alkaline phosphatase: 98 U/L (normal 30–150 U/L)

What is the most likely diagnosis?

A Osteoporosis.

B Myeloma.

C Osteomalacia.

D Paget disease.

E Potts disease (spinal tuberculosis).

2. A 58-year-old woman presents to her GP with hip pain for 3 weeks. On examination, she has bowing of her tibias. She seems to be having difficulty hearing and the doctor has to keep repeating himself. Her father had a similar issue with bowing of the tibias.

What would be the next most appropriate step in diagnosis?

A Coeliac serology.

B Bone biochemistry.

C Dual-energy X-ray absorptiometry (DEXA) scan.

D MRI of the tibias.

E Test for rheumatoid factor.

3. An 80-year-old man who has chronic renal failure starts developing bony tenderness and muscle weakness. He even finds walking with a Zimmer frame difficult due to pain. Blood tests are performed:

Calcium: 1.56 mmol/L (normal 2.12–2.65 mmol/L)

Phosphate: 0.62 mmol/L (normal 0.8–1.4 mmol/L)

Alkaline phosphatase: 198 U/L (normal 30–150 U/L)

What is not a possible consequence of his condition?

A Skeletal deformity.

B Tetany.

C Polydipsia.

D Convulsions.

E Arrhythmias.

4. A 56-year-old woman presents to her physician with pain shooting down her right leg from her back and also with sore knees. They feel warm to touch. She also has pain when walking. Bone biochemistry is checked and the results are as follows:

Calcium: 2.38 mmol/L (normal 2.1–2.65 mmol/L)

Phosphate: 1.1 mmol/L (normal 0.8–1.4 mmol/L)

Alkaline phosphatase (ALP): 220 U/L (normal 30–150 U/L)

What is the likely diagnosis?

A Osteoarthritis.

B Prolapsed vertebral disc.

C Septic arthritis.

D Paget disease.

E Gout.

5. A 68-year-old woman presents to her GP feeling tired, with myalgia and bone pain. The GP does a broad battery of blood tests and these are her results:

Calcium: 1.87 mmol/L (normal 2.12–2.65 mmol/L)

Phosphate: 0.58 mmol/L (normal 0.8–1.4 mmol/L)

Alkaline phosphatase: 202 U/L (normal 30–150 U/L)

Haemoglobin: 10.3 g/dL (normal 11.5–16.0 g/dL)

Mean cell volume: 101 fL (normal 76–96 fL)

Iron: 9 μmol/L (normal 11–30 μmol/L)

Folate: 1.9 μg/L (normal 2.1 μg/L)

Which investigation would be most useful to confirm the diagnosis?

A Anti–double-stranded DNA antibody.

B Antiphospholipid antibody.

C Anti–smooth muscle antibody.

D Anti–vitamin D_3 antibody.

E Antitissue transglutaminase antibody.

6. A 70-year-old female undergoes a dual-energy X-ray absorptiometry (DEXA) scan which revels a bone mineral density T score of –2.8. It is decided that the patient should be prescribed bisphosphonate therapy in combination with calcium supplements and vitamin D. What is the mechanism of action of bisphosphonate therapy?

A Parathyroid hormone analogue.

B Increase in osteoblast activity.

C Antibody directed against RANK ligand.

D inhibition of sclerostin.

E Inhibition of osteoclast activity.

7. A 2-year-old boy is reviewed in the paediatric department due to recurrent fractures of the tibia and humerus despite any predisposing trauma. Upon examination, there seems to be a varus deformity of his legs and a slight blue discolouration of his sclera. What is the most likely diagnosis?

A Duchenne muscular dystrophy.

B Osteogenesis imperfecta.

C Paget disease.

D Rickets.

E Osteomalacia.

8. A 55-year-old man was diagnosed with liver cirrhosis 1 year ago, secondary to alcoholic fatty liver disease. He is admitted to hospital due to an acute deterioration in his state. Blood tests are carried out to confirm he has osteomalacia attributed to his liver cirrhosis. Which of the following features would not be seen in his blood results?

A Macrocytic anaemia.

B Raised parathyroid hormone levels.

C Low serum vitamin D.

D High urinary calcium excretion.

E Low levels of folate.

Chapter 16 Gout and pseudogout

1. A 75-year-old man develops pain in his right wrist and right third metacarpophalangeal joint. The joints are red, warm, swollen and tender. He cannot do his usual activities due to pain. Aspiration of his wrist shows rhomboid calcium pyrophosphate crystals. An X-ray examination of the joint reveals chondrocalcinosis, subchondral sclerosis and osteophytes. He is given co-codamol for pain relief.

What is the next most effective step in his management?

A Antibiotics.

B Disease-modifying antirheumatic drugs.

C Joint replacement.

D Physiotherapy.

E Splinting.

2. A 59-year-old obese man presents to his physician with acute onset of pain and swelling in his left first metatarsophalangeal joint. It is red, swollen, tender and warm. He is unable to bear weight on it. The physician also finds unusual white lumps on his fingers. The joint is aspirated.

What will the fluid microscopy probably show?

A Gram-positive bacteria.

B Calcium pyrophosphate.

C Pus.

D Monosodium urate crystals.

E Clear synovial fluid.

3. A 55-year-old woman comes to her doctor with an excruciatingly painful right first metatarsophalangeal joint for 24 hours. The overlying skin is warm, shiny and the joint is swollen and immobile. She has a history of chronic kidney disease. Last year she had a similar short-lived episode that resolved and left her symptomless.

What is the most likely explanation for her condition?

A This is an autoimmune condition where T-lymphocytes attack the synovial lining of joints, eventually causing erosion of the cartilage and underlying bone.

B There is an ongoing chronic infection in the joint.

C Chronic hyperuricemia leading to the formation of sodium urate crystals that get deposited in the synovium, causing inflammation.

D Calcium pyrophosphate crystals have deposited in the joint space.

E Degeneration of the weight-bearing cartilage and subsequent eburnation of subchondral bone.

4. A 65-year-old man presents with a warm, hot, swollen and tender right ankle. He has a history of gout and has

had recurrent flares of his disease. He currently takes 200 mg of allopurinol daily. His GP treats him acutely with colchicine and his symptoms settle. Sometime later, his uric acid level is checked and is found to be 460 µg/mL. His other blood tests are normal, including renal function.

What is the next appropriate step in managing this man's gout?

A Increase allopurinol to 300 mg daily.
B Add febuxostat 120 mg daily.
C Start long-term prednisolone 10 mg daily.
D Add colchicine 500 µg twice daily.
E Start ibuprofen 400 mg three times daily.

5. A 65-year-old, obese man is diagnosed with gout after aspiration of his knee joint showed the presence of monosodium urate crystals. Before joint aspiration, a detailed history was taken by his GP. His history uncovered that he is a smoker, he drinks 20 units of alcohol per week (mainly beer) and he sometimes walks the dog, but does not do much to keep fit. He does not maintain a healthy balanced diet and admits to drinking plentiful soft drinks and eating lots of sugary snacks. He has a past medical history of hypertension which he manages with amlodipine and psoriasis for which he is prescribed methotrexate. Which feature of his history is not a risk factor for gout?

A Drinking 20 units of alcohol per week.
B Methotrexate usage.
C Being male.
D Hypertension.
E Diagnosis of psoriasis.

6. A 55-year-old male previously had a single gout attack that resolved spontaneously after a week. However, after consultation with the rheumatology team it was decided that the patient should be started on allopurinol. Which feature of his gout attack indicates the prescription of allopurinol?

A The patient is under 60 years of age.
B Tophi were present on the Achilles tendon.
C The patient was pyrexic during the first day of his gout attack.
D Prescription of NSAIDs is contraindicated in this patient due to a past medical history of peptic ulcer disease.
E A podagra was present.

7. A 78-year-old female patient presents to the GP with pain, swelling and loss of function in her left knee that has been getting worse over the past 2 months. She has a past medical history of hypothyroidism. The GP thinks that osteoarthritis is the most likely diagnosis. What

other condition would fit this clinical picture and should be considered?

A Paget disease.
B Osteoporosis.
C Fibromyalgia.
D Chronic pyrophosphate arthropathy.
E Rheumatoid arthritis.

8. A 56-year-old woman is seen at the rheumatology clinic as she is suffering from recurrent gout flares. A series of blood tests are carried out which suggest that the patient's gout is attributed to metabolic syndrome. Which of the following conditions is not associated with metabolic syndrome?

A Systemic lupus erythematous.
B Dementia.
C Polycystic ovarian syndrome.
C Type 2 diabetes mellitus.
D Psoriasis.

Chapter 17 Paediatric joint disease

1. The majority of the blood supply to the femoral head in adults arises from:

A Artery of ligamentum teres.
B Lateral femoral circumflex artery.
C Obturator artery.
D Medial femoral circumflex artery.
E Profunda femoris artery.

2. A 12-year-old boy attends the hospital with a new onset of pain in his left hip. He is overweight and has not started puberty. He is unable to bear weight on this leg and on examination all movements are generally painful. An X-ray examination reveals that he has an abnormality of the femoral neck in keeping with an SCFE. In what position is his leg most likely to lie?

A Internal rotation.
B External rotation.
C Flexion.
D Abduction.
E Adduction.

3. A baby is assessed in the birthing room after delivery at term. An abnormality is noted involving an inward-pointing foot and calf wasting. The father tells you he had the same thing as a child. What is the most likely diagnosis?

A Talipes equinovarus.
B Normal variant.
C Cerebral palsy.
D Pes planus.
E Spina bifida.

4. A 6-year-old boy attends the fracture clinic with a fracture of his wrist, which has been treated in a cast and seems to be healing. His mother tells you he also recently broke his other wrist and had a supracondylar fracture 1 year ago, all with low-energy trauma. He seems happy and well-dressed but is small in stature and on examination has a subtle scoliosis. What is the most likely underlying medical diagnosis here?

A Marfan syndrome.
B Idiopathic scoliosis.
C Nonaccidental injury.
D Osteoporosis.
E Osteogenesis imperfecta.

5. A 5-year-old boy presents to the clinic with pain in his left knee. He has had no problems in achieving his mobility milestones and walked normally up until 4 weeks ago but has gradually started to struggle. An X-ray examination shows a normal knee but an abnormality to the femoral head including loss of epiphyseal height and subchondral fracture with partial collapse. His inflammatory markers are normal. What is his likely diagnosis?

A Developmental dysplasia of the hip.
B Septic arthritis.
C Perthes disease.
D Slipped capital femoral epiphysis.
E Nonaccidental injury.

6. A 13-month-child begins to walk. Her parents notice that she has a shorter left leg than right leg. It is not painful for her to walk and she has not otherwise been unwell. She was born by planned C-section due to persistent breech positioning, however has had normal development up until now. What would be the imaging investigation of choice for her?

A X-ray.
B MRI.
C CT.
D Hip arthrogram.
E Ultrasound.

Chapter 18 Fractures

1. A patient is admitted to an orthopaedic ward with a proximal tibia fracture while awaiting surgery. During the night the patient experiences a severe increase in pain. This is initially settled with opiate analgesia but rapidly returns and eventually opiate analgesia is no longer effective. What are you primarily concerned about?

A Further displacement of the fracture.
B Deep vein thrombosis.
C Compartment syndrome.

D Embolic arterial occlusion.
E Nerve injury following the fracture.

2. A 68-year-old woman is seen 3 days after a total hip replacement. Initially progressing well, she suddenly develops sharp left-sided chest pain and shortness of breath. On examination, she has slight pyrexia (37.5°C) and is hypoxic on room air (SpO$_2$ 91%) and tachycardic (heart rate 110 bpm). What is the cause of her symptoms?

A Pulmonary thromboembolism.
B Myocardial infarction.
C Basal atelectasis.
D Fat embolism.
E Pneumothorax.

3. What is the main principle when choosing internal fixation over casting of fractures?

A Lower complication rate.
B Cheaper.
C Early mobilization.
D Ensure union of fracture.
E Less pain.

4. A young man is involved in a road traffic accident and is brought into A&E with a collar in situ. He has a Glasgow Coma Scale of 15, but after completing an ABCDE survey he is found to be unstable due to a suspected unstable pelvic fracture. What is the first step to take in dealing with this?

A Place an external fixator while in A&E.
B Urgent angiogram.
C Place a pelvic binder.
D Laparotomy and pelvic packing.
E Anteroposterior X-ray examination of the pelvis.

5. A 92-year-old lady who is normally fit and well presents to A&E with a painful hip and is not able to bear weight. She is normally mobile in the home but has chronic obstructive pulmonary disorder and a poor maximum walking distance. She is examined and her hip is found to be in external rotation and shortened. She is seen to have an intracapsular neck of femur fracture on X-ray examination. What is the best treatment for her?

A Hemiarthroplasty.
B Dynamic hip screw (DHS).
C Total hip replacement.
D Girdlestone procedure.
E Conservative management.

6. A 50-year-old man suddenly feels pain in his right thigh whilst walking outside and falls to the ground. He is alarmed to find that his leg is badly angulated and X-ray examination in the emergency department

confirms a fracture. He explains that he has had pain in this leg for some time and over the last few months has lost weight. He also mentions that he has been coughing up blood and worries that his lifelong smoking habit is the cause. What are you concerned about?

A A simple fracture.
B Compartment syndrome.
C A pathological fracture.
D Complex regional pain syndrome.
E Fat embolism.

7. A 46-year-old secretary falls from a ladder on to her forearm. Her arm is badly angulated and there is a wound over the middle part of the forearm with bone exposed. The Emergency Medicine doctor swiftly manipulates her arm and places it in a back slab. What other steps are important in her management?

A IV antibiotic prophylaxis.
B Making sure her tetanus vaccine/boosters are up to date.
C Taking a photo with a departmental camera for her notes and for discussion with the Plastics team.
D Checking her neurovascular status.
E All of the above.

8. A 28-year-old concert pianist trips and falls in their garden and unfortunately sustains an intraarticular, comminuted, distal radius fracture. Which of the following options will provide them with the best long-term outcome?

A 4 weeks in a close contact cast.
B 6 weeks in a close contact cast.
C External fixation.
D Open reduction and internal fixation.
E A wrist splint with early mobilization.

Chapter 19 Trauma

1. A man arrives in A&E following a car accident, with a suspected pelvic fracture. He is unresponsive, hypotensive and tachycardic. Which is the first step in the management of this patient?

A Obtain intravenous access and commence fluid resuscitation.
B Apply a pelvic binder.
C Get an anteroposterior pelvis X-ray examination.
D Crossmatch the patient for type-matched blood.
E Assess the airway whilst stabilizing the cervical spine.

2. A 20-year-old patient is involved in a road traffic accident, fracturing their femur. They are brought into the A&E and

assessed using an ABCDE approach. Their blood pressure is noted to be 100/60 and their pulse is 110. What is their likely percentage blood loss?

A 0%–15%.
B 15%–30%.
C 30%–40%.
D >40%.

3. An 80-year-old patient trips in her bathroom and hits her head on a toilet seat. She is admitted to A&E and undergoes evaluation using an ABCDE approach. She is found to have a bruise on the back of her head and complains of neck pain. She has a GCS of 14 and no neurological abnormalities. She is on warfarin with an INR of 3. Which is the next best investigation?

A MRI head and C-spine.
B X-ray examination of C-spine.
C CT angiogram.
D CT head and C-spine.
E Bone scan.

4. A 30-year-old man falls 6 metres from some scaffolding. On admission to A&E he complains of shortness of breath and chest pain. On examination he is cyanosed and unable to complete sentences. His trachea is deviated to the right and he has absent breath sounds on the left side. Blood pressure is low, pulse rate is 120 bpm and oxygen levels are only 80% on high-flow oxygen. What is the most important step in his immediate management?

A Insertion of a chest drain.
B Insertion of a wide bore cannula into his right 2nd intercostal space.
C Insertion of a wide bore cannula into his left 2nd intercostal space.
D Intubation and ventilation.
E Blood transfusion.

5. A heavy steel girder falls directly on to a 45-year-old man on a construction site, crushing his lower abdomen. He is rushed to the emergency department and is noted to have bruising around his lower abdomen and groin. His airway and breathing are stable, but his blood pressure is low and he has tachycardia. Intravenous fluids are started, which correct the hypotension. On secondary survey, a doctor finds blood at the urethral meatus and notes that the man has not passed urine. What is his most likely injury?

A Hip fracture.
B Pelvic fracture.
C Penile injury.
D Lumbar spine fracture/dislocation.
E Wedge fracture lumbar spine.

6. A 23-year-old woman loses control of her car at high speed and crashes. Unfortunately, she is not wearing her seat belt and is ejected from the vehicle. When the paramedic arrives, she complains of severe lower back pain and says that she cannot feel her legs. Later in hospital she is unable to pass urine, so a catheter is inserted, which drains 1000 mL of clear urine. What is your main concern?

A Lumbar spine fracture.
B Sacral spine fracture.
C Pelvic fracture.
D Traumatic cauda equina syndrome.
E Bladder injury.

Chapter 20 Infection of bones and joints

1. Which is the most common pathogen in septic arthritis in adults?

A Streptococcus sp.
B Mycobacterium tuberculosis.
C Staphylococcus aureus.
D Haemophilus influenzae.
E Enterobacter sp.

2. A 64-year-old man with a background of diabetes presents with a 24-hour history of progressive atraumatic left knee pain. He is unable to bend his knee and unable to bear weight. On examination, he is pyrexial and his left knee is hot and erythematous. He has a large effusion, virtually no range of movement and global tenderness around the knee. What is the most important step in this man's management?

A Anteroposterior and lateral X-ray examination of the knee.
B Commence intravenous antibiotics.
C Aspiration of the knee.
D Bloods for inflammatory markers.
E Ultrasound scan of the knee.

3. A 38-year-old electrician presents with a painful swollen right knee. He states that over the past week his knee has become increasingly swollen and red and he now has a decreased range of motion. On examination, there is a large erythematous swelling anterior to the patella, which is tender to palpate. There is thickened skin over the anterior of the knee. There is no effusion in the knee. He is able to flex his knee to 45 degrees before he is limited by a combination of pain and tightness in the knee. What is the likely diagnosis?

A Osteoarthritis.
B Septic arthritis.
C Baker cyst.
D Patellar fracture.
E Prepatellar bursitis.

4. In the case of septic arthritis in intravenous drug abusers, which of the following pathogens is most likely?

A Staphylococcus aureus.
B Pseudomonas.
C Fungal infections.
D Streptococcus sp.
E All of the above.

5. A farmer falls 3 metres from a ladder in his cattle yard. He sustains an open fracture of his tibia, which is heavily contaminated. Which bacteria would be most likely to contaminate the wound?

A Anaerobic bacteria.
B Staphylococcus aureus.
C Mycobacterium tuberculosis.
D Methicillin-resistant Staphylococcus aureus.
E Escherichia coli.

6. A 51-year-old Caucasian woman presents with back pain. She has not been well for the last 3 months. Recently, she has lost weight and had night sweats. She mentions that she lived in India for 10 years when she was 20. On examination, she has a gibbus in the middle region of the thoracic spine and has tenderness on palpation. Which organism are you most concerned about?

A Staphylococcus aureus.
B Staphylococcus epidermidis.
C Escherichia coli.
D Mycobacterium tuberculosis.
E Pseudomonas aeruginosa.

Chapter 21 Malignancy

1. A 30-year-old man presents with an intensely painful right proximal tibia with no history of trauma. He experiences pain during the day and night. Of note, he states that aspirin relieves his pain significantly. On examination, there is significant tenderness over the proximal tibial metaphysis. X-ray examination shows a small lucent area in the tibial metaphysis with dense sclerosis surrounding it. What is the most likely diagnosis?

A Enchondroma.
B Osteoid osteoma.
C Chondrosarcoma.
D Osteochondroma.
E Lymphoma.

2. A 24-year-old, normally fit and healthy woman presents with a 4-month history of gradually increasing pain in her left knee. There was no history of trauma. She is now having difficulty bearing weight and is frequently woken at night with pain. She also notes weight loss in the same

timeframe. X-ray examination of her knee demonstrates an expansile and lytic lesion in her distal femur, with cortical destruction and significant periosteal reaction. What is the most likely diagnosis?

A Tuberculosis.

B Osteosarcoma.

C Enchondroma.

D Osteomyelitis.

E Stress fracture.

3. An 89-year-old man presents with a painful lumbar spine and difficulty mobilizing. He tells you this has only been present for 6 weeks but that he has noticed some weight loss and feels generally unwell. He undergoes an X-ray examination of the spine, which shows sclerotic change through L5 and S1. What is the most likely underlying diagnosis?

A Prostate cancer.

B Renal cancer.

C Lung cancer.

D Thyroid cancer.

E Bowel cancer.

4. Which of these common bony structures visible on X-ray images might be an indication of malignancy?

A Looser zones.

B Periarticular erosions.

C Osteophytes.

D Periosteal reaction.

E Vertebral trabecular thickening.

5. A 55-year-old man presents with a pathological fracture of his left clavicle after lifting a suitcase. On the X-ray image, there is a diffuse area of abnormal bone. The skull X-ray shows numerous lytic lesions and his erythrocyte sedimentation rate (ESR) is 130 mm/h. What investigation is most important here in making a diagnosis?

A Bone scan.

B CT head.

C Protein electrophoresis.

D Full blood count.

E MRI clavicle.

6. A 60-year-old woman presents with a complete flaccid paralysis of the legs. Prior to this, she had 3 weeks of severe back pain. X-ray images show complete collapse of T12 vertebra. Chest X-ray examination, abdominal and thyroid ultrasound scans are normal. The ESR is 30 mm/h and serum electrophoresis is normal. What is the most appropriate diagnosis here?

A Lung metastasis.

B Kidney metastasis.

C Bowel metastasis.

D Breast metastasis.

E Thyroid metastasis.

Chapter 22 Sports injuries

1. What causes a locked knee?

A Anterior cruciate ligament tear.

B Radial meniscal tear.

C Medial collateral ligament tear.

D Bucket handle meniscal tear.

E Tibial plateau fracture.

2. An 18-year-old football player presents to A&E with a knee injury. He describes turning quickly and twisting his right knee, precipitating immediate pain. He states his knee was grossly swollen before he left the pitch. On examination, there is a tense effusion, no joint line tenderness and a poor range of motion. Lachman test is positive, but otherwise the knee is stable. What is the diagnosis?

A Medial meniscal tear.

B Posterior cruciate ligament tear.

C Medial collateral ligament tear.

D Patellar dislocation.

E Anterior cruciate ligament tear.

3. A 23-year-old man walks into A&E reporting pain in his left shoulder. He has an obvious deformity and is unable to move the shoulder. A dislocation is diagnosed. What is the most likely position for the humerus to lie, in relation to the glenoid?

A Anterior medial.

B Posterior.

C Anterior superior.

D Anterior inferior.

E Superior.

4. Which of the following conditions make a patellar dislocation more likely?

A Patella fracture.

B Cerebral palsy.

C Anterior cruciate ligament injury.

D Hypoplastic trochlea.

E Osteoarthritis.

5. A 24-year-old male is playing 5-a-side football when he twists his ankle and falls to the ground. He cannot weight bear following and attends his local minor injuries unit where he has an X-ray which shows no bony injury. Three months later he has ongoing pain and instability of his ankle. What investigation should be carried out now?

A Repeat X-ray of the ankle.
B X-ray of the foot.
C CT of the ankle.
D MRI of the ankle.
E MRI of the foot.

6. A 26-year-old professional skier, tears her ACL during a training session. This is confirmed by MRI. What is the best available management for her?
A Rest, ice, elevation and avoidance of future contact sports.
B Rest and then physiotherapy once the acute injury has settled, with targeted quads strengthening.
C ACL repair.
D ACL reconstruction.
E External knee bracing.

Chapter 23 Soft tissue disorders

1. De Quervain tenosynovitis involves inflammation of which tendon sheath?
A Extensor pollicis longus.
B Abductor pollicis longus.
C Extensor indicis.
D Flexor pollicis longus.
E Extensor carpi radialis longus.

2. A 55-year-old man presents with pain and swelling over his left elbow. He has an obvious swelling but not much redness at the olecranon and a normal range of motion. His C-reactive protein is 6 and his white cells 7.3. What is the first-line treatment for this condition?
A Nonsteroidal antiinflammatory drugs (NSAIDs) and rest.
B Aspiration and culture.
C Intravenous antibiotics.
D Open washout.
E Bursectomy.

3. Which tissue is primarily involved in the development of Dupuytren contracture?
A Flexor tendons.
B Palmar fascia.
C Metacarpophalangeal joint capsule.
D Flexor tendon sheaths.
E Skin.

4. A 52-year-old male was running in a regional athletics competition and whilst running, felt what he describes as a blow to the back of his leg. He couldn't continue running and attends the local minor injuries unit. On examination he has swelling and early bruising at the posterior aspect of his ankle and a positive Simmonds test. What is your management plan for him?

A Rest, ice, compression and elevation.
B Nonsteroidal antiinflammatory drugs (NSAIDs).
C Surgical repair.
D Below knee plaster cast in equinus
E Physiotherapy.

5. A 49-year-old cleaner presents with recurrent episodes of prepatellar bursitis. Repeated periods of rest and NSAIDs have been trialled. This most recent episode of bursitis has left him with a sinus which has been discharging for the past 6 days. What treatment would you recommend?
A Oral antibiotics.
B IV antibiotics.
C A vacuum-assisted dressing to assist with closure.
D Surgical excision of the bursa.
E Surgical laying open of the sinus tract.

Chapter 24 Principles of orthopaedic surgery

1. An 82-year-old female undergoes hemiarthroplasty after fracture of her left hip. Six hours after the operation, her pulse is 70 bpm and her blood pressure is 80/40. She is not confused but is not producing any urine. Which is the most likely cause for her condition?
A Cardiogenic shock.
B Hypovolaemia.
C Anaphylaxis.
D Sepsis.
E Neurogenic shock.

2. A 79-year-old male presents to A&E with pain in his right hip. He is unable to move and reports that he simply bent over to do up his shoelace and felt a severe pain in his hip. Of note in his history, he had a total hip replacement on the right side 9 years previously but had been functioning well. What is the most likely cause for his pain?
A Hip dislocation.
B Periprosthetic fracture.
C Implant loosening.
D Deep infection.
E Implant failure and breakage.

3. A 55-year-old female had a total hip replacement carried out 6 months previously. She has constantly struggled with pain and has leakage through the wound. She has a C-reactive protein of 110 and white cell count of 12.0. She has attended the A&E today but remains haemodynamically stable. What is the best treatment?
A Immediate intravenous antibiotics and admission.
B Admission, observation and aspiration in theatre.
C Single-stage revision total hip replacement.
D Admission and bone scan.
E Discharge and review in clinic.

4. A 69-year-old male who has a BMI of 32, underwent a total knee replacement 2 days ago, develops shortness of breath on the ward with an acute drop in his saturations from 99% on air to 88%. He complains to the nursing staff of chest pain. What is at the top of your differential diagnosis?

   A Myocardial infarction.
   B Hospital-acquired pneumonia.
   C Atelectasis.
   D Congestive heart failure.
   E Pulmonary embolus.

5. The preassessment appointment is important in the patient's care for which of the following reasons?

   A To diagnose any hitherto unknown conditions such as hypertension or aortic stenosis.
   B To record the patient's baseline bloods and observations.
   C To ascertain if the patient can be medically or physically optimized in any way prior to their surgery.
   D To ascertain if there are any new contraindications to the patient's surgery such as a local skin infection.
   E All of the above.

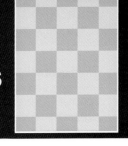

UKMLA SBA answers

Chapter 1 Taking a history

1   C. A medical history of an under-active thyroid. This is commonly associated with carpal tunnel syndrome. A family history of hypertension is important but does not clarify the diagnosis. Many patients try multiple analgesics to relieve the pain from this condition. Her social history might reveal exacerbating factors such as typing at a keyboard but does not narrow the diagnosis. Marked fatigue often occurs with hypothyroidism but is not directly associated with carpal tunnel syndrome.

2   B. Prednisolone 10 mg daily for several years. Corticosteroids are a well-recognized risk factor in developing osteoporosis. Corticosteroid use of 7.5 mg prednisolone (or equivalent) daily for more than 3 months is considered to be sufficiently high to warrant bone protection. A family history of traumatic hip fracture is unlikely to present significant increased risk of osteoporosis, as is the case of menopause at the age of 53 years, which would be considered normal. Living abroad might confer a protective effect against osteoporosis as increased sunlight exposure improves vitamin D metabolism. A personal history of type 2 diabetes does not increase your risk of osteoporosis.

3   A. A recent history of swallowing trouble. These are features of CREST syndrome (systemic sclerosis), an important cause of secondary Raynaud disease. Primary Raynaud disease does not typically ulcerate, nor is it associated with other connective tissue diseases. Alcohol misuse is not a recognized risk factor for secondary Raynaud disease, nor is a family history of osteoarthritis. Nifedipine and other calcium channel blockers are commonly used to help all forms of Raynaud phenomenon. COPD is not associated with secondary Raynaud disease.

4   D. Reactive arthritis. This inflammatory joint condition can occur after bacterial infections (such as mycoplasma pneumoniae in lower respiratory tract infections) and favours the larger joints of the lower limbs. Acute polyarticular gout is unlikely in someone as a first presentation. Rheumatoid arthritis is a symmetrical inflammatory arthritis typically affecting the hands and feet. Ankylosing spondylitis is an axial spondyloarthropathy affecting the back, although it is commonly associated with the HLA-B27 antigen, as is reactive arthritis. Polyarticular septic arthritis is rare and usually presents as life-threatening sepsis.

5   C. A past medical history of psoriasis that affects his scalp. This patient's presentation of asymmetrical oligoarthritis accompanied by dactylitis and nail pitting with a past medical history of psoriasis is indicative of psoriatic arthritis. Smoking is a risk factor for many rheumatological conditions but it is not specific. A BMI of 30 kg/m^2 supports a diagnosis of psoriatic arthritis due to its association with metabolic syndrome. However, it is not specific to the condition. His father's past medical history of probable reactive arthritis supports the diagnosis of psoriatic arthritis as both conditions have an association with a variation in HLA-B27. However, it is also associated with ankylosing spondylitis and enteropathic arthritis. A vegetarian diet would be protective against gout.

6   E. This is a likely case of reactive arthritis caused by a sexually transmitted infection. Determining if the patient is vulnerable to catching a sexually transmitted infection is an important part of the history. Exploring how the pain affects the patient's daily function is important but will not help you to obtain a diagnosis. Smoking cigarettes can be a risk factor for many conditions. A high-protein diet would be a risk factor for gout, which would present similarly. However, gout would be very unlikely to affect someone as young as 21 years of age. Trauma to the knee may explain the knee stiffness. However, it would not explain the systemic features experienced by the patient.

Chapter 2 Examining joints

1   E. High-stepping gait. This is because the leg must be lifted higher to clear the ground in patients with a foot-drop. Trendelenburg gait is seen in patients with abnormal hip abductor function. An antalgic gait is a painful gait often seen in osteoarthritis or any painful condition. A circumduction gait occurs in hemiplegia. Waddling gait is seen in patients with congenital hip dislocations, among other conditions.

2   B. Extensor pollicis longus. The tendon of EPL runs over the radial side of the wrist joint and is commonly affected by displaced wrist fractures. It controls thumb extension and can be tested by asking the patient to straighten the distal joint of the thumb or lift the thumb off a flattened surface

with the palm face-down. Adductor pollicis controls thumb adduction, abductor pollicis brevis controls abduction and opponens pollicis controls thumb opposition. Extensor digitorum is responsible for extension of the metacarpophalangeal, proximal interphalangeal and distal interphalangeal of the digits.

3   A. Carpal tunnel syndrome. Her hypothyroidism is a risk factor for the condition. The classic presentation is of pain occurring in the thumb, index and middle finger and the thumb side of the ring finger. Systemic causes of peripheral neuropathy most commonly cause a glove-and-stocking distribution of pain or anaesthesia. Peripheral vascular disease causes intermittent claudication, typically found in the legs. C8 radiculopathy would result in altered sensation over the C8 dermatome, which covers the 4th and 5th digits. Golfer's elbow is an acute swelling of the medial epicondyle, which would typically affect the ulnar nerve if any.

4   A. The Babinski reflex. This reflex is present in those with an upper motor neuron lesion (e.g., due to a stroke). Reduced power in the legs (MRC grade 3), muscle wastage and visible muscle fasciculations are all signs of a lower motor neuron lesion. Cogwheel rigidity is a characteristic finding in Parkinson disease.

5   D. The posterior cruciate ligament. This finding describes a positive posterior sag sign that is seen when testing for posterior cruciate ligament damage. The medial meniscus can be tested using McMurray's test but this is not often used in clinical practice. A popliteus muscle tendon injury is relatively uncommon and the collateral ligaments are tested by flexing the knee and applying pressure to each side. The patella grind test would be used to assess the integrity of the patellar tendon.

6   C. The sciatic nerve. In a positive straight leg raise test, pain will radiate to the foot when the leg is passively raised and the foot is dorsiflexed. This test stretches the sciatic nerve and will elicit pain with lumbar disc disease.

7   E. The axillary nerve. An axillary nerve injury can occur due to a compressive force or trauma causing anterior dislocation of the shoulder. The axillary neve innervates the deltoid muscle and damage will cause muscle wastage, loss of function and numbness over the area.

8   B. Subscapularis. This is one of the rotator cuff muscles and damage to the subscapularis will present with inability to internally rotate the shoulder against resistance. Teres minor and supraspinatus are also rotator cuff muscles but are involved in shoulder abduction and external rotation. The brachioradialis is implicated in elbow flexion and levator scapulae elevates the scapula.

Chapter 3 Investigations

1   A. Anti–double-stranded DNA antibodies. These are highly specific for systemic lupus erythematosus (SLE). ESR would be elevated, but it is nonspecific. Skin biopsy can be useful for cutaneous lupus but in a classic photosensitive malar rash it would be unlikely to help confirm the diagnosis. Thyroid disease is important to consider but would not confirm the diagnosis of SLE.

2   B. Methotrexate hepatotoxicity. It is important that a patient's blood is closely monitored when increasing doses of methotrexate. Signs of toxicity include flu-like symptoms, nausea, diarrhoea, fatigue and recurrent mouth ulcers. Blood shows a hepatitic pattern of derangement. Primary biliary cirrhosis is associated with rheumatoid arthritis but presents insidiously with itching and cholestatic blood. Acute viral hepatitis is unlikely and typically the derangement would be far more severe. Gallstones cause painful jaundice with elevated alkaline phosphatase, GGT and bilirubin. Alcohol abuse is a possibility, but there is nothing in her history to suggest overuse.

3   C. Anti-SCL-70. This woman has systemic sclerosis with secondary Raynaud phenomenon, sclerodactyly and telangiectasia. Jo-1 is associated with antisynthetase syndrome. Anti-dsDNA is very specific for SLE. p-ANCA is associated with vasculitis. Histone antibodies are seen in drug-induced lupus.

4   D. MRI. The twisting mechanism with a popping sensation suggests a meniscal tear for which MRI is the best investigative procedure. Joint aspiration, in the context of trauma, is likely to show haemarthrosis but will not facilitate the diagnosis. X-ray examination is limited to diagnosing bony issues. Ultrasound is useful for looking at soft tissue, but it is technically difficult to get deep views of the knee. ESR will be nonspecifically elevated in the context of injury and inflammation

5   B. Cyclic citrullinated peptide antibody (anti-CCP). This is the most specific factor for RA. When strongly positive, it has a high predictive value for the development of RA. Rheumatoid factor is sensitive for RA but not as specific. Jo-1 autoantibodies will be present in myositis and dermatomyositis. Antibodies to MPO will be present in microscopic polyangiitis and eosinophilic granulomatosis with polyangiitis. C-reactive protein will be raised due to inflammation and is nonspecific.

6   A. Systemic lupus erythematous (SLE). The urinalysis results and evident hypertension are signs of nephritic syndrome. Connective tissue disease (e.g., SLE) can cause damage to the kidneys which can present as nephritic syndrome.

7   C. Needle-shaped monosodium urate crystals. This finding is indicative of monosodium urate crystal arthropathy (i.e., gout). These crystals will show a strong negative birefringence. Rhomboid-shaped calcium pyrophosphate crystals with a weak positive birefringence will be present in pseudogout.

8   C. Heavy menstrual periods. Iron-deficiency anaemia is a microcytic anaemia that is most commonly due to heavy menstrual bleeding in someone who is menstruating and is otherwise fit and well. However, in those that are not menstruating, iron-deficiency anaemia is due to blood loss from the gastrointestinal tract until proven otherwise. Long-term NSAID use is a risk factor for gastric ulcer formation. Thalassemia is a hereditary cause of microcytic anaemia, however it is symptomatic and the patient in this scenario would be aware that she had the condition before the age of 19. Low levels of folate would cause a macrocytic anaemia.

9   E. Complement. Systemic lupus erythematous is a condition of complement consumption, therefore during an active SLE flare, levels of C3 and C4 will be low.

Chapter 4 Regional musculoskeletal pain

1   A. A history of urinary incontinence. This is a red flag feature of back pain and an urgent MRI should be carried out to exclude cord compression. An elevated ESR is nonspecific for inflammation but does not imply an urgent cause for concern. A family history of psoriasis may predispose the patient to psoriatic arthritis with sacroiliitis, but it does not require an urgent investigation. Abnormal TFTs may explain fatigue but are not usually implicated in back pain. A positive ANA is a common nonspecific finding in the general population, particularly at low titres.

2   B. A ruptured ACL. The history here is classical for an ACL rupture and the description of a fluid level seen on the radiograph suggests a lipohaemarthrosis, which usually indicates a fracture or ruptured ACL. With the history of acute injury, a rheumatoid knee or a septic arthritis are not likely. A patellar dislocation is extremely painful but would not show a lipohaemarthrosis on X-ray. Pseudogout is a crystal arthropathy seen in the elderly which can show chondrocalcinosis, but not lipohaemarthrosis.

3   C. Spinal stenosis. The pain is bilateral, radiates and is relieved by flexing the spine (hence the patient's stooped gait). Extension aggravates his symptoms. Prolapsed intervertebral discs give pain in response to an acute injury, which is usually unilateral. Mechanical back pain does not usually give radiating neurological symptoms.

Spondylolisthesis pain usually improves on lying flat. The patient does not have red flag features suggesting malignancy.

4   D. ESR. This gentleman has polymyalgia rheumatica, a common cause of bilateral shoulder pain, fatigue and stiffness in the elderly. Treatment is with steroids. Nerve conduction studies are unlikely to yield useful results, nor will X-ray images as his history does not suggest a bony cause for his symptoms. The history is not typical of multiple myeloma, the test for which is a urinary Bence Jones protein. MRI of the neck is helpful in neuropathic disorders to exclude nerve root compression but would not be helpful here.

5   E. Complex regional pain syndrome is characterized by severe pain after an injury, skin changes, hypersensitivity and occasional swelling. Arterial insufficiency causes claudication and ulceration. Upper limb DVT would not normally cause hypersensitivity. Factitious pain is rare and we should be wary of labelling patients with this. Phantom-limb pain is seen postamputation.

6   D. Pelvic and hip plain radiographs. By listening to this man's history he is most likely to be suffering from hip osteoarthritis. It is not unusual that many people in the same family have osteoarthritis; just because there is a family history, it doesn't mean that the arthritis is familial! You should come to a diagnosis by history and examination alone, but an X-ray is still required to prove your diagnosis, grade the severity of the arthritis and help to plan future treatment. A CT or MRI is unnecessary, all the relevant information described can be gained from the plain radiographs. There is no suggestion that this is inflammatory and so inflammatory markers are not needed.

7   B. A meniscal tear. This chronic pain which has developed gradually does not tie in with a diagnosis of septic arthritis, gout or an ACL rupture. Instead, when considering his history as an athlete, his history of pain with movement and of locking, and also his examination finding of tenderness along one side of the joint line, a meniscal tear is the likely diagnosis here. If his pain was more global, then generalized osteoarthritis could also be considered as a diagnosis, however he would not have symptoms of locking with osteoarthritis alone. In reality, it is likely that he would have a degree of both some OA and some degenerative meniscal pathology!

8   C. Plantar fasciitis. This history and the location of this patient's pain is classical for plantar fasciitis. The patient is most tender at the medial tuberosity of the calcaneus on palpation. In the setting of a fit and healthy 22 year old, diabetic neuropathy is unlikely and would not affect the hindfoot preferentially. Achilles' tendinopathy would affect

the hindfoot, but would not cause point tenderness over the patient's heels. Morton neuroma causes forefoot pain and there is no indication in the question that the patient has an inflammatory condition.

Chapter 5 Widespread musculoskeletal pain

1   A. CT thorax, abdomen and pelvis. This woman has an atypical presentation of PMR with overlapping inflammatory joint disease; the possibility of a paraneoplastic rheumatic syndrome must be considered. A CT scan of the thorax, abdomen and pelvis is the first-line test when considering an occult malignancy. Abnormal vitamin D levels would not explain the synovitis or elevated ESR. Muscle biopsy is usually only undertaken for the diagnosis of myositis. Rheumatoid factor is nonspecific and steroids would normally improve standard rheumatoid arthritis. Skeletal survey is a test for multiple myeloma; it may be undertaken later but would not be a first-line test.

2   C. Pregabalin. This woman has fibromyalgia. A multitherapy approach to treatment is required involving physiotherapy/graded exercise, addressing trigger stressors and analgesia (anticonvulsants are often used). Naproxen is a nonsteroidal antiinflammatory drug and therefore not useful. Adalimumab is a monoclonal antibody used in severe inflammatory arthritis. Methotrexate is similarly reserved for inflammatory arthritis. Opiates such as oxycodone are generally avoided in the management of fibromyalgia.

3   D. Reassurance. This woman has fibromyalgia. Her initial tests are normal and she has no neurological deficits. She needs reassurance and referred to services such as physiotherapy, cognitive behavioural therapy and occupational therapy. In the absence of neurological features, MRI is unlikely to have any diagnostic use. Immunology is normal in fibromyalgia. Electromyography is reserved predominantly for disorders affecting the neuromuscular junction. IV immunoglobulins are used in a variety of severe autoimmune conditions but have no role here.

4   E. Foot drop. This usually indicates an L5/S1 nerve root lesion. Altered sleep pattern, pain in multiple tender points, alternating bowel habits and headache are all common features of fibromyalgia.

5   C. High serum calcium. Bony metastases will increase serum calcium due to their influence on osteoclast activity. Alkaline phosphatase is a marker of bone turnover and would also be raised. Serum parathyroid hormone is raised in hypocalcemic states. Anti-CCP antibodies would be detectable in rheumatoid arthritis. P-ANCA would be detectable in the case of vasculitis.

6   A. Fibromyalgia. This condition most commonly affects middle-aged women and presents as wide spread pain that responds poorly to analgesia. It is closely associated with tiredness, insomnia and poor concentration. It is often triggered by a difficult emotional period. The patient has no cutaneous signs of SLE and does not complain of pain in specific joints as would be seen in osteoarthritis or rheumatoid arthritis. Polymyalgia rheumatica rarely affects patients under the age of 60.

7   D. Acute myeloid leukaemia. Paraneoplastic rheumatic syndrome describes widespread musculoskeletal pain that is most commonly attributed to a haematological malignancy. Less frequently it can be due to metastasis of primary tumours, most commonly tumours of the lung, breast, kidney, thyroid (follicular) or prostate.

8   D. Palpation of trigger points. Pain produced upon light palpation of trigger points is suggestive of fibromyalgia. Palpation of the spinous processes is nonspecific. A positive Schober test would suggest ankylosing spondylitis. Tinel test will elicit a tingling sensation in the case of carpal tunnel syndrome. The straight leg raise test is used to assess compression of the sciatic nerve.

Chapter 6 An acute, hot, swollen joint

1   A. Gram-positive cocci. This woman has septic arthritis and the most common organism is *Staphylococcus aureus*, a common skin bacterium. Gram-negative bacilli tend to inhabit the GI tract. Crystal arthropathy is unlikely because she is clinically exhibiting signs of infection. Blood would indicate a haemarthrosis, but she is not known to be on anticoagulants or to have suffered trauma.

2   B. DMARDs. This man has psoriatic arthritis, a common cause of acute inflammatory monoarthritis in young men. His rash is characteristic of the skin symptoms caused by psoriatic arthritis. Methotrexate or leflunomide are usually first-line DMARDs. Antibiotics will not help. Paracetamol may help his pain but not the underlying condition. Systemic steroids often worsen skin symptoms of psoriasis. Topical emollients will help treat the skin symptoms but not the arthritis.

3   C. A previous history of right ankle swelling and pain. This suggests recurrence of a gout flare. Septic arthritis does not typically happen episodically. A low-grade fever can be a feature of either condition as can a high CRP level. A history of immunosuppression favours the diagnosis of septic arthritis. A family history of rheumatoid arthritis is not particularly relevant to either condition.

4   A. Reducing alcohol intake of all types of alcohol. Drinking alcohol of any type can increase a person's likelihood of a

sudden attack of gut. Alcohol increases the level of uric acid in the blood. Beer is worse than spirits or wine but no alcohol is safe from causing the drinker a bout of gout. This lady's diuretics may well be precipitating her gout, but just stopping them is unlikely to help her other comorbidities. A considered approach to her polypharmacy is needed. Losing weight is recommended to prevent attacks of gout, but this should be done in a measured way as rapid weight loss can also cause an acute attack. Seafood (in particular mussels, crab, shrimp and other shellfish) can trigger an attack of gout.

5   D. IV antibiotics. This patient has a septic arthritis of her knee and is systemically unwell with it. She needs antibiotics as soon as possible (definitely within an hour) and only after a joint aspiration so that an organism can be identified and her antibiotics tailored from empirical antibiotics, once her cultures are back. Blood cultures are investigations not management. IV fluids and oxygen are important facets of managing her sepsis, but will not treat her infection. Paracetamol is important as part of her analgesia regime but again, will not treat her septic arthritis.

6   E. Hyperparathyroidism. All the conditions listed here cause hypercalcaemia, but hyperparathyroidism is most likely of the conditions listed to be associated with pseudogout.

Chapter 7 A child with a limp

1   B. Hypothyroidism. Hypothyroidism conveys no risk to developing Perthes disease. Hypothyroidism and other hormonal conditions are risk factors in slipped upper femoral epiphysis. Delayed bone age, low socioeconomic group, low birth weight and a family history are all risk factors of developing Perthes disease.

2   E. Slipped capital femoral epiphysis. This condition occurs in adolescents aged 11 to 14 years and is more common in boys than girls. A background of chronic pain prior to the slip is common.

3   A. Transient synovitis. With the history of a recent viral illness and normal radiology and inflammatory markers, transient synovitis is most likely.

4   D. Immediate resuscitation. While the other steps may be important in the management of the patient, they should not delay resuscitation and should be part of an ongoing process of reassessment.

5   C. Nonaccidental injury. There are many red flags in this scenario for nonaccidental injury. The child is too young to be walking and so cannot have hurt themselves significantly if under appropriate supervision. She is in significant pain and so a fracture is likely. She was in the

care of someone new for the first time when the symptoms began. NAI should be your first thought in cases such as these.

6   B. Developmental dysplasia of the hip. Late-presenting developmental dysplasia of the hip presents with a painless limp and leg-length discrepancy. Slipped capital femoral epiphysis and osteomyelitis would cause pain, and pes planus and congenital talipes equinovarus would not cause a leg length discrepancy.

7   E. Juvenile idiopathic arthritis. Presentation with monoarthritis is common, with other joints involved later. Generalized symptoms suggest a systemic disorder. The presence of eye symptoms is worrying as blindness can result.

8   A. Osgood-Schlatter disease. The disease is often bilateral and occurs during the adolescent years. Tender, swollen tibial tuberosities are present bilaterally. Patellar tendon rupture bilaterally is unlikely and the patient would not be walking. Patellar tendinitis would give pain palpating along the tendon rather than at its insertion. Chondromalacia patellae gives anterior knee pain rather than pain at the tibial tuberosity. Perthes' can give referred pain to the knee, but again, would not give pain at the tibial tuberosities.

9   D. Perthes disease. The boy is the right age to have Perthes' and the history of knee pain is typical. The loss of abduction is worrying as it could mean impending joint subluxation. The sclerosis of the femoral head is due to avascular necrosis.

10 B. Osteomyelitis. A diagnosis of osteomyelitis is difficult in a very young child such as this one. In this case, the child clearly has an infection. In the absence of an obviously swollen joint and with a normal hip ultrasound scan, the most likely cause is osteomyelitis.

Chapter 8 Back pain

1   D. Nucleus pulposus. A disc prolapse occurs when part of the nucleus pulposus herniates through the annulus fibrosus and presses on a spinal nerve root.

2   D. Bilateral sciatic-type pain. Bilateral leg symptoms are suggestive of impending cauda equina syndrome.

3   B. MRI scan. In order to assess for compression of the nerve roots at the cauda equina, MRI is the best investigative procedure. This must be done urgently if clinical suspicion is high. A CT scan can be useful in cases where an MRI is contraindicated and with modern scanners can give lots of information; however, MRI is gold standard.

4   C. Metastatic prostate cancer. This is the most likely cause: the spread of tumour into the spine is thought to made

more likely by backflow through the venous complex. It has the classic sclerotic appearance on X-ray images.

5   E. Discitis. This condition often presents later after the patient has had a number of normal investigations as X-ray changes are not immediately apparent. This patient is at a higher risk of developing sepsis having diabetes and chronic renal failure. The X-ray changes seen on the X-ray 1 week after the onset of his symptoms are typical for discitis.

6   A. Advise antiinflammatories, stretching and to continue gentle activity in the first instance. This man has acute low back pain. This is very common and usually resolves. Note the absence of red flags. In the first instance some general advice on how to manage the pain should be given with worsening advice on what symptoms should alert the patient to go to the emergency department (cauda equina red flags). If the pain does not settle in the next 6 weeks then further tests may be warranted at that point.

7   E. Spondylolisthesis. Fast bowlers in cricket are at increased risk. The features seen on the X-ray image in this case are diagnostic. Scoliosis is not painful. Ankylosing spondylitis would cause a restriction in movement at the lumbar spine. A prolapsed intervertebral disc and spinal stenosis would both be uncommon in this age and would cause radiation of symptoms down the patient's legs.

8   D. Ankle-brachial pressure index. While this case initially sounds like it might be spinal stenosis, this man does not get any relief from bending over when his symptoms come on. Vascular claudication is the diagnosis to further investigate here and so the next test to do would be an ankle-brachial pressure index. If the diagnosis was still in doubt, a Doppler ultrasound or CT angiogram could be requested.

Chapter 9 Altered sensation and weakness

1   D. Median nerve. A dorsally angulated distal radius fracture can cause compression of the median nerve, giving symptoms of carpal tunnel syndrome.

2   D. Carpal tunnel syndrome. This woman has carpal tunnel syndrome. Her symptoms and their distribution are typical of carpal tunnel syndrome. Percussion at the wrist crease is Tinel sign.

3   C. Nerve conduction studies. These studies can be useful when planning surgery for carpal tunnel disease and will give a grading from 1 to 4 as to how severe it is. Ultimately, the decision to decompress is still being made clinically.

4   A. Transient ischaemic attack. This story is much more acute and concerning than that of a simple nerve

entrapment and should be investigated for stroke or TIA with a central cause far more likely than a peripheral cause.

5   E. Axillary nerve. This man has sustained an anterior dislocation of his shoulder. The axillary nerve leaves the brachial plexus and winds around the surgical neck of the humerus to supply sensation to the 'regimental badge patch area' over the upper lateral aspect of the the upper arm, and motor function to the deltoid. This injury is usually the result of a neuropraxia.

6   A. Pancoast tumour. An apical lung tumour has resulted in compression of the sympathetic nerves that arise from T1 and run up to supple the eye and forehead. This results in Horner syndrome (ipsilateral miosis, ptosis and facial anhidrosis) on the affected side. The tumour is also compressing the T1 myotome.

7   A. Radial nerve. The radial nerve runs in the spiral groove on the posterior aspect of the midshaft of the humerus. It is in direct contact with the bone at this point, which makes it prone to injury. In the majority of humeral shaft fractures, the injury to the nerve is a neuropraxia and resolves with time. In some cases, the nerve is trapped in the fracture or has a more serious injury and in these instances, the nerve must be explored.

8   C. MRI. This lady has suffered a C6/7 cervical disc prolapse. A disc at this level would compress the C7 nerve root, causing numbness and/or pain in the middle finger. C7 supplies the triceps and flexor carpi radialis and there is resultant weakness of elbow extension and flexion of the wrist.

Chapter 10 Osteoarthritis

1   A. Lytic bone lesions. This suggests malignant infiltration of the bone. The other four findings are all classic signs of osteoarthritis.

2   B. Osteophytes. This gentleman is suffering from osteoarthritis. Erosions are a feature of inflammatory arthritis. A hairline fracture would have a quicker scale of onset. Osteopenia is usually incidental and not usually a primary cause of pain. Soft tissue swelling is clinically discernible on examination; X-ray examination is primarily an investigation of bony structures.

3   C. Heberden nodes. The patient's clinical history and age are suggestive of osteoarthritis. Ulnar deviation and boutonniere deformity are suggestive of rheumatoid arthritis. A Dupuytren contracture is common with advancing age, but it is not typically painful. MCP swelling is suggestive of inflammatory arthritis.

4   D. Physiotherapy. This man has osteoarthritis (OA). The evidence for glucosamine is poor. Joint replacement may

be warranted but most patients explore nonsurgical options first. Systemic steroids do not have a role to play in managing OA, although joint injection can help with pain; however, the hip joint is a challenging joint to inject and must be done under ultrasound or X-ray guidance.

5   D. Having previous partial meniscectomy surgery. Loss of part of the meniscus will reduce load distribution and shock absorption. This is a key risk factor in the development of osteoarthritis (OA). Being a professional cyclist will increase muscle strength and will be protective against OA. Being female and having a lack of osteoporosis are risk factors for OA. The evidence is unclear on the link between vegetarianism and OA.

6   B. No further testing is required to diagnose the patient with OA. NICE guidelines state that a patient can be diagnosed with OA without further investigation if they are 45 or over, have activity-related joint pain and have either no morning-related stiffness or morning stiffness that lasts no longer than 30 minutes.

7   A. Tramadol. This is the only weak opioid in the list. Oxycodone and hydromorphine are strong opioids. Ibuprofen and paracetamol are nonopioid analgesic options.

8   D. Aspiration of the knee joint. All acute monoarthritis is septic until proven otherwise. A diagnosis of septic arthritis is backed up by the fact that the patient is systemically unwell. The joint should be aspirated and the synovial fluid should be cultured to look for bacterial strains.

Chapter 11 Rheumatoid arthritis

1   A. Splinting. The patient is developing carpal tunnel syndrome, a recognized complication of RA. Steroids and methotrexate have no place in the treatment of this: they are disease-modifying antiinflammatory drugs. Vitamin B$_{12}$ can cause peripheral paresthesia but would not be aligned only to the median nerve and would therefore not be useful for treatment. Physiotherapy tends not to be helpful. Surgery may be a late consideration if conservative measures fail.

2   C. Start DMARDs. In the absence of other issues, methotrexate would be the drug of choice. Physiotherapy has a role to play in the management of rheumatoid arthritis but will not quickly alleviate the synovitis. MRI of the hands is unnecessary and will delay treatment. Hydrotherapy again may have a role to play, but the focus on early disease is inducing remission. NSAIDs are good for treating symptoms but do not treat the cause.

3   D. Naproxen. This is a nonsteroidal antiinflammatory drug with an associated risk of gastrointestinal bleeding. Hydroxychloroquine, methotrexate and sulfasalazine are disease-modifying antirheumatic drugs used to treat rheumatoid arthritis, while paracetamol is an analgesic used for pain relief. In the context of nodulosis, the patient should be warned that methotrexate might make it worse, but it would not be considered a contraindication to taking it.

4   E. HLA-DR4. Genetic variation in human leucocyte antigen DR4 appears to be the most significant in the development of rheumatoid arthritis. Therefore, taking a family history when you suspect rheumatoid arthritis is important. HLA-DQ2.5 variation is associated with the development of coeliac disease and variation in HLA-B27 is associated with the spondyloarthropathies. PALB2 variants can lead to the development of familial breast cancer and variations in the MLH1 gene are associated with Lynch syndrome and ovarian cancer.

5   C. X-ray imaging of the cervical spine. It is important to take lateral flexion X-ray images or magnetic resonance imaging of the cervical spine in patients with rheumatoid arthritis requiring general anaesthesia due to the associated risk of atlantoaxial subluxation. The anaesthetist must be aware of neck instability so that precautions can be taken during intubation.

6   A. A 10-year history of methotrexate usage. Methotrexate decreases folate levels in the body, thereby leading to a macrocytic anaemia. Hashimoto thyroiditis may also lead to a macrocytic anaemia but given that the patient showed no obvious signs of hypothyroidism, this is less likely. NSAID usage may cause gastric bleeding and iron-deficiency anaemia but this will lead to a microcytic anaemia. Heavy menstrual periods are a common cause of iron-deficiency anaemia but again, this is a microcytic anaemia and at the age of 60 it is unlikely that the patient still has menstrual periods. Anaemia of chronic disease will cause a microcytic or normocytic anaemia.

7   E. B cells. Rituximab is a biological therapy that is targeted against B cells. Ustekinumab is a biological therapy used in psoriatic arthritis that targets IL-23. Tocilizumab and sarilumab block IL-6 and JAK inhibitors such as Upadacitinib target the Janus kinase family of enzymes. Etanercept, infliximab and adalimumab target TNF-α.

8   D. Check HIV, tuberculosis, varicella and hepatitis status. Biological therapies cause immunosuppression and carry an increased risk of infection. Starting these drugs may reactive a dormant condition. Rituximab is the first-line biological therapy and should be coprescribed with methotrexate. Biological therapies can also increase the risk of haematological malignancies and this risk should be communicated to the patient. Hydroxychloroquine is a DMARD that carries a risk of retinal damage.

Chapter 12 Spondyloarthropathies

1 A. *Haemophilus influenzae*. This is a respiratory pathogen. The man has reactive arthritis, which is associated with gut infections and sexually transmitted infections.

2 B. Corticosteroids. These will act fast to settle both the bowel and joint symptoms. They can be given systemically or via rectal foam in the first instance. NSAIDs often aggravate gastrointestinal symptoms. Panproctocolectomy is the surgery of last choice in patients with IBD who fail with medical management. Biological specimens are useful but are not indicated first-line in the absence of severe disease; they are very useful in axial disease involvement. Sulfasalazine is commonly used as maintenance therapy in inflammatory bowel disease and enteropathic arthritis, but steroids are more appropriate acutely to induce remission.

3 C. Onycholysis. This occurs in psoriatic arthritis. Keratoderma blennorrhagica is associated with reactive arthritis. Koilonychia (spoon-shaped nails) is associated with iron-deficiency anaemia. Leuconychia is a generally benign condition of white marks on the nail due to trauma or injury to the growing nail. Paronychia is an infection of the skin adjacent to the nail.

4 D. Anticardiolipin antibody. This is associated with connective tissue disease and antiphospholipid syndrome. Ankylosing spondylitis is a seronegative spondyloarthropathy. The other four are the four As associated with ankylosing spondylitis.

5 E. Ankylosing spondylitis. 90% of patients are HLA-B27 positive. Around 60% to 80% of patients with psoriatic and reactive arthritis are positive. 60% for enteropathic arthritis and 25% for undifferentiated spondyloarthritis.

6 C. The patient is 30 years old or older. Ankylosing spondylitis normally develops in the teenage years and in early adulthood with a peak age of onset in the mid-20s but, still affecting patients into their 30s. It is very unusual for patients to present with ankylosing spondylitis over the age of 45. The remaining options are key features that clinicians should be aware of when ankylosing spondylitis is suspected.

7 A. BASMI. This is the Bath AS Metrology index that is used to assess spinal mobility in patients with ankylosing spondylitis. The Bath AS functional index (BASFI) score is also used in patients with ankylosing spondylitis but assesses how the disease affects daily life. The CHA_2DS_2-VASc score assesses the risk of stroke in patients diagnosed with atrial fibrillation. The PEST Questionnaire is a screening tool to detect psoriatic arthritis in patients with psoriasis. The DAS 28 score is used to determine the severity of rheumatoid arthritis.

8 D. Arthritis mutilans. This is a rapid, extremely destructive pattern of psoriatic arthritis seen in the hands and feet. A key feature is the 'pencil-in-cup' deformity visualized on X-ray imaging. Thankfully, it is rare. Reactive arthritis is preceded by infection and permanent joint damage is rare. Symmetrical polyarthritis is often indistinguishable from rheumatoid arthritis and asymmetrical oligoarthritis describes pathology in very few joints. Enteropathic arthritis would occur in conjunction with inflammatory bowel disease.

9 B. Ustekinumab. This is an anti IL23 therapy that is used as a last-line treatment in psoriatic arthritis. Infliximab targets TNF-α, tocilizumab targets IL6 and rituximab targets B cells. Methotrexate has an antiinflammatory effect by altering folate metabolism.

Chapter 13 Connective tissue diseases

1 B. Systemic sclerosis. This patient has evidence of widespread multisystem sclerosis and fibrosis with pulmonary hypertension, pulmonary fibrosis, Raynaud phenomenon, scleroderma and calcinosis in the hands and telangiectasia. Linear scleroderma is a limited cutaneous pattern of the disease. SLE presents differently and would not give calcinosis. Paraneoplastic syndrome is generally associated with few signs and would not give pulmonary fibrosis. Multiple sclerosis is a neurological disorder characterized by progressive weakness and spasticity.

2 C. Schirmer test. This test is used in the diagnosis of Sjögren syndrome. An HIV test is a reasonable second-line test if no cause is found for these symptoms. Schober test measures lumbar spine mobility. Transoesophageal echography is used to exclude valvular lesions such as endocarditis. Trendelenburg test is used to assess hip muscle weakness.

3 E. Serum creatine kinase levels. Dermatomyositis will produce inflamed muscles, which leak enzymes due to oedema in the cells. Elevated creatine kinase levels are seen, usually several orders of magnitude compared with normal. ESR may be elevated but is nonspecific and positive antinuclear antibodies are seen in many connective tissue diseases. Chest X-ray examination should be performed to exclude malignancy but is not diagnostic of dermatomyositis and X-ray examination of the affected joints does not normally reveal erosions.

4 A. Antiphospholipid antibody. A stillbirth and two vascular events suggest antiphospholipid syndrome, which is also associated with levido, migraines, low platelets and systemic lupus erythematosus. Other antibodies should be checked given the association, but the primary antiphospholipid syndrome must be confirmed. A prothrombin time may be checked after thrombolysis to

monitor coagulation but is nondiagnostic. Syphilis serology is occasionally checked in unusual cases of thrombosis and arteritis but is a very unlikely cause.

5   E. Eosinophilia. Haematological features of severe SLE may include lymphopenia, neutropenia and a normocytic anaemia of chronic disease. Raised AST and ALT may reflect liver damage due to lupus hepatitis. ST-segment elevation may be seen on electrocardiogram due to serositis. Heavy proteinuria will occur in nephrotic syndrome due to glomerulonephritis caused by SLE.

6   A. Calcinosis, Raynaud phenomenon, oesophageal disease, sclerodactyly, telangiectasia (CREST syndrome). Limited disease in systemic sclerosis or scleroderma makes up around 70% of cases. Involvement of the internal organs is less common.

7   C. Systemic sclerosis. This scenario illustrates a systemic sclerosis or scleroderma renal crisis. This is a life-threatening medical emergency characterized by renal failure associated with severe hypertension. It tends to occur in patients with diffuse cutaneous disease within the first 5 years of diagnosis. Patients present with headaches, blurred vision and sometimes seizures. Mortality is high and rapid treatment is essential.

8   E. Sarcoidosis. Sarcoidosis is a multisystem disease that mainly affects the lungs and intrathoracic lymph nodes. However, it can also cause arthralgia, erythema nodosum, heart block, optic neuritis, kidney stone formation and other constitutional symptoms. Granuloma formation is the key feature of sarcoidosis and therefore, a lung biopsy is the gold standard diagnostic procedure for sarcoidosis. A chest X-ray will also show hilar lymphadenopathy.

Chapter 14 The vasculitides

1   A. Temporal artery biopsy. This is the gold standard test for giant cell arteritis. ESR should be elevated but this is nonspecific. ANCA screening is likely to be negative Ultrasound scans are becoming an effective way of diagnosing giant call arteritis. They may become the most useful form of investigation in the future in centers with experienced operators. MRI of the aortic arch is a sensitive test for aortic vasculitis, but there is no guarantee that any lesions would be visible.

2   D. Administer prednisolone. This woman has polymyalgia rheumatica with features of giant cell arteritis. It requires urgent treatment to preserve vision and reduce the risk of stroke. Checking ESR is an important part of diagnosis, as is arranging a temporal artery biopsy, but it should not obstruct treatment. Muscle biopsy is not required in this scenario. Nonsteroidal antiinflammatory drugs are good for treating the symptoms of inflammation but will not alter the disease process.

3   A. Granulomatosis with polyangiitis (formerly Wegener granulomatosis). This condition is strongly linked to the presence of PR3 ANCA and affects multiple body systems, particularly the lungs and kidneys. Giant cell arteritis is associated with polymyalgia rheumatica and characteristically presents with a temporal, unilateral headache that shows poor improvement with analgesia. Polyarteritis nodosa causes aneurysm formation and presents with skin ulceration. Eosinophilic granulomatosis with polyangiitis is strongly linked with myeloperoxidase (MPO) ANCA. The classic symptoms of Behçet disease are oral and genital ulceration.

4   B. Give IV hydrocortisone and saline. The presentation of acute dehydration and hypotension is seen in an adrenal crisis. An adrenal crisis most commonly occurs due to secondary adrenal insufficiency. When a patient takes prescribed steroids for a long period of time, the body stops production of endogenous steroids and the patient is reliant on prescribed steroids. Immediate cessation of prescribed steroids would result in an adrenal crisis. This is a life-threatening medical emergency that must be treated with prompt corticosteroid replacement (hydrocortisone) and IV fluids. Fludrocortisone release is maintained in secondary adrenal insufficiency as it is controlled by the renin-angiotensin-aldosterone system.

5   E. Intravenous immunoglobulins and low-dose aspirin. This presentation describes Kawasaki disease (also known as mucocutaneous lymph node syndrome). This disease normally affects children under the age of 5 and presents with a persistent high fever and a vasculitis rash. Key features of the disease are the strawberry tongue appearance, cervical lymphadenopathy and desquamation of the skin on the hands and feet.

6   C. Streptococcus throat infection. This presentation is characteristic of Henoch-Schonlein purpura. This is a form of vasculitis that normally presents in children and adolescents with a purpuric rash across the legs and buttocks, abdominal pains, asymmetrical arthritis and self-limiting glomerulonephritis. It is strongly associated with IgA deposition and is normally precipitated by a streptococcus throat infection (i.e., tonsilitis, usually group A β-haemolytic).

7   A. Eosinophils. This presentation of weight loss, night sweats, diarrhoea and atopy with allergic rhinitis is characteristic of eosinophilic granulomatosis (formerly Churg Strauss syndrome). The eosinophilic stage of the disease will show high eosinophil levels in peripheral blood samples. This condition is also strongly linked to the presence of MPO ANCA.

Chapter 15 Metabolic bone disease

1 A. Osteoporosis. Vertebral height loss, back pain from a probable vertebral fracture and previous history of low-energy fracture all suggest osteoporosis. Myeloma would cause back pain for weeks or months, hypercalcaemia and weight loss. Osteomalacia is a disorder of low vitamin D levels. It results in low calcium levels/low phosphate and raised alkaline phosphatase. Paget disease would cause an elevated alkaline phosphatase level and is not associated with vertebral height loss. Potts disease is very rare and is associated with systemic upsets including weight loss, night sweats and unexplained persistent pyrexia.

2 B. Bone biochemistry. The patient has Paget disease of bone and this simple blood test will show an elevated alkaline phosphatase level. Coeliac serology should be tested if vitamin D deficiency is thought to be the cause. DEXA is used for diagnosing osteoporosis. MRI would give the diagnosis but is costly and will take time to organize. Isotope bone scanning is therefore the imaging modality of choice. Rheumatoid factor will not help in this diagnosis

3 C. Polydipsia. The patient has renal osteomalacia where vitamin D fails to be metabolized into the active form by chronically failing kidneys. Polydipsia is a commonly seen symptom in hypercalcaemia but is not associated with low calcium or low phosphate levels. The other features are all possible.

4 D. Paget disease. Back pain, knee pain with increased blood flow and high levels of alkaline phosphatase suggest this. Osteoarthritis should not cause an increase in ALP. A prolapsed disc may explain her back pain but not the biochemical changes of the knee warmth. Septic arthritis rarely involves so many joints in a patient who seems otherwise well. Gout would again not explain the biochemistry picture.

5 E. Antitissue transglutaminase antibody. Coeliac disease is a common malabsorptive cause of osteomalacia causing low levels of iron, folate, vitamin D and other essential vitamins and minerals. Anti–double-stranded DNA is found in lupus. Antiphospholipid antibodies are seen in patients with recurrent venous and arterial thrombus. Anti–smooth muscle antibody is found in lupus and autoimmune liver disease. Anti–vitamin D_3 antibodies is not a readily available test, but the picture remains more complex than straightforward osteomalacia due to isolated vitamin D deficiency.

6 E. Inhibition of osteoclast activity. Bisphosphonates are the first-line therapeutic drugs in combination with calcium supplements and vitamin D for the treatment of osteoporosis. Teriparatide is a parathyroid hormone analogue and strontium ranelate inhibits osteoclast activity

and increases osteoblast activity. Denosumab is an antibody directed at RANK ligand (a ligand produced by osteoblasts that upregulates osteoclast formation) and romosuzumab is a monoclonal antibody that inhibits sclerostin, increasing bone formation and reducing bone resorption.

7 B. Osteogenesis imperfecta. Also known as brittle bone disease, this is a genetic condition that presents as recurrent childhood fractures (without predisposing trauma), low muscle tone, varus deformity of the legs and possible blue discolouration of the sclerae. Duchenne muscular dystrophy is also a genetic childhood condition, however, this disease primarily affects the muscles. Rickets is another paediatric condition that affects the mineralization of cartilage of the epiphyseal growth plates. It too could present with a varus deformity of the legs however, other signs of rickets would be swelling of the epiphyses of the wrists and at the costochondral junctions. Both Paget disease and osteomalacia affect an adult population.

8 D. High urinary calcium excretion. Osteomalacia causes low levels of serum calcium, therefore there would be very little calcium excreted in the urine. Hypocalcemia is due to low levels of serum vitamin D. The liver is an important organ in the biological activation of vitamin D, therefore a history of liver cirrhosis will see decreased levels of active vitamin D. The low levels of calcium in the blood would trigger secondary hyperparathyroidism, explaining the raised levels of serum parathyroid hormone. Alcoholic fatty liver disease is associated with low levels of folate which would cause a macrocytic anaemia.

Chapter 16 Gout and pseudogout

1 E. Splinting. This will allow the joint time to rest and pain relief to be given. Aspiration has not grown organisms and antibiotics are therefore not required. DMARDs are not indicated in pseudogout. Joint replacement is not performed in an acute setting such as this. Physiotherapy is likely to be required, but only once the inflammation has settled.

2 D. Monosodium urate crystals. These are found in acute gout. The white lumps are tophi. Bacteria need to be excluded from an acute hot joint but the presence of tophi make septic arthritis less likely. Calcium pyrophosphate crystals occur in pseudogout, mainly seen in the elderly in knees and wrists. Pus is possible, but white tophus is more likely given the finger deposits. Clear synovial fluid is unlikely; fluid tends to be slightly cloudy when inflammation is present.

3 C. Chronic hyperuricemia. This leads to the formation of sodium urate crystals that are deposited in the synovium,

causing inflammation. This is the underlying process in gout. Chronic kidney disease often leads to asymptomatic hyperuricemia and gout develops when these crystals are deposited in tissue. The patient's history is not suggestive of rheumatoid arthritis, chronic septic arthritis, pseudogout or osteoarthritis.

4   A. Increase allopurinol to 300 mg daily. The patient's blood should be rechecked within 12 weeks and the dose increased as required to maintain serum uric acid below 360 μg/mL. There is no indication for changing to febuxostat at this time. Steroids can be useful in the acute setting but are avoided long term. Colchicine and nonsteroidal drugs such as ibuprofen are typically used for acute flares but are sometimes continued in the medium term in difficult-to-manage cases.

5   B. Methotrexate usage. Methotrexate is not a drug associated with an increased risk of gout. Although, ciclosporin which may also be used in the treatment of psoriasis is. Psoriasis is associated with metabolic syndrome which is linked to the development of gout. Male sex, a past medical history of hypertension and drinking more than the recommended weekly alcohol intake are all risk factors for gout.

6   B. Tophi were present on the Achilles tendon. The presence of tophi, recurrent gout attacks, renal impairment, uric acid renal stones and evidence of bone/joint damage are all indications for prophylactic therapy in gout. Age does not determine whether allopurinol should be prescribed, nor does the inability to prescribe NSAIDs. A podagra describes gout affecting the first metatarsophalangeal joint and pyrexia is a common feature in an acute gout attack.

7   D. Chronic pyrophosphate arthropathy. Chronic pyrophosphate arthropathy is associated with, and can present similarly to osteoarthritis with a history of gradual onset pain, swelling and loss of joint function. It is most commonly seen in elderly women and is associated with hypothyroidism. Paget disease would present as bony pain, normally affecting the spine, pelvis, femurs, skull and tibia. Osteoporosis most commonly affects postmenopausal women but is asymptomatic until a low-impact trauma fracture occurs. Fibromyalgia typically presents in middle-aged women and sees widespread pain. Rheumatoid arthritis would normally present before the age of 78 and typically affects multiple small joints of the hands and feet.

8   A. Systemic lupus erythematous. This is an autoimmune condition and is not associated with metabolic syndrome. The remaining conditions are all associated with metabolic syndrome. Metabolic syndrome describes a collection of risk factors that mostly increase the risk of cardiovascular disease and type 2 diabetes mellitus.

Chapter 17 Paediatric joint disease

1   D. Medial femoral circumflex artery. The majority of the blood supply to the femoral head in adults arises from the medial femoral circumflex artery. There is a lesser contribution from the lateral femoral circumflex artery. The artery of the ligamentum teres supplies a negligible blood supply in adults.

2   B. External rotation. The classic position for a leg to lie after SCFE is in external rotation and on flexion. This will persist due to the impingement of the displaced anterior-lateral femoral metaphysis (Drehmann sign). The hip will be painful on all movements and it is likely to have lost internal rotation, flexion and abduction.

3   A. Talipes equinovarus. This baby has a deformity that is commonly called a clubfoot. The initial treatment is a cast and then further assessment should be made if this is unsuccessful. It is likely that the foot will always appear abnormal but this often does not affect the quality of life.

4   E. Osteogenesis imperfecta. There is a chance that this child is the victim of NAI and this should be explored. However, given the scoliosis, short stature and multiple low-energy fractures, a diagnosis of osteogenesis imperfecta should be considered and investigated.

5   C. Perthes disease. This boy has findings consistent with Perthes disease on his X-ray examination. This can commonly present with knee pain. Abnormal inflammatory markers would suggest possible septic arthritis.

6   B. X-ray. A similar question was asked in Chapter 7 which asked you about the diagnosis which is DDH. This question asks of you two things, what the diagnosis is and, knowing that, how best to investigate the patient. As the patient is 13 months, an X-ray is the most appropriate initial investigation. If the child was younger (<4 months) and its hip had not started to ossify (and therefore would not be seen on X-ray), then an ultrasound would be indicated.

Chapter 18 Fractures

1   C. Compartment syndrome. The principal symptom of compartment syndrome is pain. Any patient who has a severe increase in pain following a fracture should be assessed for compartment syndrome. Proximal tibial fractures are at increased risk of developing compartment syndrome.

2   A. Pulmonary thromboembolism. Although rare, pulmonary thromboembolism is a recognized complication of arthroplasty surgery. The onset and nature of the patient's symptoms are highly suggestive of this condition.

3   C. Early mobilization. The main principle of internal fixation is to allow early mobilization.

4 C. Apply a pelvic binder. While the others are sensible options, a pelvic binder can be quickly and simply applied by anybody and should be the FIRST step taken if it has not already been done. Blood samples should also be taken.

5 A. Hemiarthroplasty. Fixation with DHS is not an option because the blood supply to the femoral head will be compromised. The patient is not fit enough for total hip replacement. Girdlestone is a complete disarticulation of the hip and is a last resort if all other options have failed. Conservative treatment in a previously mobile patient would be a poor option, committing her to several months of pain and immobility.

6 C. A pathological fracture. This is a fracture of abnormal bone. The history alone is suspicious of this with clinical features pointing towards a lung primary with metastasis to his femur. The lesion was initially only causing pain, but now has weakened to the bone to such a degree that it broke with only the minimal force generated by walking. Other primary malignancies that metastasize to bone are thyroid, kidney, breast and prostate.

7 E. All of the above. As per the British Orthopaedic Association Standards for Trauma, all of the steps mentioned must be carried out for open fractures. This patient needs an urgent washout and debridement of her wound, stabilization of her fracture and antibiotics to help prevent osteomyelitis.

8 D. Open reduction and internal fixation. This fracture needs to be reduced anatomically to give the patient the best chance at retaining good function in their wrist. This needs to be done open with internal fixation to hold the reduction. Anatomical reduction cannot be achieved by a wrist splint, by casting or by external fixation.

Chapter 19 Trauma

1 E. Assess the airway while stabilizing the cervical spine. In the assessment of any trauma patients, follow the ABCDE pathway and assess systems in order of importance. Do not become distracted by the perceived main issue. All patients should be assumed to have a cervical spine injury until proven otherwise.

2 B. They are likely to have lost 15% to 30% of blood volume. Their blood pressure has fallen in response to volume depletion and their pulse rate has gone up in order to attempt to maintain perfusion of end organs.

3 D. A CT scan should be obtained of the head and C-spine. It is likely this patient also has an intracranial abnormality. If the patient already needs to undergo a CT scan and has symptoms, C-spine X-ray examination will be an extra, unhelpful step. While an MRI is informative, it is difficult to obtain in an emergency situation, unlike a CT scan.

4 C. Insertion of a wide bore cannula into his left 2nd intercostal space. This man is suffering a tension pneumothorax. This can occur after trauma, creating a one-way valve in the lung or chest wall. This means that air flows into the chest cavity, but not out again, which collapses the lung, causing hypoxia. The mediastinum is displaced to one side, which reduces venous return to the heart and therefore cardiac output. The patient therefore becomes hypotensive. This is life-threatening and requires immediate decompression with a large-bore needle (before chest X-ray), followed by insertion of a chest drain.

5 B. Pelvic fracture. The mechanism here suggests that this man has had a heavy crush injury to his pelvis. Venous bleeding can be massive with pelvic fractures and can be fatal. The man's hypotension and tachycardia are signs of hypovolaemic shock. Associated bladder and urethral injuries are not uncommon and this man may have either a ruptured bladder or a urethral tear, which would explain the blood at his urethral meatus and his inability to pass urine. He should have a retrograde urethrogram before attempted catheterization.

6 D. Traumatic cauda equina syndrome. This is a high-energy injury and the clinical examination findings point towards a diagnosis of a traumatic cauda equina syndrome. This is likely due to a lumbar fracture and she may have an associated pelvic fracture, but the most concerning thing here which needs immediate attention, is the traumatic cauda equina syndrome.

Chapter 20 Infection of bones and joints

1 C. *Staphylococcus aureus*. *S. aureus* is the most common pathogen in septic arthritis in adults, followed by *Streptococcus* and *Enterobacter*. *S. aureus* is the most common pathogen in all ages.

2 C. Aspiration of the knee. This man has septic arthritis until proven otherwise. It is important that this is confirmed via joint aspiration as soon as possible. X-ray examination and blood tests can be performed first, but joint aspiration is the most important investigation. When possible, antibiotics should be withheld until after joint aspiration has been performed.

3 E. Prepatellar bursitis. Prepatellar bursitis is common in patients who kneel when working (e.g., electricians, plumbers). This patient's signs and symptoms suggest an obvious bursitis and do not highlight an intraarticular pathology.

4 E. All of the above. Intravenous drug abusers inject themselves with potentially contaminated drugs through a dirty needle. They are also frequently immunosuppressed and undernourished; consequently,

they are at risk of a wide range of infections. As a result, they will require a broad range of antibiotics to cover potential pathogens.

5   A. Anaerobic bacteria. This man has an open fracture that is potentially contaminated by cattle manure, among other things. Anaerobic bacteria and *Clostridium perfringens* (gas gangrene) infections are important to consider here based on the history. The fracture site should be irrigated and debrided urgently in theatre. Heavily soiled wounds should be covered with high-dose intravenous antibiotics, including an intravenous cephalosporin, penicillin and metronidazole. Tetanus prophylaxis should be given if vaccinations are not up to date.

6   D. *Mycobacterium tuberculosis.* Living in India for a number of years may have exposed this woman to tuberculosis, which has remained dormant for many years. This has now become activated, however, and caused collapse of one of her thoracic vertebral bodies, resulting in a gibbus (sharp angulated kyphosis). She will need an MRI scan and then biopsy of the lesion to confirm the diagnosis.

Chapter 21 Malignancy

1   B. Osteoid osteoma. Osteoid osteoma presents insidiously, giving rise to intense pain and tenderness over the affected area, sometimes with a history of night pain. A central lucent nidus surrounded by a dense area of reactive bone will be seen on X-ray image. Salicylates greatly reduce the pain.

2   B. Osteosarcoma. Osteosarcoma is most common between the ages of 10 and 40 years and frequently occurs around the knee. The symptoms of night pain and weight loss are suspicious of malignancy. The X-ray findings are typical of osteosarcoma.

3   A. Prostate cancer. The finding of a sclerotic lesion makes prostate cancer the most likely cause for this metastatic deposit. Prostate cancer often metastasizes to the spine due to the venous drainage connection.

4   D. Periosteal reaction. This is the Codman triangle appearance on an X-ray image whereby, in aggressive lesions, the cortex does not have time to remodel and there is a raised multilayered edge of periosteum. Looser zones are present in osteomalacia, vertebral trabecular thickening is seen in Paget disease and the other changes are in keeping with osteoarthritis.

5   C. Protein electrophoresis. The fracture under normal loads should raise suspicion and the X-ray features (those of multiple lytic lesions in the skull) are typical of myeloma, as is the high ESR. Out of the available answers, protein electrophoresis, of serum and urine, will diagnose myeloma.

6   D. Breast metastasis. You were not told that she had a breast lump, however she has a malignant spinal lesion causing acute spinal cord compression. The normal investigations exclude all the other potential sources of primary malignancy (except bowel carcinoma, but this rarely metastasizes to the spin), leaving breast carcinoma as the most likely.

Chapter 22 Sports injuries

1   A. Bucket handle meniscal tear. The handle part of a bucket handle tears and flips over, becoming trapped in the joint and preventing full extension.

2   E. Anterior cruciate ligament tear. An anterior cruciate ligament tear is normally caused by a twisting injury to the knee. Patients will describe immediate pain and rapid swelling. Examination will reveal a large effusion, due to the haemarthrosis, and laxity in the AP axis. Lachman test and anterior drawer test are used for diagnosis.

3   D. The majority of dislocations come out anterior inferior due to the weakness of the muscle cover in this position.

4   D. Hypoplastic trochlea. A shallow trochlea will increase the risk of patellar dislocation, which is particularly common in young women and can be difficult to treat.

5   MRI of the ankle. From the history this patient likely has an ankle ligament injury which will show up on MRI better than any of the other imaging modalities listed.

6   ACL reconstruction. This professional sportswoman will benefit from an ACL reconstruction, which will lower the risk of future meniscal or chondral injury. Grafts can be a bone-patella-bone or hamstring autograft or a cadaveric allograft.

Chapter 23 Soft tissue disorders

1   B. Abductor pollicis longus. De Quervain tenosynovitis is inflammation of the tendon sheaths of abductor pollicis longus and extensor pollicis brevis.

2   A. This is olecranon bursitis and should initially be treated with a period of rest and NSAIDs.

3   B. almar fascia. Dupuytren contracture is a disease in which palmar fascia undergoes fibrosis and contracture.

4   D. Below knee plaster cast in equinus. This man has suffered an Achilles tendon rupture. While surgery is an option, in the first instance, conservative management in an equinus cast or in a walking boot with heel wedge raises, avoids the complications associated with surgery. Professional athletes and patients who present with a delayed presentation may be offered surgical repair.

5   D. Surgical excision of the bursa. The patient has chronic bursitis which will not get better without excision of the sinus tract.

Chapter 24 Principles of orthopaedic surgery

1   B. Hypovolaemia. The patient is likely to be still very hypovolaemic postoperatively. This should be corrected but not too aggressively in an older patient.

2   A. Hip dislocation. Given the patient's history, he is most likely to have suffered a dislocation of his hip replacement. This normally happens with a low-impact mechanism; a periprosthetic fracture would usually require more force.

3   B. Admission, observation and aspiration in theatre. This is a problem frequently encountered on the orthopaedic ward. If the patient is well, antibiotics should be withheld until samples have been taken. Immediate single-stage revision would be unwise in the presence of likely infection. A bone scan would add little as infection is extremely likely with this history. This patient clearly requires investigation and should not be discharged.

4   E. Pulmonary embolus. This overweight gentleman is in the immediate postop phase and so is at an increased risk of venous thromboembolus on at least two accounts.

5   E. All of the above. The preassessment appointment is a very important point in the patient journey to make sure the patient's surgery can go ahead in the safest way possible.

OSCEs and Short Clinical Cases

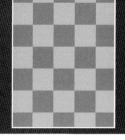

OSCE 1 – A hot swollen knee

Mr Smith has presented with a hot, painful, swollen knee. Please take a history from him.

Checklist

- Introduce yourself and check the patient's details. The demographics of the patient can be important in determining a likely cause.
- Use the SOCRATES method to elicit the history of the pain the patient has been experiencing – site, onset, character, radiation, associated features, timing, exacerbating/ relieving factors and severity.
- Establish whether the patient is ill, or has features in keeping with a systemic upset.
- Ask about previous episodes, and what the patient was doing prior to this current episode.
- Explore the patient's past medical history; is there anything to suggest autoimmune conditions, chronic kidney disease or immunocompromised?
- A drug history can be important, particularly if the patient is on anticoagulants or diuretics. Always ask if the patient has any allergies.
- Take a social history and explore and functional limitations that the patient has. Sexual history is important in considering reactive causes.
- Ask about family history, including any HLA B27-associated diseases.
- Give the patient time to explore their ideas, concerns and expectations.
- Summarize the findings of your history taking, give the patient a final opportunity to offer additional information ('*is there anything else you would like to tell me?*'), and report your findings to the examiner with a sensible differential.

Questions for reflection

1. What are the possible causes of an acute monoarthritis of the knee?
   - Septic arthritis
   - Crystal arthropathy – gout or pseudo-gout
   - Inflammatory arthritis (reactive arthritis, rheumatoid or a seronegative spondyloarthropathy)
   - Transient synovitis
   - Haemarthrosis
2. What is your gold standard test of choice in establishing the diagnosis?
   - Joint aspiration with fluid sent for microscopy, culture and crystal microscopy.

3. What may his blood tests show?
   - Inflammatory markers (CRP and ESR) may be generally raised, but are nonspecific, as is a transient rise in white cell count.
   - Urate may be raised in gout, though it can be normal during acute attacks.
   - Patients on warfarin can have spontaneous bleeds when their INR is raised.
   - Procalcitonin is a very useful test in differentiating between bacterial sepsis and inflammation; it is raised in the former.
4. What antibiotics would you consider using in septic arthritis?
   - *Staphylococcus* and *Streptococcus* species are the most common causes of septic arthritis; therefore treatment is usually with flucloxacillin and benzylpenicillin. If gram-negative organisms are being considered then gentamycin is usually added.

OSCE 2 – Painful, stiff, swollen hands

Mrs Martin, a 37-year-old woman, has painful, stiff hands. Examine them.

Checklist

- Remember to ensure the patient is comfortable and well exposed. Ensure the patient's upper limbs are visible to the elbows. Warn the patient before touching them or moving their joints.
- **Look:** check for skin conditions such as psoriasis, rheumatoid nodules and tight skin. Observe if there are any scars present. Check the nails for onycholysis and splinter haemorrhages. Look for deformity, swelling and erythema over the joints. Check both sides of the hands – is there evidence of muscle wasting?
- **Feel:** palpate each joint systemically for the boggy/spongy feeling of synovitis. Bony overgrowth (osteophytes) feel hard. Use a bimanual approach. Feel the tendons for thickening. Check sensation in the medial, ulnar and radial nerve distribution.
- **Move:** move the joints actively and passively assessing for any impedance or loss of function. The 'prayer' sign is useful when assessing hand and wrist function, as is the simple task of making a fist. Straighten the fingers against resistance and abduct the fingers. Use functional tests such as holding paper to check interossei function or abduction of the thumb to check medial nerve innervation.
- **Special tests:** Tinel and Phalen tests should be performed in patients who have symptoms of carpal tunnel.

257

- Offer to examine the joint above (wrist), and to check the neurovascular integrity of the limb.
- Present your positive findings to the examiner and offer a differential diagnosis.

Questions for reflection

1. What are the classical patterns of joint swelling in the hands?
   - Rheumatoid arthritis; typically affects the PIP/MCP joints in a symmetrical fashion. Late complications include boutonnière and swan-neck deformities with ulnar deviation and Z-thumb.
   - Psoriatic arthritis; PIP and DIP joint swelling with associated nail changes and skin lesions.
   - Osteoarthritis; hard, bony DIP and PIP swelling (Heberden and Bouchard nodes) with CMC pain and a lack of inflammatory features.
2. What X-ray findings might you find in a patient with rheumatoid arthritis?
   - Soft tissue swelling
   - Juxta-articular osteoporosis
   - Joint space narrowing – usually symmetrical and concentric
   - Marginal erosions
3. What drugs are used in the management of rheumatoid arthritis?
   - Synthetic DMARDs – hydroxychloroquine, sulphasalazine, methotrexate and leflunomide
   - Corticosteroids
   - NSAIDs
   - Biologic DMARDs
4. What are the extraarticular features of rheumatoid arthritis?
   - Eyes – keratoconjunctivitis, episcleritis and scleritis
   - Lungs – pleural effusions, pulmonary fibrosis
   - Skin – rheumatoid nodules, vasculitis
   - Neurology – peripheral neuropathy
   - Renal – amyloidosis
   - Heart – pericarditis, myocarditis, accelerated coronary artery disease
   - Spleen – Felty syndrome
5. What antibodies can be used in establishing a diagnosis of rheumatoid arthritis?
   - Rheumatoid factor – present in at least 5% of the health population, 70% of RA patients
   - Anticyclical citrullinated peptide (anti-CCP) – more specific for RA, sensitivity similar to RF

OSCE 3 – Treatment of giant-cell arteritis

Mr Jones, a 78-year-old man, has been diagnosed with giant-cell arteritis. Discuss treatment for this condition with him.

Checklist

- Introduce yourself and check the patient's details.
- Establish the patient's baseline level of knowledge on the condition. Ask '*what have you been told so far?*'.
- Explain in simple terms the aetiology of the condition, for example, talking about '*swelling of the blood vessels in the neck and head*', causing headache, blurred vision and pain on chewing.
- Ask if the patient has received any treatment so far.
- Discuss with the patient the reason for giving high doses of steroids – these reduce the swelling in the vessels.
- Explain the treatment regimen – many patients take a long time to wean off steroids (18–36 months). The steroid dose will be reduced gradually.
- Discuss monitoring measures; inflammatory markers will be checked regularly to ensure treatment response/ monitor for relapse.
- Inform the patient of potential complications – impaired glucose tolerance, osteoporosis and discuss how these will be managed (baseline DEXA +/– bisphosphonates and calcium supplement; oral glucose tolerance test).
- Give the patient ample opportunity to raise concerns, question the plan and ask for clarity on specific points. Explore their ideas, concerns and expectations.
- Summarize your consultation, asking the patient to repeat back to you the information they have retained, and use this opportunity to reinforce any gaps in knowledge/ understanding.

Questions for reflection

1. What are the diagnostic criteria for giant-cell arteritis?

   For diagnostic purposes, at least 3 of the 5 following criteria should be met:
   - Age at onset >50 years
   - New headache
   - Temporal artery abnormality (beading, nonpulsatile, etc.)
   - Elevated ESR >50 mm/h
   - Abnormal artery histology from biopsy
2. What does a 'positive' biopsy show?
   - Infiltration of the artery wall by mononuclear cells, or granulomatous inflammation, usually with multinucleated giant cells.
3. What is a typical 'starting' dose of steroids?
   - Usually steroids are started at 60 mg prednisolone OD and are reduced on a fortnightly basis by 10 mg until reaching a level of 20 mg. Reduction from this level is normally slower. If blurred vision/jaw claudication is present initial treatment is often with IV methylprednisolone.
4. Are there any additional medications you should consider using?

- Low-dose aspirin is indicated to reduce the risk of thrombotic events.
5. If the patient relapses multiple times are there any additional measures you would consider?
   - Adding a steroid-sparing agent, such as methotrexate, is indicated in the situation of multiple relapses or difficulty in weaning steroids.

OSCE 4 – Back stiffness

Mr Smith has been referred with back pain and stiffness. Examine his spine.

Checklist

- Ensure the patient is fully exposed. For this examination, they should be wearing an open gown, or just their underwear. Introduce yourself and check the patient's details. Informed consent and use of a chaperone are very important in this situation.
- Remember that movement of an acutely tender back can be extremely painful. Ask the patient beforehand if any specific regions are tender.
- **Look:** assess the patient's posture, noting cervical lordosis, thoracic kyphosis or lumbar lordosis. If the patient has sciatica they are often stooped, or the affected leg is lifted and flexed. Muscle wasting, asymmetry and scoliosis are often present. Note any scars.
- **Feel:** palpation is best performed with the patient standing. Start by palpating down the bony midline, then the paraspinal muscles and finally the sacroiliac joints.
- **Move:** this should be broken down into specific areas of the spine:
  I. Cervical spine: check flexion, extension, lateral flexion and rotation.
  II. Thoracolumbar spine: flexion (mark two points on the spine and observe the change in distance between them, noting reduced flexion). Extension, rotation and lateral flexion should also be checked.
- **Special tests:** straight-leg raise – this is done to identify nerve root irritation.
- Offer to examine the peripheral joints if symptoms are present. Also note any additional areas you may wish to examine (skin for rashes, GI system for evidence of IBD) if appropriate.

Questions for reflection

1. What are the extra-axial features of ankylosing spondylitis?
   - Acute anterior uveitis
   - Aortic incompetence
   - Apical lung fibrosis
   - Amyloidosis

   These are commonly referred to as the 4-As of AS.
2. What human leucocyte antigen is implicated in AS?

- HLA-B27 (92% of cases are HLA-B27 positive)
3. What might you expect to find on a plain radiograph of the patient's lumbosacral spine?
   - Sacroiliitis may be present.
   - Syndesmophyte formation is a commonly found sign in patients with advanced AS.
   - Occasionally 'bamboo' spine is still seen.
4. What treatment options are available?
   - Physiotherapy is an important part of the management of AS.
   - NSAIDs are used as initial therapy and help to reduce pain and stiffness.
   - Biologics such as TNF-inhibitors and anti-IL-17a.

OSCE 5 – Hip pain

Mrs Todd is a 72-year-old woman with a history of hip pain. Take a history.

Checklist

- Introduce yourself and check the patient's details.
- Approach the case using the SOCRATES model. Site is particularly important when exploring the hip – many patients talk about 'hip pain' but actual mean pain over the greater trochanter. Onset is important as duration of symptoms can reveal a lot about potential pathology. Is the pain sharp or dull? Is their radiation, and if so does it follow a neuropathic route? Are their associated features, or a specific time of the day it comes on (morning/rest pain is more indicative of inflammatory pain, evening/postactivity pain is more likely to relate to degenerative joint disease)? Exacerbating and relieving factors should be discussed as should severity of pain.
- Ask about stiffness, grinding/clicking and systemic features.
- Discuss the patient's past medical history. Are there conditions that would suggest an underlying inflammatory cause?
- Examine the patient's medication use. What is being used for analgesia? Is there a history of allergy?
- When considering social history, ask about occupation, functional status and social support. How have they been managing with tasks of daily living recently?
- What are the patient's concerns, ideas and expectations; give them time to explore these during the consultation.

Questions for reflection

1. What are the cardinal X-ray features of osteoarthritis?
   - Joint space narrowing
   - Sclerosis
   - Cyst formation
   - Osteophyte formation
2. What are the primary and secondary causes of OA?

- **Primary:** increasing age, obesity, family history, female gender.
- **Secondary:** preexisting joint damage, systemic diseases (haemophilia, neuropathy, etc.), metabolic causes (chondrocalcinosis, acromegaly).

3. What are the management options available?
   - Conservative – physiotherapy, analgesia, weight loss, walking aids.
   - Invasive – intraarticular joint injections, joint replacement surgery.
4. What are the risks involved in total-hip replacement?
   - Thromboembolic disease
   - Infections
   - Fracture
   - Dislocation
   - Change in limb length
   - Loosening of implant
5. What measures are taken to reduce the risk of blood clots post surgery?
   - Mechanical antithrombotic measures (antiembolic stockings)
   - Anticoagulant medication (low-molecular-weight heparin), continued for 4 to 5 weeks post surgery.

OSCE 6 – Hand pain

Mrs Allen is a 42-year-old woman with a history of hand pain, worse at night. Examine the hands.

Checklist

- Introduce yourself to the patient, check their details and ensure they are exposed to at least the elbow on either side.
- The history here offers some clue as to the diagnosis, night pain is a particular feature of a relatively small number of conditions.
- **Look:** inspect the hands with the patient resting comfortably. Check for skin conditions, nail changes, joint swelling, deformity or the presence of scars. Pay particular attention to the presence of any muscle wasting in the hand, and ensure you examine the palmar surface for this.
- **Feel:** palpate the joints in a systematic fashion using a bimanual approach. Feel for the difference between bony nodularity and synovial swelling. Assess if there is any warmth or tenderness. Examine for sensory disturbance in the distribution of the medial, ulnar and radial nerves.
- **Move:** assess the function of the hand by systematically moving through the particular motions of the hand joints. Check movement actively and passively and note any resistance, pain, weakness and fixed deformity. Ask about activities of daily living, such as picking up small objects and fastening buttons/buckles, etc.

- **Special tests:** Tinel and Phalens test should be performed in patients with symptoms suggestive of carpal tunnel syndrome.

Questions for reflection

1. What is the distribution of sensory impairment in carpal tunnel syndrome?
   - Sensation is affected over the thumb, index, middle and lateral side of the ring finger on the affected side.
2. Which conditions predispose to carpal tunnel syndrome?
   - Diabetes
   - Hypothyroidism
   - Rheumatoid arthritis
   - Acromegaly
   - Pregnancy
   - Trauma (wrist fracture)
3. What investigations may be undertaken to establish/confirm the diagnosis?
   - Nerve conduction studies show reduced nerve condition velocities at the wrist and can often grade the neuropathy as mild/moderate/severe.
4. How is carpal tunnel syndrome managed?
   - **Conservative:** lifestyle modification (avoiding repetitive tasks, weight loss), wrist splinting, physiotherapy, analgesia.
   - **Invasive:** corticosteroid injections, decompression surgery.
5. What is the recurrence rate of carpal tunnel syndrome?
   - Literature suggests up to 25% of patients have had recurrent symptoms even after decompression.

OSCE 7 – X-ray of a painful knee

Mrs Buxton is a 73-year-old woman with a painful knee. Her GP suspects she has osteoarthritis. Review the X-ray.

Checklist

- Confirm the patient details, the correct image and the orientation of the film.
- Demonstrate a systematic approach to examining the film.
- Your opening statement should sound like this; *'This is a plain knee radiograph of Mrs Buxton taken on [date] at [time]. It is an AP and lateral image, and I note the side marker is correct…'*
- Comment on the image quality, *'The image is of adequate quality'*, unless it clearly is not.
- Next move onto the obvious abnormalities; for osteoarthritis, it may include the following, *'The radiograph shows loss of joint space, with subchondral sclerosis, marginal osteophytes and cyst formation.'*
- If you are unable to see any abnormalities then say so, but demonstrate your systematic approach to image review by talking through your examination of the anatomy of the knee.

- If you are unsure if something is normal or abnormal describe it equivocally and offer a potential explanation.
- Summarize by revisiting your findings; '*In conclusion this image shows multiple radiological features in keeping with a diagnosis of osteoarthritis*'.

Questions for reflection

1. What is the underlying pathological process in OA?
   - Biomechanical forces causing abnormal stress on articular cartilage are thought to interact with biochemical and genetic factors leading to degradation in articular cartilage. A mismatch between cartilage breakdown and repair occurs resulting in progressive loss of the protective articular cartilage eventually leading to bony destruction.
2. What are the surgical options for dealing with OA?
   - Arthroscopy; a thin tube with a camera is inserted into the knee joint to inspect the interior articular surface. If damaged, the operator can remove the damaged cartilage, or floating pieces of bone/cartilage can be removed to improve pain.
   - Knee replacement; this involves removing part or all of the knee joint and replacing it with a prosthetic joint.
3. How long does a knee replacement last?
   - For newer knee replacements, the lifespan of the joint is around 20 years. Around 1/10 need replacing after 10 years.
4. What medications would you consider using in someone with OA?
   - NSAIDs can be useful for pain and swelling.
   - Stronger analgesia (opiates are often used in severe OA).
   - Intra-articular steroid injections can offer relief to patients reluctant to have surgery, or in whom the risk of an anaesthetic is high, but evidence is increasing that this is a poorly effective treatment.

OSCE 8 – A stiff shoulder

Mr Phillips has come to see you with a stiff shoulder. Examine the joint.

Checklist

- Introduce yourself to the patient, check their details and ensure adequate exposure (in this case the gentleman should be bare above the waist).
- **Look:** Inspect the shoulders, back and upper limbs for any evidence of asymmetry. Examine from the front, back and side. Swelling of the shoulder is uncommon, but is best seen anteriorly. Muscle wasting may be present due to nerve damage or chronic rotator cuff tendinopathies. Scars from shoulder replacement or arthroscopy are usually located anteriorly.
- **Feel:** palpate for tenderness, warmth and swelling over the acromioclavicular, sternoclavicular and glenohumeral joints. Previous shoulder dislocation often results in a palpable gap at the acromioclavicular joint line. Feel the surrounding muscles for tenderness and check for sensory disturbance in the limb.
- **Move:** examine active and passive movements of the shoulder joint. Check abduction, forward flexion, and internal and external rotation. Loss of passive external rotation and abduction are highly suggestive of a frozen shoulder, and the patient may display the 'hitch-up' sign on active abduction as a compensatory mechanism (see Chapter 2). A normal range of passive movements makes glenohumeral disease unlikely.
- **Special tests:** closer examination of the rotator cuff muscles is often undertaken. *Supraspinatus* is tested with the arm abducted to 30 degrees, flexed to 30 degrees and internally rotated with the thumb pointing downward; abduction is then resisted. Resisted internal rotation tests *subscapularis,* and resisted external rotation tests *infraspinatus* and *teres minor.*
- Present your findings to the examiner like so; '*Mr Phillips is a [age] year old gentleman who presents with a stiff shoulder. On examination, he has some wasting of the deltoid muscle. There was no warmth or swelling over the joint. There was marked reduction in active and passive shoulder abduction and external rotation. The likely diagnosis is of a frozen shoulder. I would consider the following tests to confirm my diagnosis… and would also like the opportunity to examine the joints above and below*'.

Questions for reflection

1. What conditions are associated with a frozen shoulder?
   - Diabetes mellitus
   - Thyroid disorders
   - Previous injury/surgery
   - Prolonged immobilization
2. Which four muscles make up the rotator cuff?
   - Supraspinatus
   - Infraspinatus
   - Subscapularis
   - Teres minor
3. What are the potential X-ray findings in adhesive capsulitis?
   - Diffuse osteopenia
   - Osteoarthritis
   - Calcific tendonitis
4. What treatment options are available?
   - Nonoperative: NSAIDs, physiotherapy and intraarticular steroid injections.
   - Operative: manipulation under anaesthesia, arthroscopic surgical release.

Index

Note: Page numbers followed by *f* indicate figures and *t* indicate tables.